Contents

1

General

8   **ULTRASONOGRAPHY OF THE ROTATOR CUFF: A Comparison of Ultrasonographic and Arthroscopic Findings in One Hundred Consecutive Cases**
Teefey, Sharlene A. | JBJS. Vol 82A, April 2000, pages 498-504

15   **SHOULDER INJURIES IN THE THROWING ATHLETE**
Altchek, David W. | JAAOS. Vol 3, May/June 1995, pages 159-165

22   **THE EFFECT OF SURGERY FOR ROTATOR CUFF DISEASE ON GENERAL HEALTH STATUS: Results of a Prospective Trial**
McKee, Michael D. | JBJS. Vol 82A, July 2000, pages 970-979

Basic Research

34   **STRENGTH OF FIXATION WITH TRANSOSSEOUS SUTURES IN ROTATOR CUFF REPAIR**
Caldwell, George L., Jr. | JBJS. Vol 79A, July 1997, pages 1064-1068

39   **EXPERIMENTAL ROTATOR CUFF REPAIR: A Preliminary Study**
Gerber, Christian | JBJS. Vol 81A, September 1999, pages 1281-1290

49   **THERMAL MODIFICATION OF CONNECTIVE TISSUES: Basic Science Considerations and Clinical Implications**
Arnoczky, Steven P. | JAAOS. Vol 8, September/October 2000, pages 305-313

Evaluation and Treatment

60   **PARTIAL-THICKNESS TEARS OF THE ROTATOR CUFF: Evaluation and Management**
McConville, Owen R. | JAAOS. Vol 7, 1999, pages 32-43

73   **DÉBRIDEMENT OF PARTIAL-THICKNESS TEARS OF THE ROTATOR CUFF WITHOUT ACROMIOPLASTY: Long-term Follow-up and Review of the Literature**
Budoff, Jeffrey E. | JBJS. Vol 80A, May 1998, pages 733-748

89   **ARTHROSCOPIC MANAGEMENT OF ROTATOR CUFF DISEASE**
Gartsman, Gary M. | JAAOS. Vol 6, July/August 1998, pages 259-266

98   **ARTHROSCOPIC REPAIR OF FULL-THICKNESS TEARS OF THE ROTATOR CUFF**
Gartsman, Gary M. | JBJS. Vol 80A, June 1998, pages 832-840

How to Reach Us

The Journal of Bone and Joint Surgery
Editorial and Business offices: JBJS, 20 Pickering Street, Needham, Massachusetts 02492-3157. Telephone: (781) 449-9780
www.jbjs.org · e-mail: edit@jbjs.org · Editorial Fax: (781) 449-9787 · Advertising Fax: (781) 449-449-3485 · Subscription Fax: (781) 449-449-3485

Journal of the American Academy of Orthopaedic Surgeons
Editorial offices: JAAOS, 6300 N. River Road, Rosemont, IL 60018-4262; e-mail: jaaos@aaos.org
Customer Service Telephone: (800) 626-6726, ++(847) 823-8025

THE JOURNAL OF BONE & JOINT SURGERY | JOURNAL OF THE AMERICAN ACADEMY OF ORTHOPAEDIC SURGEONS

BS

Articles reprinted from the *Journal of the American Academy of Orthopaedic Surgeons* and *Instructional Course Lectures 47*
© 2001 American Academy of Orthopaedic Surgeons

Articles reprinted from *The Journal of Bone and Joint Surgery*
© 2001 The Journal of Bone and Joint Surgery, Incorporated

Journal of the American Academy of Orthopaedic Surgeons

Alan M. Levine, MD
Editor-in-Chief

Peter Jokl, MD
Associate Editor, Sports Medicine

The Journal of Bone and Joint Surgery

James D. Heckman, MD
Editor-in-Chief

Robin R. Richards, MD
Deputy Editor for the Upper Extremity

ISBN 0-89203-263-4

Editorial Staff
Journal of the American Academy of Orthopaedic Surgeons

Vice President, Education Programs
Mark W. Wieting

Director, Department of Publications
Marilyn L. Fox, PhD

Managing Editor
Judith A. McKay

Manager, Production and Archives
Mary C. Steermann

Assistant Production Managers
David R. Wiegand, David M. Stanley

Manuscript Coordinator
Adria R. Landy

Editorial Assistant
Laura E. Goetz

Desktop Publishing Assistant
Dena M. Lozano

Editorial Staff
The Journal of Bone and Joint Surgery

Managing Editor
Mady Tissenbaum

Desktop Publishing
Kristin Burati
Carla Hillyard
So Yuk Wong

Focus on the Rotator Cuff

10/18/04

Contents

Continued

107 FULL-THICKNESS ROTATOR CUFF TEARS: Factors affecting surgical outcome
Iannotti, Joseph P. | JAAOS. Vol 2, March/April 1994, pages 87-95

116 TRANSFER OF THE PECTORALIS MAJOR MUSCLE FOR THE TREATMENT OF IRREPARABLE RUPTURE OF THE SUBSCAPULARIS TENDON
Resch, H. | JBJS. Vol 82A, March 2000, pages 372-382

127 LONG-TERM FUNCTIONAL OUTCOME OF REPAIR OF LARGE AND MASSIVE CHRONIC TEARS OF THE ROTATOR CUFF
Rokito, Andrew S. | JBJS. Vol 81A, July 1999, pages 991-997

135 THE RESULTS OF REPAIR OF MASSIVE TEARS OF THE ROTATOR CUFF
Gerber, Christian | JBJS. Vol 82A, April 2000, pages 505-515

146 CONTINUOUS PASSIVE MOTION AFTER REPAIR OF THE ROTATOR CUFF: A Prospective Outcome Study
Lastayo, Paul C. | JBJS. Vol 80A, July 1998, pages 1002-1011

Specific Conditions

158 FROZEN SHOULDER: Diagnosis and Management
Warner, Jon J. P. | JAAOS. Vol 5, May/June 1997, pages 130-140

169 CALCIFIC TENDINOPATHY OF THE ROTATOR CUFF: Pathogenesis, Diagnosis, and Management
Uhthoff, Hans K. | JAAOS. Vol 5, July/August 1997, pages 183-191

178 ROTATOR CUFF TEAR ARTHROPATHY
Jensen, Kirk L. | JBJS. Vol 81A, September 1999, pages 1312-1324

191 THE ROTATOR CUFF–DEFICIENT ARTHRITIC SHOULDER: Diagnosis and Surgical Management
Zeman, Craig A. | JAAOS. Vol 6, November/December 1998, pages 337-348

Complications and Salvage Procedures

204 CLINICAL OUTCOME AFTER STRUCTURAL FAILURE OF ROTATOR CUFF REPAIRS
Jost, Bernhard | JBJS. Vol 82A, March 2000, pages 304-314

215 FAILED REPAIR OF THE ROTATOR CUFF: Evaluation and Treatment of Complications
Karas, Evan H. | JAAOS Instructional Course Lectures. Vol 47, 1998, pages 87-95

224 TRANSFER OF THE LATISSIMUS DORSI MUSCLE AFTER FAILED REPAIR OF A MASSIVE TEAR OF THE ROTATOR CUFF: A Two to Five-year Review
Miniaci, Anthony | JBJS. Vol 81A, August 1999, pages 1120-1127

233 PAINFUL SHOULDER AFTER SURGERY FOR ROTATOR CUFF DISEASE
Williams, Gerald R., Jr. | JAAOS. Vol 5, March/April 1997, pages 97-108

245 MANAGEMENT OF CHRONIC DEEP INFECTION FOLLOWING ROTATOR CUFF REPAIR
Mirzayan, R. | JBJS. Vol 82A, August 2000, pages 1115-1121

THE ROTATOR CUFF:
CURRENT THINKING AND TREATMENT

In the United States the annual incidence of musculoskeletal problems affecting the upper extremity is greater than seventeen per one thousand individuals in the general population. Rotator cuff problems are amongst the most common of upper extremity disorders. Most orthopedists have patients in their practices with rotator cuff complaints. The rotator cuff is a complex structure consisting of the tendinous insertions of the supraspinatus, infraspinatus, teres minor and subscapularis muscles. The rotator cuff contributes in a substantive way to the dynamic kinesiology of the shoulder by maintaining both appropriate alignment and mechanical efficiency of the glenohumeral joint.

The purpose of assembling this compendium of recent articles in one publication is to update and enhance the practitioner's understanding of treatment and outcomes pertaining to rotator cuff pathology. This volume presents selected recent articles which define the causes of rotator cuff failure from biomechanical, histologic and metabolic perspectives. The subject material includes partial thickness rotator cuff tears, cuff tear arthropathy, calcific tendinopathy, the role of ultrasonography, the effect of thermal modification on connective tissue, arthroscopic rotator cuff surgery, cuff debridement, repair techniques, pectoralis major and latissimus transfers, frozen shoulder, failed surgery, rehabilitation techniques and outcome. Diagnostic methods including the application of medical history, appropriate physical examination and imaging techniques are presented.

With a clear understanding of the pathology appropriate treatment strategies, both operative and nonoperative, can be entertained. Proper patient selection and a treatment strategy based on the data provided within these pages will allow the practitioner and the patient to predict outcome following a defined treatment protocol with some degree of certainty. Comprehension of this compendium of materials should allow the practitioner to accurately diagnose the specific condition causing rotator cuff dysfunction in his or her patient.

With future research an understanding of rotator cuff tissue healing mechanisms, together with factors that enhance healing and their potential limitations, will become part of our knowledge base. With this information more effective procedures to correct the deficiencies of the large, presently irreparable, tears of the rotator cuff can be developed. Factors which affect the expected outcomes and treatment choices such as patient selection and patient physician expectation need definition. Our ultimate goal should be to define methods to prevent incapacitating rotator cuff dysfunction through effective interventional regimens which can prevent or reverse the most common causes of rotator cuff pathology, including overuse and degenerative processes.

The glenohumeral articulation is considered one of the most complex and poorly understood articulations. In treating abnormalities of the rotator cuff further research defining the biomechanical and physiological function of the rotator cuff is needed. Based on this information precise definitions of the etiology and diagnosis of rotator cuff pathology will be developed. This compendium defines the state of the art at the present time. The orthopedic surgeon armed with this knowledge will be able to plan treatment appropriately.

We both hope that you will enjoy reading and learning from this collection of current articles as much as we have in collecting them for your review.

PETER JOKL, MD
Journal of the American Academy of
Orthopaedic Surgeons
Yale University School of Medicine,
New Haven, CT

ROBIN R. RICHARDS, MD, FRCSC
The Journal of Bone and Joint Surgery
St. Michael's Hospital and
the University of Toronto,
Toronto, Ontario, CANADA

JBJS

THE JOURNAL OF BONE & JOINT SURGERY

JAAOS

JOURNAL OF THE AMERICAN ACADEMY OF ORTHOPAEDIC

section one

General

Ultrasonography of the Rotator Cuff

A Comparison of Ultrasonographic and Arthroscopic Findings
in One Hundred Consecutive Cases*

BY SHARLENE A. TEEFEY, M.D.†, S. ASHFAQ HASAN, M.D.†, WILLIAM D. MIDDLETON, M.D.†,

MIHIR PATEL, M.D.†, RICK W. WRIGHT, M.D.†, AND KEN YAMAGUCHI, M.D.†

*Investigation performed at the Mallinckrodt Institute of Radiology and the Department of Orthopaedic Surgery,
Washington University School of Medicine, St. Louis, Missouri*

Abstract

Background: There has been limited acceptance of shoulder ultrasonography by orthopaedic surgeons in the United States. The purpose of this retrospective study was to determine the diagnostic performance of high-resolution ultrasonography compared with arthroscopic examination for the detection and characterization of rotator cuff tears.

Methods: One hundred consecutive shoulders in ninety-eight patients with shoulder pain who had undergone preoperative ultrasonography and subsequent arthroscopy were identified. The arthroscopic diagnosis was a full-thickness rotator cuff tear in sixty-five shoulders, a partial-thickness tear in fifteen, rotator cuff tendinitis in twelve, frozen shoulder in four, arthrosis of the acromioclavicular joint in two, and a superior labral tear and calcific bursitis in one shoulder each. All ultrasonographic reports were reviewed for the presence or absence of a rotator cuff tear and a biceps tendon rupture or dislocation. All arthroscopic examinations were performed according to a standardized operative procedure. The size and extent of the tear and the status of the biceps tendon were recorded for all shoulders. The findings on ultrasonography and arthroscopy then were compared for each parameter.

Results: Ultrasonography correctly identified all sixty-five full-thickness rotator cuff tears (a sensitivity of 100 percent). There were seventeen true-negative and three false-positive ultrasonograms (a specificity of 85 percent). The overall accuracy was 96 percent. The size of the tear on transverse measurement was correctly predicted in 86 percent of the shoulders with a full-thickness tear. Ultrasonography detected a tear in ten of fifteen shoulders with a partial-thickness tear that was diagnosed on arthroscopy. Five of six dislocations and seven of eleven ruptures of the biceps tendon were identified correctly.

Conclusions: Ultrasonography was highly accurate for detecting full-thickness rotator cuff tears, characterizing their extent, and visualizing dislocations of the biceps tendon. It was less sensitive for detecting partial-thickness rotator cuff tears and ruptures of the biceps tendon.

The use of high-resolution ultrasonography in North America for the detection of rotator cuff tears has achieved only limited acceptance by orthopaedic surgeons compared with other modalities such as magnetic resonance imaging. Uncertainty about the accuracy of this modality may have contributed to its low utilization rate. Although initial studies, published in the mid-1980s, that compared ultrasonographic and surgical findings showed a high rate of accuracy (92 to 94 percent in series of fifty-one and forty-seven patients[5,7]) for the detection of rotator cuff tears, later studies showed somewhat lower rates (60 to 84 percent in series of thirty-eight, ten, and forty-nine patients[1,3,9]). Additionally, only a few studies have compared the accuracy of ultrasonography with that of arthroscopy for determining the presence or absence of rotator cuff tears[2,8,12,13] and fewer have correlated the tear size with the surgical findings[2,13]. Brenneke and Morgan, in a study of sixty-one patients, found that ultrasonography had a sensitivity of 95 percent and a specificity of 93 percent for the detection of full-thickness tears[2]. They also found that it accurately predicted the size of full-thickness tears in 89 percent of patients who had a tear that was greater than four centimeters, in 43 percent of those who had a tear that was two to four centimeters, and in 70 percent of those who had a tear that was less than two centimeters. Wiener and Seitz, in a study of 225 patients, demonstrated that ultrasonography had a sensitivity of 95 percent and a specificity of 94 percent for the detection of full-thickness tears and a sensitivity of 91 percent and a specificity of 94 percent for predicting the size of the tear[13].

The purpose of the current study was to compare the diagnostic performance of ultrasonography with that of arthroscopic surgery to determine its accuracy for detecting rotator cuff tears and biceps tendon pathology.

Materials and Methods

The study comprised 100 shoulders in ninety-eight consecutive patients with shoulder pain who had under-

*No benefits in any form have been received or will be received from a commercial party related directly or indirectly to the subject of this article. No funds were received in support of this study.

†Mallinckrodt Institute of Radiology (S. A. T. and W. D. M.) and Department of Orthopaedic Surgery (S. A. H., M. P., R. W. W., and K. Y.), Washington University School of Medicine, 510 South Kingshighway, Box 8131, St. Louis, Missouri 63110.

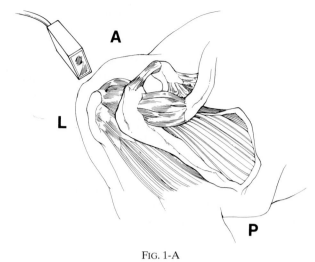

FIG. 1-A

Drawing of a left shoulder, viewed from above with the arm in extension, showing the transducer oriented in a plane parallel to the longitudinal axis of the rotator cuff. A = anterior, L = lateral, and P = posterior.

gone standardized preoperative ultrasonography and subsequent arthroscopy between January 1996 and September 1997. The interval of time between the ultrasonographic and the arthroscopic examination ranged from one to 417 days (mean, sixty days). There were fifty-four female patients and forty-four male patients, and their ages ranged from fourteen to eighty-two years (mean age, fifty-six years).

The primary arthroscopic or final clinical diagnosis was a full-thickness tear of the rotator cuff in sixty-five shoulders, a partial-thickness tear in fifteen, rotator cuff tendinitis in twelve, frozen shoulder in four, arthrosis of the acromioclavicular joint in two, and a superior labral tear and calcific bursitis in one shoulder each. Two patients with a full-thickness tear had a large partial-thickness component.

In general, the indications for the surgery and the arthroscopic examination included shoulder pain of more than six months' duration and a lack of a response to nonoperative treatment including physical therapy, nonsteroidal anti-inflammatory medications, and at least one cortisone injection. For the patients with a full-thickness tear, the indications for the operation included severe pain of more than three months' duration despite the nonoperative measures just mentioned. Patients with a full-thickness tear who had a recent loss of shoulder elevation or a recent injury (sustained less than three months before the time of presentation) were offered the option of an operation at earlier than three months.

Ultrasonographic Technique

All ultrasonograms were obtained in real time with use of an ATL HDI 3000 scanner (Advanced Technologies Laboratories, Bothell, Washington) or a Siemens Elegra scanner (Siemens Medical Systems, Issaquah, Washington) and a variable high-frequency linear-array transducer (7.5 to ten megahertz). All patients had stan-

dardized bilateral ultrasonography of the shoulder, performed by one of two radiologists who were very experienced with the technique and who had conducted more than 2500 examinations during a ten-year period.

The ultrasonographic examination was performed with the patient seated on a stool and the radiologist standing behind the patient. First, the biceps tendon was examined in the transverse plane from the level of the acromion inferiorly to the point where the tendon merged with the biceps muscle. The transducer then was rotated 90 degrees in order to examine the tendon longitudinally. Next, images of the subscapularis tendon were made with the patient's arm externally rotated; the transducer was placed in a transverse anatomical orientation at the level of the lesser tuberosity and was moved medially.

Images of the supraspinatus tendon were made with the shoulder extended, the elbow flexed, and the hand placed on the iliac wing. This position was necessary in order to expose as much of the supraspinatus tendon as possible from under the acromion. The transducer was oriented parallel to the tendon (approximately 45 degrees between the coronal and sagittal planes) in order to visualize the fibers in a longitudinal plane (Figs. 1-A and 1-B), and it was moved anteriorly to posteriorly in order to visualize the supraspinatus and infraspinatus tendons. The transducer was rotated 90 degrees in order to examine the tendons in the transverse plane (Figs. 2-A and 2-B).

Ultrasonographic Criteria

A finding of a full-thickness rotator cuff tear was recorded when the rotator cuff could not be visualized because of complete avulsion and retraction under the acromion or when there was a focal defect in the rotator cuff created by a variable degree of retraction of the torn tendon ends. In the latter case, either joint fluid or thickened bursal tissue and the deep surface of the del-

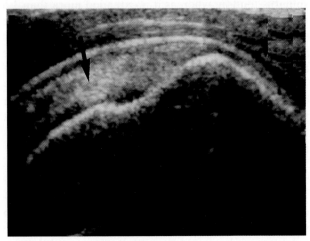

FIG. 1-B

Corresponding ultrasonographic image showing the rotator cuff (arrow) in the longitudinal plane.

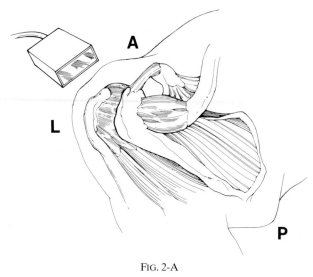

FIG. 2-A

Drawing of a left shoulder, viewed from above with the arm in extension, showing the transducer oriented in a plane perpendicular to the longitudinal axis of the rotator cuff. A = anterior, L = lateral, and P = posterior.

toid muscle occupied the defect created by the tear. If no tear was visualized, the deltoid muscle was compressed against the cuff with the transducer in an attempt to separate the torn tendon ends at the site of a nonretracted tear.

A finding of a partial-thickness tear was recorded when there was minimal flattening of the bursal side of the rotator cuff (a bursal-side partial-thickness tear) or a distinct hypoechoic or mixed hyperechoic and hypoechoic defect visualized in both the longitudinal and the transverse plane at the deep articular side of the rotator cuff (an articular-side partial-thickness tear).

The extent of the rotator cuff tear was determined with transverse measurements. According to empirical guidelines instituted prior to the inception of this study, if the tear extended posteriorly 1.5 centimeters or less from the intra-articular portion of the biceps tendon it was recorded as involving only the supraspinatus tendon, whereas if it extended more than 1.5 to 3.0 centimeters it was recorded as involving both the supraspinatus and the infraspinatus tendon. The teres minor tendon was not evaluated when the extent of the tear was determined.

A finding of a rupture of the biceps tendon was recorded when the tendon was not identified within or medial to the intertubercular sulcus. Dislocation of the biceps tendon was recorded when the tendon was anterior or medial to the lesser tuberosity.

Surgical Technique and Criteria

All arthroscopic examinations and operative procedures were performed by a single orthopaedic surgeon who recorded all findings in a standardized manner. The presence or absence of a rotator cuff tear and the size and extent of the tear, when present, were recorded. Specifically, the presence or absence of a full-thickness

tear or of a bursal or articular-side partial-thickness tear and the width (perpendicular to the long axis of the cuff fibers) of any tear that was found were recorded. The biceps tendon was examined arthroscopically for dislocation or rupture. Representative arthroscopic images were made of all tears and other pathological findings, such as abnormalities of the biceps tendon.

In shoulders in which a partial-thickness tear was present or the arthroscopic findings were discrepant from those recorded on ultrasonography, or both, a tagging suture (number-1 PDS [polydioxanone]) was placed, from the bursal side without a knot, through the suspected area of the rotator cuff to guide arthroscopic bursal imaging. In shoulders in which a full-thickness tear was recorded on ultrasonography but was not visualized on arthroscopy, an extensive partial-thickness tear was present. In these shoulders, a mini-open deltoid split (a three to four-centimeter skin incision with approximately a three-centimeter deltoid split without any takedown of the deltoid origin) was performed to directly visualize the involved area of the rotator cuff and to verify the arthroscopic findings. Additionally, as all full-thickness tears were repaired through a mini-open deltoid-splitting approach, the size and extent of the tear were determined by direct visualization. If a partial-thickness tear was recorded on ultrasonography but was not seen on arthroscopy, a mini-open deltoid split was not performed.

Data Analysis

The ultrasonographic and arthroscopic findings were correlated with regard to the presence or absence of a full or partial-thickness rotator cuff tear, the size and extent of the tear, and the presence or absence of a dislocation or rupture of the biceps tendon. When there was disagreement between the findings, representative arthroscopic and ultrasonographic images were reevalu-

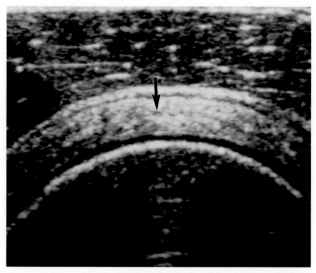

FIG. 2-B

Corresponding ultrasonographic image showing the rotator cuff (arrow) in the transverse plane.

TABLE I
FULL-THICKNESS ROTATOR CUFF TEARS:
ULTRASONOGRAPHIC VERSUS ARTHROSCOPIC FINDINGS*

	Arthroscopy		
	Positive	Negative	Total
Ultrasonography			
Positive	65	3	68
Negative	0	17	17
Total	65	20	85

*The values are given as the numbers of shoulders. When true-positive indicated a full-thickness tear and true-negative, no tear, ultrasonography had a sensitivity of 100 percent (sixty-five of sixty-five), a specificity of 85 percent (seventeen of twenty), a positive predictive value of 96 percent (sixty-five of sixty-eight), a negative predictive value of 100 percent (seventeen of seventeen), and an accuracy of 96 percent (eighty-two of eighty-five).

ated jointly to explain the discrepancy.

Only the full-thickness tears were analyzed with regard to their size and extent. The subscapularis was classified only as intact or torn. Two of the sixty-five shoulders with a full-thickness tear were excluded from the analysis; one shoulder had a very limited range of motion and indeterminate findings regarding the extent of the tear on ultrasonography, and the other shoulder had had the arthroscopic examination one year after the ultrasonographic study.

Results

Detection of Rotator Cuff Tears

Ultrasonography correctly identified all sixty-five full-thickness rotator cuff tears that were diagnosed on arthroscopy (Figs. 3-A and 3-B, and Table I). There were no false-negative studies. Ultrasonography incorrectly identified a full-thickness rotator cuff tear in three shoulders that were found to have a partial-thickness tear on arthroscopy; one of the three tears was extensive (more than 50 percent of the cuff thickness) and involved the entire supraspinatus tendon.

Ultrasonography correctly identified seven of fifteen partial-thickness rotator cuff tears that were diagnosed on arthroscopy (Figs. 4-A and 4-B, and Table II). In three additional shoulders, it identified a full-thickness rather than a partial-thickness tear. Because a tear was identified, these studies were considered to be true-positive. There were five false-negative studies. Ultrasonographic visualization of the rotator cuff was limited by a decreased range of motion in two of these shoulders, and arthroscopy showed only mild fraying of the supraspinatus tendon in a third. There were three false-positive ultrasonograms, one of which showed an ill defined hypoechoic region, suggestive of a partial tear, on the deep capsular side of the cuff near its insertion. Another of the false-positive studies showed subtle flattening of the bursal side of the supraspinatus tendon. Ultrasonography correctly predicted the absence of a tear in seventeen of twenty shoulders that had no evidence of a tear on arthroscopy.

In six shoulders for which the arthroscopic findings were discrepant from those recorded on ultrasonography, a tagging suture was placed through the suspicious area of the rotator cuff to guide arthroscopic bursal imaging. In three of these shoulders, ultrasonography revealed a full-thickness tear but a partial-thickness tear was detected on arthroscopy. In the other three shoulders, a partial-thickness tear was recorded on ultrasonography but the cuff was normal on arthroscopy.

Size and Extent of the Tears

Of the sixty-three full-thickness rotator cuff tears that were analyzed for these parameters, twenty-six were

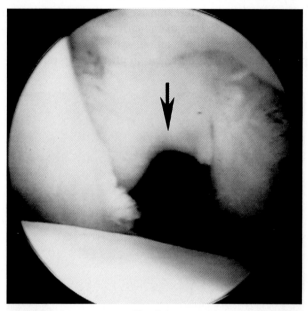

FIG. 3-A

Arthroscopic image showing a small full-thickness tear of the left supraspinatus tendon (arrow).

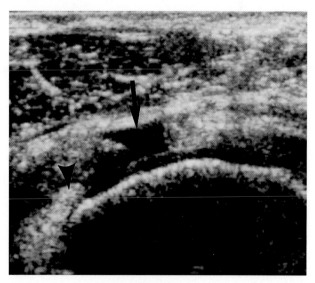

FIG. 3-B

Corresponding ultrasonographic image showing the small tendon tear. Fluid separates the torn tendon ends (arrow). The image is oriented in a plane perpendicular to the longitudinal axis of the tendon. The biceps tendon is to the left of the tear (arrowhead).

found on arthroscopy to involve only the supraspinatus tendon and to be less than 1.5 centimeters wide, and thirty-seven involved both the supraspinatus and the infraspinatus and were more than 1.5 centimeters wide. In addition, seven shoulders had a tear of the subscapularis tendon. Transverse measurement with ultrasonography correctly predicted the extent of the tear in twenty-one (81 percent) of the twenty-six shoulders with an isolated tear of the supraspinatus tendon. In three shoulders, ultrasonography overestimated the width of the tear by 0.5 centimeter or less and in two, by 1.1 and 1.3 centimeters. In the latter two shoulders, arthroscopy confirmed the presence of a full-thickness tear of the supraspinatus but also showed an extensive partial-thickness tear (more than 50 percent of the cuff thickness) extending into the infraspinatus tendon, which had been interpreted as a full-thickness tear on ultrasonography.

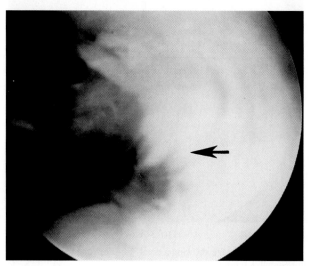

FIG. 4-A

Arthroscopic image showing a small partial-thickness tear of the right supraspinatus tendon (arrow).

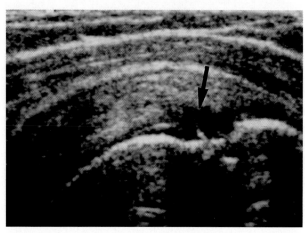

FIG. 4-B

Corresponding ultrasonographic image showing the small hypoechoic tendon tear, located on the deep capsular side of the cuff (arrow). The image is oriented in a plane parallel to the longitudinal axis of the tendon.

TABLE II
PARTIAL-THICKNESS ROTATOR CUFF TEARS:
ULTRASONOGRAPHIC VERSUS ARTHROSCOPIC FINDINGS*

	Arthroscopy		
	Positive	Negative	Total
Ultrasonography			
Positive	10	3	13
Negative	5	17	22
Total	15	20	35

*The values are given as the number of shoulders. When true-positive indicated a partial-thickness tear and true-negative, no tear, ultrasonography had a sensitivity of 67 percent (ten of fifteen), a specificity of 85 percent (seventeen of twenty), a positive predictive value of 77 percent (ten of thirteen), a negative predictive value of 77 percent (seventeen of twenty-two), and an accuracy of 77 percent (twenty-seven of thirty-five).

Transverse measurement with ultrasonography correctly predicted the extent of the tear in thirty-three (89 percent) of the thirty-seven shoulders that had a combined tear of the supraspinatus and infraspinatus tendons. In the four remaining shoulders, ultrasonography underestimated the extension of the tear into the infraspinatus tendon by one to 1.5 centimeters. In three of these shoulders, arthroscopy showed that the infraspinatus component was a midsubstance extension of the tear medial to the supraspinatus portion of the tear. Ultrasonography correctly identified six of the seven tears of the subscapularis tendon. Overall, ultrasonography correctly predicted the size and extent of the tear in 86 percent of the shoulders with a full-thickness tear.

Five of the thirty-seven shoulders had a massive tear with retraction of the torn tendon underneath the acromion. The edge of the torn tendon could not be visualized at the time of the ultrasonographic study.

Dislocation of the Biceps Tendon

Ultrasonography correctly identified five of six dislocations of the biceps tendon that were diagnosed on arthroscopy. The one false-negative study, which showed an absence of the biceps tendon, was interpreted as demonstrating a rupture rather than a dislocation. There were ninety-four true-negative ultrasonograms and no false-positive ultrasonograms.

Rupture of the Biceps Tendon

Ultrasonography correctly identified seven of eleven ruptures of the biceps tendon that were diagnosed on arthroscopy. There were four false-negative studies. Two of the false-negative ultrasonograms showed the normal echogenic fibrillar pattern of the tendon within the groove. There was one false-positive ultrasonogram, and there were eighty-eight true-negative ultrasonograms.

Discussion

High-resolution shoulder ultrasonography has not been widely utilized by orthopaedic surgeons to diagnose and characterize rotator cuff and biceps tendon pathology. This limited acceptance may be due in part to the paucity of shoulder ultrasonographic studies in the orthopaedic literature compared with magnetic resonance imaging studies, the frequent lack of local radiological expertise, and difficulty in recognizing the relevant anatomy and pathology on hard-copy ultrasonographic images. In addition, wide ranges of sensitivity (57 to 100 percent) and specificity (50 to 100 percent) have been reported, in series ranging from ten to 225 patients, for the ultrasonographic detection of rotator cuff tears, causing further uncertainty about the true accuracy of this modality[1-3,5,7-9,12,13]. Investigators who reported poor results for the diagnosis of rotator cuff tears used ultrasonographic criteria that either are no longer accepted or have been refined, employed a scanning technique that has since been modified to improve visualization of the cuff, and used older equipment and transducers with a lower frequency than is currently available[1,3,8,9].

In the present study, the accuracy of shoulder ultrasonography was reinvestigated in the context of modern refinements in the scanning technique, improvements in the resolution capabilities of the equipment, and clarification of the criteria for diagnosing a rotator cuff tear. In contrast to many of the earlier studies, in which the findings on ultrasonography were correlated with those on arthrography or open surgery, we compared the findings on ultrasonography with those on arthroscopy, which is a procedure with several potential advantages. Magnified arthroscopic images can provide accurate intra-articular and bursal visualization of the rotator cuff and, in contrast to arthrography, can delineate partial-thickness and midsubstance tears as well as intra-articular pathology of the biceps tendon.

We found that ultrasonography was highly accurate for detecting full-thickness rotator cuff tears and for characterizing their extent in the transverse plane. It led to a misdiagnosis of a full-thickness tear in only three shoulders, all of which had a partial-thickness tear on arthroscopy, with one of the tears involving more than 50 percent of the cuff substance. Our sensitivity rate of 100 percent and our specificity rate of 85 percent compare favorably not only with the rates reported in recent previous studies on ultrasonography (in which sensitivity or specificity, or both, has been as high as 95 percent[12,13]) but also with those reported in numerous magnetic resonance imaging studies[6,8,10,11].

Only a few studies have evaluated the use of ultrasonography for determining the size and extent of the tear[2,13]. Brenneke and Morgan reported that ultrasonography was accurate for predicting the size of large tears but less so for moderate and small tears[2]. We found that ultrasonography was very accurate in predicting the extent of any tear in the transverse plane. Our findings substantiate those reported by Wiener and Seitz[13]. Two of the shoulders in which we overestimated the extent of the tear by more than one centimeter had a full-thickness tear with an extensive partial-thickness com-

ponent on arthroscopy. The partial-thickness component was misinterpreted as a full-thickness tear. In both of these shoulders, a focal defect was produced by compression of the deltoid muscle against the rotator cuff with the transducer, an integral part of our examination. Like full-thickness tears, partial-thickness tears involving more than 50 percent of the cuff substance appear to demonstrate a focal defect (a criterion used to define a full-thickness tear) when the deltoid muscle is compressed into the tear. While this maneuver increased the sensitivity of ultrasonography for detecting small, non-retracted, full-thickness tears, it lowered the specificity; ultrasonography may not be able to differentiate extensive partial-thickness tears from full-thickness tears.

In three shoulders in which ultrasonography underestimated the extent of the tear, arthroscopy showed a medial midsubstance extension of the supraspinatus tear into the infraspinatus tendon. The midsubstance component of the tear was not detected when we viewed only the more lateral aspect of the rotator cuff near its insertion, which demonstrates the importance of proper positioning of the arm to visualize the rotator cuff not only at its insertion but more medially.

Our ability to detect partial-thickness rotator cuff tears with ultrasonography was limited; however, two of the five shoulders that had a false-negative study had a decreased range of motion (the patient was unable to externally rotate and extend the shoulder past the level of the buttock) that prevented a thorough evaluation of the cuff, and in a third the partial-thickness tear that was identified on arthroscopy consisted only of mild fraying of the supraspinatus tendon, which may not be detectable with ultrasonography. While Brenneke and Morgan also reported a low sensitivity for the detection of partial-thickness tears[2], two other recent studies demonstrated a sensitivity of more than 90 percent[12,13].

Biceps tendon abnormalities frequently are associated with rotator cuff tears. In the current study, the prevalence of rupture of the biceps tendon was 11 percent and that of dislocation was 6 percent. The dislocations, whether anterior or medial to the lesser tuberosity, were recognized easily on ultrasonography; we correctly diagnosed five of the six dislocations. On the other hand, we identified only seven of the eleven biceps tendon ruptures. Adhesion of a ruptured biceps tendon at the articular entrance to the groove was the most likely cause of a false-negative ultrasonogram. Two of the false-negative ultrasonographic studies showed the normal echogenic fibrillar pattern of the tendon within the groove, creating the false impression of an intact tendon.

Our study was limited by its retrospective design; however, when the operative and ultrasonographic findings were in disagreement, representative ultrasonographic hard-copy and arthroscopic images were reviewed jointly to explain the discrepancy. Additionally, prior to the inception of this study, standardized criteria for determining the presence, location, and extent of a rotator cuff tear in the transverse plane had been established, and the statistical analysis was based on the original interpretation of the ultrasonographic study rather than on a retrospective review of the images.

Although diagnostic arthroscopy was performed in an unblinded fashion, the surgeon's knowledge of the ultrasonographic results prior to the operation was advantageous to the patient as it led to a more focused evaluation of the rotator cuff, particularly when the arthroscopic findings did not correlate with the ultrasonographic report. In all shoulders for which a discrepant ultrasonographic finding was reported, the area in question was tagged with a suture intraoperatively to allow focused intra-articular and bursal-side viewing of the cuff.

Patients with a normal ultrasonogram who had resolution of the symptoms did not have arthroscopy and were not included in the study. Hence, it is possible that the actual number of false-negative studies may have been greater than what our study showed. On the other hand, patients with normal ultrasonograms but persistent symptoms frequently had arthroscopy and thus were included in the study. Since patients with persistent symptoms are more likely to have a tear than patients in whom the symptoms have resolved, it is unlikely that the sensitivity would have decreased markedly had we included all patients with normal ultrasonograms.

We found that ultrasonography was a highly accurate and reliable technique for detecting full-thickness rotator cuff tears and biceps tendon dislocations in painful shoulders. The high accuracy is in part attributable to improved image resolution, optimization of the scanning technique, and reliance on well defined criteria. However, more than with almost any other imaging modality that is employed to evaluate the shoulder, the success of an ultrasonographic examination depends heavily on the experience of the operator.

In summary, our findings indicate that shoulder ultrasonography can be a valuable noninvasive procedure for imaging of the rotator cuff. Not only is it comparable with magnetic resonance imaging in terms of accuracy for detecting full-thickness tears; it provides bilateral information, is better tolerated, allows patient viewing of real-time information, and is less expensive. Improvements in image resolution have allowed for more intuitive anatomical and correlative pathological interpretation of the hard-copy images by orthopaedic surgeons. Increased awareness of the important role that ultrasonography can play in the diagnosis of rotator cuff pathology may foster acceptance and increase the availability of this imaging modality to the orthopaedic community.

References

1. **Brandt, T. D.; Cardone, B. W.; Grant, T. H.; Post, M.;** and **Weiss, C. A.:** Rotator cuff sonography: a reassessment. *Radiology,* 173: 323-327, 1989.
2. **Brenneke, S. L.,** and **Morgan, C. J.:** Evaluation of ultrasonography as a diagnostic technique in the assessment of rotator cuff tendon tears. *Am. J. Sports Med.,* 20: 287-289, 1992.
3. **Burk, D. L., Jr.; Karasick, D.; Kurtz, A. B.; Mitchell, D. G.; Rifkin, M. D.; Miller, C. L.; Levy, D. W.; Fenlin, J. M.;** and **Bartolozzi, A. R.:** Rotator cuff tears: prospective comparison of MR imaging with arthrography, sonography, and surgery. *AJR: Am. J. Roentgenol.,* 153: 87-92, 1989.
4. **Clark, J. M.,** and **Harryman, D. T., II:** Tendons, ligaments, and capsule of the rotator cuff. Gross and microscopic anatomy. *J. Bone and Joint Surg.,* 74-A: 713-725, June 1992.
5. **Hodler, J.; Fretz, C. J.; Terrier, F.;** and **Gerber, C.:** Rotator cuff tears: correlation of sonographic and surgical findings. *Radiology,* 169: 791-794, 1988.
6. **Iannotti, J. P.; Zlatkin, M. B.; Esterhai, J. L.; Kressel, H. Y.; Dalinka, M. K.;** and **Spindler, K. P.:** Magnetic resonance imaging of the shoulder. Sensitivity, specificity, and predictive value. *J. Bone and Joint Surg.,* 73-A: 17-29, Jan. 1991.
7. **Mack, L. A.; Matsen, F. A., III; Kilcoyne, R. F.; Davies, P. K.;** and **Sickler, M. E.:** US evaluation of the rotator cuff. *Radiology,* 157: 205-209, 1985.
8. **Nelson, M. C.; Leather, G. P.; Nirschl, R. P.; Pettrone, F. A.;** and **Freedman, M. T.:** Evaluation of the painful shoulder. A prospective comparison of magnetic resonance imaging, computerized tomographic arthrography, ultrasonography, and operative findings. *J. Bone and Joint Surg.,* 73-A: 707-716, June 1991.
9. **Paavolainen, P.,** and **Ahovuo, J.:** Ultrasonography and arthrography in the diagnosis of tears of the rotator cuff. *J. Bone and Joint Surg.,* 76-A: 335-340, March 1994.
10. **Quinn, S. F.; Sheley, R. C.; Demlow, T. A.;** and **Szumowski, J.:** Rotator cuff tendon tears: evaluation with fat-suppressed MR imaging with arthroscopic correlation in 100 patients. *Radiology,* 195: 497-500, 1995.
11. **Rafii, M.; Firooznia, H.; Sherman, O.; Minkoff, J.; Weinreb, J.; Golimbu, C.; Gidumal, R.; Schinella, R.;** and **Zaslav, K.:** Rotator cuff lesions: signal patterns at MR imaging. *Radiology,* 177: 817-823, 1990.
12. **Van Holsbeeck, M. T.; Kolowich, P. A.; Eyler, W. R.; Craig, J. G.; Shirazi, K. K.; Habra, G. K.; Vanderschueren, G. M.;** and **Bouffard, J. A.:** US depiction of partial-thickness tear of the rotator cuff. *Radiology,* 197: 443-446, 1995.
13. **Wiener, S. N.,** and **Seitz, W. H., Jr.:** Sonography of the shoulder in patients with tears of the rotator cuff: accuracy and value for selecting surgical options. *AJR: Am. J. Roentgenol.,* 160: 103-107, 1993.

Shoulder Injuries in the Throwing Athlete

David W. Altchek, MD, and David M. Dines, MD

Abstract

The throwing athlete with shoulder pain presents a diagnostic and treatment challenge to the orthopaedic surgeon. Because pitching a baseball requires the arm to accelerate at 7,000 degrees per second, tremendous forces are experienced at the shoulder joint. Electromyographic studies have shown that the larger scapular and trunk muscles are primarily responsible for arm acceleration. The smaller and more fragile rotator cuff muscles play a significant role in decelerating the arm. During the entire throwing mechanism, the rotator cuff and the capsulolabral complex act to stabilize the humeral head on the glenoid fossa. As a result, the labrum, the capsule, and the rotator cuff are frequently the site of shoulder injury in throwers. The diagnosis of injury to these structures is based on the findings from the history, physical examination, and imaging studies. The majority of throwing injuries respond well to a carefully designed rehabilitation program. Athletes who do not improve within 6 months are candidates for surgical repair. The procedure is planned so as to minimize the amount of surgical trauma and thereby to facilitate an early return to sport. Arthroscopy is a valuable first step to confirm the pathologic diagnosis. The arthroscope alone is used to perform subacromial debridement, labral repair, or debridement of undersurface partial-thickness rotator cuff tears. If the athlete has clinical evidence of shoulder instability and arthroscopic evidence of capsular stretch, an open stabilization procedure is performed.

J Am Acad Orthop Surg 1995;3:159-165

The act of throwing places extreme demands on the shoulder. The athlete must maximally accelerate and decelerate the arm over a short period of time and at the same time maintain precise control over the object being thrown. It is not surprising that such an activity, when performed repetitively, can lead to shoulder injury. All structures that restrain the humeral head in the glenoid fossa are at risk.

This article will review the biomechanics of the throwing mechanism. We will describe a clinical approach to the problem of shoulder pain in the throwing athlete, including the details of the physical examination, the use of diagnostic tests, and the role of rehabilitation. We will also discuss the role of arthroscopy and open surgical procedures when the rehabilitation program has failed.

Biomechanics of Throwing

The four primary stages of throwing—windup, cocking, acceleration, and follow-through—have been extensively studied. Recent studies using high-speed digital video recording have illustrated the three-dimensional patterns of motion during the throw.[1] These data reveal that the shoulder is maintained in an abducted position of approximately 100 degrees throughout the throw. In the horizontal plane, the arm at maximal cocking is horizontally abducted 30 degrees and finishes in a position of 10 degrees of adduction at follow-through. External rotation has been measured to maximize at approximately 175 degrees, but combines additional movement of the scapula and hyperextension of the trunk.

The speed of arm rotation has also been measured with the use of high-speed video technology. The shoulder, which is maximally externally rotated at 175 degrees during the late cocking phase, moves to 105 degrees of internal rotation during the throwing mechanism at an astonishing speed of 7,000 degrees per second. Using a mathematical model, the

Dr. Altchek is Assistant Attending Orthopaedic Surgeon, Sports Medicine and Shoulder Service, The Hospital for Special Surgery, New York; Assistant Professor of Surgery (Orthopaedics), Cornell University Medical College, New York; and Team Physician, New York Mets. Dr. Dines is Chief of Orthopaedic Surgery, North Shore University Hospital, Manhasset, NY; Associate Attending Orthopaedic Surgeon, Sports Medicine and Shoulder Service, The Hospital for Special Surgery; Associate Professor of Surgery (Orthopaedics), Cornell University Medical College; and Associate Team Physician, New York Mets.

Reprint requests: Dr. Altchek, The Hospital for Special Surgery, 535 East 70th Street, New York, NY 10021.

torque forces occurring in the shoulder during the throw have been estimated. The highest torques, approaching 52 newton-meters, are observed at follow-through, when the arm is being decelerated. [2]

Electromyography has permitted the evaluation of the muscular firing patterns about the shoulder during the throwing sequence. [3] The rotator cuff musculature and biceps are relatively inactive during the acceleration phase of the throw, whereas the pectoralis major, serratus anterior, latissimus dorsi, and subscapularis muscles show the highest activity during this phase of the throw. In contrast, deceleration is accomplished by the rotator cuff musculature and the larger trunk muscles acting in concert. It is during this phase of follow-through that the highest forces are measured, and the rotator cuff must act eccentrically. This information is important in understanding the possible mechanisms of rotator cuff failure and the methods of injury rehabilitation in the throwing athlete. [3]

In addition to the events that occur during throwing, it is important to understand the stabilizing effects of the joint and its surrounding soft tissues. The rotator cuff tendon units have been shown to provide direct compression of the humeral head into the glenoid fossa. Presumably, effective synchronized muscle firing helps to limit abnormal translation of the humeral head on the glenoid. [1,4] Abnormal motion is further limited by the glenohumeral ligaments and the glenoid labrum (the capsulolabral complex). [4-6]

Sequential cutting studies in cadaveric specimens have evaluated the specific role of the glenohumeral ligaments in limiting glenohumeral translation. The anterior superior portion of the capsule limits inferior and posterior motion of the humeral head on the glenoid when the shoulder is adducted. The inferior gleno-humeral ligament complex limits anterior and posterior translation of the humeral head on the glenoid when the shoulder is abducted. The inferior glenohumeral ligament complex is defined by anterior and posterior bands, which are visible when the capsule is placed under tension. [6]

The labrum, which serves as the attachment site of the glenohumeral ligaments, plays an uncertain role in limiting glenohumeral motion, but may add to stability by increasing the depth of the glenoid. [4] In traumatic anterior shoulder instability, detachment of the anterior inferior labrum has been commonly noted. A cadaveric study that reproduced this type of labral detachment found that dislocation did not occur. [7] The results of that study suggest that in order for dislocation to occur, additional plastic deformation of the glenohumeral ligaments must also occur. This hypothesis is further supported by the work of Bigliani et al, [8] who demonstrated permanent deformation of the glenohumeral ligament prior to labral detachment in a cadaveric model of shoulder instability.

Ligamentous injury in the overhead-throwing athlete is frequently microtraumatic in nature. A classic Bankart lesion is rarely observed. This is in direct contrast to traumatic anterior instability, in which Bankart lesions, accompanied by a variable degree of capsular laxity, are commonly seen. The microtraumatic injury in the throwing athlete frequently results in stretch or plastic deformation of the capsular ligaments.

All of this information demonstrates that there are a number of systems that control the position of the humeral head on the glenoid. Muscular tension, ligamentous support, proprioceptive neuromuscular control, and osseous architecture all play a role. Muscular control is a dynamic system of control, while ligamentous support is a static sys-tem. A normally functioning asymptomatic shoulder requires a balance between these two systems and the osseous architecture, which is of particular importance in throwing. The ligamentous system allows the motion required to accelerate the ball, while the stability of the humeral head on the glenoid is maintained by muscular contraction and ligamentous tension. In the microtraumatic model of throwing injury, overload or injury to one portion of this restraint system shifts the burden to the other portion. This may account for the frequently observed combination of a partial-thickness rotator cuff tear and capsulolabral injury. One must keep in mind that in throwing athletes there is a fine line between the normal laxity that allows them to propel objects at high speeds and the pathologic instability that leads to their symptoms.

Clinical Evaluation of the Throwing Athlete

With this background information, a clinical approach to shoulder dysfunction in the throwing athlete has been developed. Beginning with a careful history, the examiner should identify the primary symptoms. The vast majority of throwing athletes will present with a chief complaint of pain, despite a wide range of underlying pathologic conditions. Instability may be subtle and may not be apparent from the history. Instability symptoms may include a feeling of the arm going dead or "coming apart" or a frank sensation of subluxation. However, throwers with occult subluxation often present with pain without any distinct symptoms of instability.

The examiner should determine which phase of the throwing mechanism or arm position is most likely to reproduce symptoms, which can be helpful in defining the type of instability pattern that is present. Patients with anterior instability typically will complain of pain, "dead arm," or coming-apart symptoms during the late cocking phase or early acceleration phase. Patients with posterior subluxation typically will complain during the follow-through phase. In either case, there may be, in addition, pain or symptoms during other phases of throwing.[9]

In the thrower with microtraumatic injury to the shoulder, rotator cuff injury is not uncommon. Although full-thickness tears are unusual, partial tears, particularly those affecting the articular surface, occur frequently. Detecting such injuries on the basis of the history is difficult, however.

If the rotator cuff injury is significant, a component of night pain often will exist. The location of pain can be of some help in localizing the lesion. Anterior pain may be associated with injury to the subscapularis or biceps tendon or with capsulolabral injury. Anterolateral pain is commonly seen with supraspinatus tendon injury, while posterior pain can be related to infraspinatus tendon problems or capsulolabral injury.

The physical examination is directed toward attempting to isolate the portions of the restraint system that are responsible for producing symptoms. Atrophy, particularly of the infraspinatus fossa, should be noted. This represents chronic rotator cuff dysfunction or suprascapular nerve injury. Palpation should be carried out to identify specific areas of tenderness.

The range of rotation is assessed in various degrees of shoulder adduction and 90 degrees of abduction. Increased external rotation of the dominant shoulder compared with the nondominant shoulder can be expected as a manifestation of normal laxity. In addition, some

throwers will exhibit losses of internal rotation. Whether this represents a normal adaptive response to the repetitive stress of throwing or a pathologic contracture is not clear at present. On the basis of our clinical observations, we think that throwers with losses of internal rotation are more likely to experience shoulder pain than those athletes with symmetric internal rotation. Loss of internal rotation can result from contracture of the posterior capsule, which, when simulated in cadaveric models, results in excessive anterior and superior translation of the humeral head.[10] Conceivably, this abnormal movement could cause symptoms by producing impingement of the humeral head on the coracoacromial arch.

The rotator cuff is assessed both by testing for signs of impingement and by attempting to elicit symptoms or weakness on resistance maneuvers in abduction and external rotation.

Ligamentous stability is tested in the anterior, posterior, and inferior directions. These tests are performed on both shoulders, and the results are compared. In the injured throwing athlete, the examiner should expect to find increased laxity on the dominant side. Therefore, the goal of the examination is to determine whether translation of the humeral head on the glenoid has increased markedly, whether distinct subluxation can be produced, and whether these maneuvers reproduce the patient's symptoms.

With the patient seated, we attempt to elicit a sulcus sign. The scapula is stabilized by grasping the acromion while the humerus is adducted. The examiner then applies distal traction to the arm. We grade the inferior displacement of the humeral head on the glenoid by the size of the sulcus seen on the skin. Throwers normally exhibit 1 to 2+ displacement (evidenced by a

sulcus measuring 1 to 3 cm), whereas 3+ inferior displacement (sulcus measuring more than 3 cm) is usually associated with pathologic instability.[11] If the patient states that reproduction of his or her symptoms occurs when the sulcus sign is elicited, the examiner should consider the possibility of inferior instability.

We examine for anterior or posterior instability with the patient supine. The arm is supported in neutral rotation in the plane of the scapula. With one hand, the examiner applies an axial load at the elbow to center the humeral head on the glenoid; with the other hand, the examiner translates the humeral head anteriorly and posteriorly on the glenoid. Our grading system is as follows: 1+, increased translation compared with the opposite shoulder is observed without distinct subluxation of the humeral head over the glenoid; 2+, distinct subluxation can be produced; 3+, the humeral head can be displaced and locked over the glenoid rim.

It is expected that a thrower will have 1+ anterior laxity, while 2+ posterior laxity is not uncommon as a normal finding in the absence of symptoms. Anterior laxity of 2+ or greater is usually evidence of a pathologic condition. Throwers with labral tears will often have 1+ translation, which will cause grinding or clicking and reproduction of painful symptoms.[12]

Jobe has popularized the so-called relocation test to further evaluate patients with subtle forms of instability.[13] To perform this maneuver, the patient is placed supine with the arm abducted 90 degrees and maximally externally rotated. This position should reproduce the patient's symptoms of pain or apprehension if there is symptomatic instability. The examiner then places a posteriorly directed load on the proximal humerus, relocating the humeral head and preventing anterior subluxation. If this relieves the patient's symptoms, the test is considered diagnostic for anterior instability.

Speer et al[14] evaluated the sensitivity and specificity of the relocation test. They found that although it was highly sensitive, specificity was poor if pain alone was evaluated. The specificity of the test improved markedly if the examiner was able to reproduce and relieve the symptoms of apprehension. In clinical practice, the relocation test and its modifications should be confirmed by other portions of the examination to make a firm diagnosis of instability.

The information obtained from the history and physical examination is then supplemented by findings from diagnostic tests. Radiographs are obtained in several planes, including anteroposterior, axillary, and outlet views. On the anteroposterior view, the glenohumeral joint should be clearly visible and should be assessed for signs of instability (Hill-Sachs lesion). The acromioclavicular joint will also be visible and should be assessed for undersurface spurring or degenerative changes. The axillary view is inspected for bone reaction along the glenoid margin. The outlet view is used to assess the subacromial osseous morphology. In most cases, plain views will rarely be diagnostic in this group of patients.

Magnetic resonance imaging is frequently used to further refine the diagnosis. Currently available software and the use of a shoulder coil should allow accurate imaging of the rotator cuff, but complete identification of labral injuries remains less precise.[15] At the present time, no imaging technique can measure capsular stretch.

Once the history, physical examination, and imaging studies are complete, the physician should be able to make a provisional diagnosis.

A final diagnosis may not be possible, however. Coexisting pathologic changes, such as capsular injury resulting in subtle instability with a simultaneous partial-thickness rotator cuff tear, are not uncommon.

The athlete's response to rehabilitation often allows the physician to further refine the diagnosis. Rehabilitation is directed toward strengthening the rotator cuff and scapular musculature and improving any mechanical flaws in the throwing mechanism. In general, minor to moderate degrees of capsular stretch resulting in a small pathologic increase in glenohumeral translation can be compensated for by improved dynamic stabilization. In this situation, no further studies are required.

Treatment of Shoulder Injuries in the Throwing Athlete

Conservative Treatment

Initial treatment is directed toward decreasing pain and restoring strength and motion. Pain relief is achieved by avoidance of aggravating activities and by use of cryotherapy and nonsteroidal anti-inflammatory medications. It is our opinion that cortisone injections are not indicated in the youthful athletic population because of the possibility of tendon damage.

The most common loss of motion is that of internal rotation, due to contracture of the posterior capsule. Graduated stretching in adduction and internal rotation is performed by the therapist and the patient until motion is symmetric.

The strengthening phase of rehabilitation is directed toward the musculature needed for throwing. Because the trunk muscles play a significant role in throwing, our strengthening program is directed simultaneously at the lower extremities and the shoulder girdle. During strengthening of the shoulder girdle, the therapist must avoid overloading and thereby irritating the rotator cuff musculature. The data have shown that rotator cuff firing occurs primarily during the follow-through phase, when eccentric muscle contraction decelerates the arm.[16] Rehabilitation of the rotator cuff musculature must involve exercises that mimic this eccentric firing pattern. As a rule, we tend to avoid exercises that attempt to isolate a single muscle group, such as those performed on isokinetic devices. Instead, we recommend exercises that mimic the throwing activity, addressing the muscles of the lower extremities as well as the shoulder musculature. As pain diminishes and function improves, emphasis is placed on improving throwing mechanics by working with a coach. The capabilities necessary for a return to play are measured functionally, rather than by use of isokinetic testing devices. In our experience, this conservative treatment program can be helpful in a large percentage of throwing athletes.

Failure is defined as a lack of definitive progress by 3 months or an inability to return to competition by 6 months. If the rehabilitation program fails, a surgical solution must be considered.

Surgical Treatment

Surgical treatment of shoulder injury in the throwing athlete begins with a careful examination under anesthesia to confirm the direction of any occult instability. Such an examination, carried out as already described for the initial office examination, is crucial in deciding whether glenohumeral instability is present. For example, if we suspect instability and are considering the patient as a candidate for capsular repair, we require that the examination under anesthesia confirm the presence of excessive differences in the degree of translation between the shoulders. The minimum requirement for stabilization is the reproduction of 2+ translation.

Following this examination, the patient is positioned in a modified beach-chair position for arthroscopy.[17] We feel that this position has several advantages over the lateral decubitus position. It is well tolerated by patients who have undergone regional anesthesia (scalene block). In addition, the absence of traction on the arm allows the surgeon to assess capsular tension without distortion. Also, without having to prepare the area again and redrape, the surgeon can convert arthroscopy to an open procedure, which is a necessary next step in many cases.

Posterior and anterior arthroscopic portals are created initially to allow complete examination of the joint. The diagnostic arthroscopy begins with evaluation of the biceps attachment and the superior labrum. Labral injury in this zone may include detachment or tearing or both. The biceps tendon may be involved and should be carefully examined as well. The surgeon must be familiar with the variations of normal anatomy that exist in this area. Cooper et al[18] have demonstrated that the superior labrum is characterized by considerable variation in both attachment and shape. The anterior superior labrum in particular displays great variation: it may be absent, confluent with the superior portion of the middle glenohumeral ligament, or present but not attached to the glenoid margin.[18]

Before proceeding with labral repair in this area, the surgeon must demonstrate the presence of tissue injury. This will differentiate labral detachments that are due to injury from those that are merely anatomic variants. The anterior inferior labrum has little variability and is firmly attached to the glenoid neck.

Tears or detachments in this region are significant and are usually associated with an anterior glenohumeral instability.

The anterior capsular ligaments are next evaluated. The superior glenohumeral ligament rarely is distinct, while the middle glenohumeral ligament usually is clearly present, draped over the subscapularis tendon. The inferior glenohumeral ligament is attached to the labrum by a normally robust anterior band.[19] This capsular ligament is frequently involved in the microtraumatic instability observed in throwing athletes.

Injury frequently causes plastic deformation of the inferior glenohumeral ligament, with a resulting loss of normal tension. Pagnani and Warren[19] have described the "drive-through" sign as an arthroscopic method of evaluating this ligamentous tension. When the ligament is uninjured, external rotation of the humerus will create tension in the anterior ligaments, and the surgeon will be unable to drive the arthroscope through into the anterior portion of the joint. As deformation of the ligament increases from capsular stretch, the resting length of the ligament elongates, allowing the arthroscopic drive-through to increase.

Next, the entire undersurface of the rotator cuff is examined. Partial articular-surface tears are commonly seen in this patient population.[19,20] To assess the bursal surface of the cuff in the same region as the partial undersurface tear, a spinal needle is placed percutaneously through this area. A monofilament suture is then passed and pulled out the anterior portal. Later, during the bursal examination, this suture is identified, and the superior surface of the rotator cuff in the area of the inferior partial tear is examined. As the posterior aspect of the cuff is viewed, the arm is externally

rotated, and the posterolateral humeral head is examined for the presence of a Hill-Sachs lesion.

The posterior labrum is best viewed with the arthroscope placed in the anterior portal. Fraying of the posterior labrum is common in throwing athletes. Frank tears or detachments may occur and are recognizable.

Once the glenohumeral joint has been completely examined, the arthroscope is inserted into the subacromial space through the posterior portal. Evidence of bursal scarring or injury to the superior surface of the cuff should become evident.

After arthroscopic confirmation of the cause and direction of instability has been made, the definitive surgical procedure is carried out (Figs. 1 and 2). The choice of procedure is determined on the basis of the findings from the history, physical examination, imaging studies, examination under anesthesia, and diagnostic arthroscopy.

During arthroscopy, partial-thickness articular-side rotator cuff tears are debrided of all torn flaps. This is performed with the hope of stimulating a healing response; however, no long-term data exist at present to confirm that this treatment is efficacious. If no distinct shoulder instability exists, pathologic labral detachments are repaired arthroscopically with use of an absorbable implant designed to allow fixation of soft tissue to bone (Suretac, Acufex Microsurgical, Mansfield, Mass). There are other techniques for arthroscopic labral repair, but we prefer the use of this material. Superior labral degenerative tears without labral detachment may be debrided; however, all labral detachments should be repaired in the manner already described. It has been documented that labral debridement without repair has a poor success rate when the labrum is detached.[12]

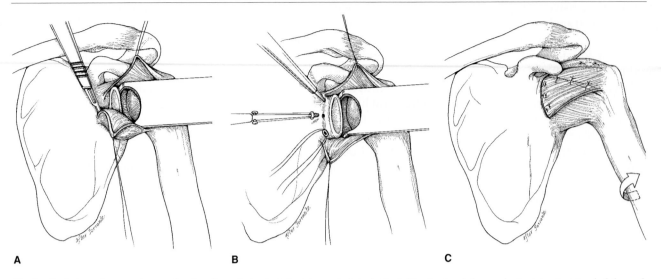

Fig. 1 Technique for capsular repair when the anterior inferior labrum is detached. **A,** The horizontal capsular incision is extended through the labrum into the glenoid neck. **B,** Suture anchors are placed at the glenoid articular margin. **C,** The completed capsular repair.

When bursitis is encountered in the subacromial space, an arthroscopic bursectomy is carried out. If the surgeon encounters a hypertrophic coracoacromial ligament that demonstrates evidence of an undersurface injury, the proximal portion of the ligament should be excised. In our experience, bone decompression or acromioplasty is rarely indicated in this youthful athletic population, in whom impingement is primarily a secondary phenomenon.[21]

If there is instability in the throwing athlete, in most cases there will be a plastic deformation of the anterior ligamentous complex. Large Bankart lesions of traumatic instability are rarely seen. For this reason, the majority of these athletes will not be candidates for arthroscopic stabilization. The goal of open stabilization is to restore capsular tension, thus eliminating pathologic translation without limiting motion.

Open anterior repair is performed selectively on the basis of the pathologic changes present.[22] The following technique is our preferred method:

The shoulder is exposed by means of a typical deltopectoral approach. The capsule is exposed by splitting the subscapularis, rather than by vertically transecting the tendon. This approach, which was described by Jobe,[23] minimizes the risk that postoperative shortening of the subscapularis will occur. A horizontal incision is made in the lower third of the muscle. Once the capsule has been identified, the incision is extended laterally into the tendon and medially past the glenoid margin. The resultant musculotendinous flaps are undermined bluntly, exposing the underlying capsule. The capsule is divided hor-

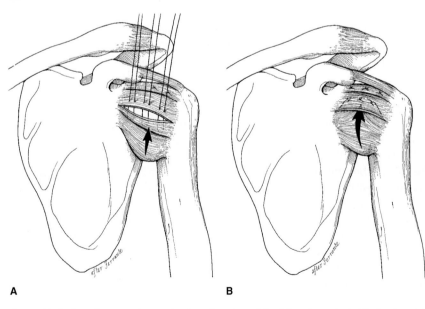

Fig. 2 Technique for capsular repair when there is no labral detachment. **A,** The horizontal capsular incision is plicated using mattress sutures. **B,** The completed capsular plication.

izontally, superior to the anterior band of the inferior glenohumeral ligament.

If the anterior inferior labrum is detached, the horizontal incision is continued through the labrum onto the glenoid neck. A subperiosteal flap, which contains in continuity the periosteum, the inferior labrum, and the inferior glenohumeral ligament (Fig. 1, A), is then elevated. After abrasion of the glenoid neck, the labrum is secured to the articular margin with the use of suture anchors (Fig. 1, B). Residual capsular laxity is eliminated by imbricating the horizontal capsular incision. The inferior flap is brought superiorly under the superior flap with use of a horizontal mattress suture. In our surgical protocol, the capsule

is tensioned with the arm in at least 60 degrees of abduction and 90 degrees of external rotation in the plane of the scapula. The shoulder is reexamined before the capsular sutures are tied. Anterior instability should be eliminated, and 90 degrees of external rotation should be possible (Fig. 1, C), which will ensure enough laxity to return to normal throwing. If there is no labral detachment, the horizontal interval is simply imbricated, shifting the inferior capsular flap superiorly (Fig. 2).

Postoperative care is directed at gradual restoration of motion and strength over a 6-week period. Return to throwing is not allowed for at least 4 months. The throwing program is graduated, beginning with

light tossing and progressing over a period of 4 to 6 months to full-velocity activity.

Summary

The diagnosis and treatment of shoulder dysfunction in the throwing athlete requires an in-depth analysis of the patient's symptoms and physical findings, which may be quite subtle. The physician must understand the role of the system of static and dynamic restraints that function to keep the shoulder stable during the complex throwing motion. Treatment is directed toward restoring the equilibrium between shoulder laxity and dynamic stabilization of the rotator cuff and scapular musculature.

References

1. Dillman CJ, Fleisig GS, Werner SL, et al: Biomechanics of the shoulder in sports: Throwing activities, in Matsen FA III, Fu FH, Hawkins RJ (eds): *The Shoulder: A Balance of Mobility and Stability.* Rosemont, Ill: American Academy of Orthopaedic Surgeons, 1993, pp 621-633.
2. Pappas AM, Zawacki RM, Sullivan TJ: Biomechanics of baseball pitching: A preliminary report. *Am J Sports Med* 1985;13:216-222.
3. Jobe FW, Moynes DR, Tibone JE, et al: An EMG analysis of the shoulder in pitching: A second report. *Am J Sports Med* 1984;12:218-220.
4. Matsen FA III, Harryman DT II, Sidles JA: Mechanics of glenohumeral instability. *Clin Sports Med* 1991;10:783-788.
5. Warner JJ, Deng XH, Warren RF, et al: Static capsuloligamentous restraints to superior-inferior translation of the glenohumeral joint. *Am J Sports Med* 1992;20:675-685.
6. O'Brien SJ, Neves MC, Arnoczky SP, et al: The anatomy and histology of the inferior glenohumeral ligament complex of the shoulder. *Am J Sports Med* 1990;18:449-456.
7. Speer KP, Deng X, Torzilli PA, et al: A biomechanical evaluation of the Bankart lesion. *Orthop Trans* 1993;18:135.

8. Bigliani LU, Pollock RG, Soslowsky LJ, et al: Tensile properties of the inferior glenohumeral ligament. *J Orthop Res* 1992;10:187-197.
9. Rowe CR, Zarins B: Recurrent transient subluxation of the shoulder. *J Bone Joint Surg Am* 1981;63:863-872.
10. Harryman DT II, Sidles JA, Clark JM, et al: Translation of the humeral head on the glenoid with passive glenohumeral motion. *J Bone Joint Surg Am* 1990; 72:1334-1343.
11. Altchek DW, Warren RF, Skyhar MJ, et al: T-plasty modification of the Bankart procedure for multidirectional instability of the anterior and inferior types. *J Bone Joint Surg Am* 1991;73:105-112.
12. Altchek DW, Warren RF, Wickiewicz TL, et al: Arthroscopic labral debridement: A three-year follow-up study. *Am J Sports Med* 1992;20:702-706.
13. Jobe FW, Kvitne RS, Giangarra CE: Shoulder pain in the overhand or throwing athlete: The relationship of anterior instability and rotator cuff impingement. *Orthop Rev* 1989;18:963-975.
14. Speer KP, Hannafin JA, Altchek DW, et al: An evaluation of the shoulder relocation test. *Am J Sports Med* 1994;22:177-183.
15. Rafii M, Firooznia H, Bonamo JJ, et al: Athlete shoulder injuries: CT arthrographic findings. *Radiology* 1987;162:559-564.

16. Kennedy K, Altchek DW, Glick IV: Concentric and eccentric isokinetic rotator cuff ratios in skilled tennis players. *Clin Res* 1993;3:155-159.
17. Skyhar MJ, Altchek DW, Warren RF, et al: Shoulder arthroscopy with the patient in the beach-chair position. *Arthroscopy* 1988;4:256-259.
18. Cooper DE, O'Brien SJ, Arnoczky SP, et al: The structure and function of the coracohumeral ligament: An anatomic and microscopic study. *J Shoulder Elbow Surg* 1993;2:70-77.
19. Pagnani MJ, Warren RF: Arthroscopic shoulder stabilization. *Operative Techniques Sports Med* 1993;1:276-284.
20. Tibone JE, Elrod B, Jobe FW, et al: Surgical treatment of tears of the rotator cuff in athletes. *J Bone Joint Surg Am* 1986;68:887-891.
21. Tibone JE, Jobe FW, Kerlan RK, et al: Shoulder impingement syndrome in athletes treated by an anterior acromioplasty. *Clin Orthop* 1985;198:134-140.
22. Altchek DW, Dines DM: The surgical treatment of anterior instability: Selective capsular repair. *Operative Techniques Sports Med* 1993;1:285-292.
23. Rubenstein DL, Jobe FW, Glousman RE, et al: Anterior capsulolabral reconstruction of the shoulder in athletes. *J Shoulder Elbow Surg* 1992;1:229-237.

The Effect of Surgery for Rotator Cuff Disease on General Health Status

RESULTS OF A PROSPECTIVE TRIAL*

BY MICHAEL D. McKEE, M.D., F.R.C.S.(C)†, AND DANIEL J. YOO, B.SC.†

*Investigation performed at the Division of Orthopaedics, Department of Surgery,
Upper Extremity Reconstructive Service, St. Michael's Hospital and the University of Toronto, Toronto, Ontario, Canada*

Abstract

Background: Previous studies of the effect of rotator cuff surgery have concentrated on limb-specific or surgeon-based outcome criteria. We conducted a prospective trial to determine the effect of surgery for rotator cuff disease on general health status.

Methods: Seventy-one patients (fifty of whom were men and twenty-one of whom were women) with a mean age of 56.1 years were enrolled in the study. In addition to routine clinical and radiographic evaluation, all patients completed the Short Form-36 (SF-36) health-status questionnaire and five limb-specific questionnaires preoperatively and at six, twelve, eighteen, and twenty-four months postoperatively. All patients had a standard open acromioplasty and resection of the subacromial bursa. Thirty-one patients had repair of an associated rotator cuff tear. Sixty-seven patients (94 percent) completed the study; the remaining four patients were lost to follow-up.

Results: The preoperative SF-36 scores for physical function (60.6, p = 0.02), role function-physical (20.8, p = 0.001), pain (38.6, p = 0.003), physical component summary (37.0, p = 0.001), and mental component summary (45.6, p = 0.02) were significantly decreased compared with normative data. The preoperative limb-specific scores also were low. At the time of the most recent follow-up evaluation, there was improvement that approached or reached significance both in the limb-specific scores (p ≤ 0.0026) and in the general-health-status scores for pain (p = 0.0001), role function-physical (p = 0.06), vitality (p = 0.01), and physical component summary (p = 0.01). The presence of a rotator cuff tear had a significant negative effect on limb-specific scores both preoperatively (p = 0.04) and postoperatively (p = 0.05). Although operative treatment of rotator cuff disease led to improved scores, patients who had filed a Workers' Compensation claim had lower limb-specific and SF-36 scores both preoperatively (p = 0.02 and p = 0.01, respectively) and postoperatively (p = 0.01 and p = 0.005, respectively).

Conclusions: Surgery for chronic rotator cuff disease reliably and significantly improves general health status.

Previous reports have described the effectiveness of surgical intervention for the treatment of rotator cuff disease that has not responded to conservative care[4,5,8-10,15,17]. The outcome measures used in most studies have been joint or limb-specific[1,2,30,35]. Those studies clearly demonstrated the debilitating effect that rotator cuff disease has on limb function. Recently, it has been shown that a variety of pathological conditions of the shoulder, including rotator cuff impingement, have a negative effect on general health status as determined with use of validated patient-oriented questionnaires[3,13,14,29,31,36,37]. Improvements in general health status following orthopaedic intervention have been well described, although many reports have lacked preoperative data or have had a short duration of follow-up[6,7,19,20,25-28]. Recently, the effectiveness of arthroscopic shoulder surgery was demonstrated by Gartsman et al., but patients who were receiving Workers' Compensation were excluded from that study[13]. Little is known regarding the impact of open rotator cuff surgery on general health status.

It is not clear whether general-health-status instruments are as sensitive to changes in a specific orthopaedic condition as limb or disease-specific instruments are. It also is not clear which components of these outcome measures are most responsive[2].

As competition for the health-care dollar increases and as economists and politicians focus on the cost-effectiveness and efficacy of various medical and surgical interventions, generic health-status instruments can be used to evaluate the effectiveness of various treatments and to compare interventions across a wide range of diseases[14,40]. The importance of the development, validation, and use of these tools has been well described in the orthopaedic literature[26-29].

In the present prospective study, we sought to determine the effect of surgery for rotator cuff disease on general health status as measured with the Short Form-36 (SF-36). We also sought to determine the prognostic

---

*No benefits in any form have been received or will be received from a commercial party related directly or indirectly to the subject of this article. No funds were received in support of this study.

†Division of Orthopaedics, Department of Surgery, Upper Extremity Reconstructive Service, St. Michael's Hospital and the University of Toronto, 55 Queen Street East, Suite 800, Toronto, Ontario M5C 1R6, Canada. E-mail address for M. D. McKee: mckee@the-wire.com.

TABLE I
PREOPERATIVE AND POSTOPERATIVE LIMB-SPECIFIC SCORES*

Outcome Measure†	Preoperative	Postoperative			
		6 Mos.	12 Mos.	18 Mos.	24 Mos.
SPADI					
Score *(points)*	34.2	69.7	74.2	69.9	74.5
P value		0.0001	0.0001	0.0001	0.0001
SSRS					
Score *(points)*	47.3	58.6	71.8	70.4	72.9
P value		0.147	0.0001	0.0001	0.0001
SST					
Score *(points)*	31.6	54.5	60.9	53.1	61.8
P value		0.0042	0.0001	0.0007	0.0001
M-ASES					
Score *(points)*	46.1	70.4	59.5	59.8	67.3
P value		0.0075	0.0718	0.0516	0.0026
SSI					
Score *(points)*	45.6	78.9	75.2	70.5	75.8
P value		0.0001	0.0001	0.0001	0.0001

*The p values pertain to the comparison between the postoperative score at each time-point and the preoperative score.
†SPADI = Shoulder Pain and Disability Index, SSRS = Subjective Shoulder-Rating Scale, SST = Simple Shoulder Test, M-ASES = Modified American Shoulder and Elbow Surgeons Patient Self-Evaluation Form, and SSI = Shoulder Severity Index.

factors associated with outcome, the time-course of improvement following surgical intervention, and which components of general health status are most likely to be affected.

Materials and Methods

Inclusion and Exclusion Criteria

Between December 1993 and May 1995, seventy-one consecutive patients were enrolled in a prospective trial to investigate the effect of surgery for rotator cuff disease (defined as impingement or tearing, or both) on general health status. All procedures were performed by the senior one of us (M. D. McK.). The clinical diagnosis of rotator cuff disease was made on the basis of patient history (pain with overhead work or activity, pain when sleeping on the involved shoulder, discomfort with internal rotation), physical findings (subacromial grinding or

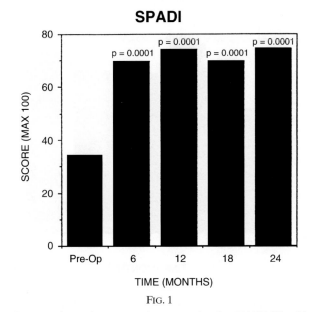

SPADI

FIG. 1
Preoperative and postoperative scores for the SPADI (Shoulder Pain and Disability Index).

crepitus, tenderness in the anterior part of the acromion, positive impingement signs, limited terminal flexion or abduction, weak external rotation, supraspinatus or infraspinatus atrophy), and radiographic findings (acromial spurs, cystic or sclerotic changes at the greater tuberosity, inferior clavicular osteophytes). Patients were considered to be candidates for surgery if they had (1) a clinical diagnosis of rotator cuff disease, (2) shoulder symptoms that had been present for a minimum of six months, (3) a history of failure of conservative care, and (4) substantial relief of pain during abduction and flexion following an injection of local anesthetic into the subacromial space (a decrease of 5 points or more on a 10-point visual analog scale)[35]. For the purposes of this study, an adequate course of conservative care was defined as treatment with at least three of the following: (1) physiotherapy, (2) anti-inflammatory medication, (3) injection of cortisone into the subacromial space, and (4) modification of work or overhead activity, or both.

All of the patients who were entered into the trial fulfilled all four criteria for surgical intervention. Patients with rotator cuff tear arthropathy, instability-associated impingement, glenohumeral arthritis, or other pathological problems involving the shoulder were excluded from the study. Eight patients who had a massive, irreparable rotator cuff tear (more than five centimeters in size) were excluded from the study. Patients who were unable to complete the questionnaires because of a psychological disorder, illiteracy, or lack of command of the English language also were excluded.

Evaluation

Preoperatively, all patients were evaluated with a complete history, physical examination, and radiographs (including a transaxillary view). Patients who were involved in an active Workers' Compensation Board claim were identified. Ancillary investigations, such as magnetic resonance imaging or arthrography of the shoulder, were performed on an individualized basis and were not done routinely. All patients completed five limb-specific questionnaires, including the Simple Shoulder Test (SST)[24], the Shoulder Pain and Disability Index (SPADI)[34], the Subjective Shoulder-Rating Scale (SSRS)[21], the Modified American Shoulder and Elbow Surgeons (M-ASES) Patient Self-Evaluation Form[33], and the Shoulder Severity Index (SSI)[32] prior to surgery[2,12,23]. For the purpose of comparison, all scores were transformed so that 100 points indicated the most positive state of health[2]. During the same sitting, all patients also completed the Short Form-36 (SF-36) general-health-status questionnaire[38,39]. The same five shoul-

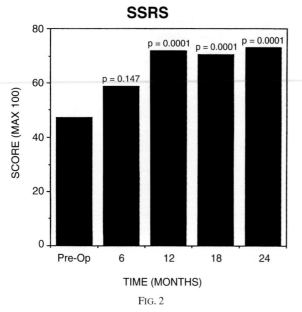

FIG. 2

Preoperative and postoperative scores for the SSRS (Subjective Shoulder-Rating Scale).

der questionnaires and the SF-36 questionnaire were completed at the time of routine clinical follow-up examinations at six, twelve, eighteen, and twenty-four months postoperatively. Demographic data regarding the patient's type of work, level of education, marital status, and medical comorbidities was also collected. A comorbidity was defined as a chronic condition for which the patient had received active treatment from a physician during the year prior to surgery.

The preoperative questionnaire package was completed in the office or clinic at the time of enrollment in the study. Postoperative questionnaires usually were completed while the patient waited in the clinic for medical assessment. If sufficient time was not available for completion during the clinic visit, the patient could take the questionnaire home and return it later; this occurred approximately 10 percent of the time. Completion of the questionnaire package took approximately thirty minutes. Patients were enthusiastic about completing the package once its purpose had been explained to them; they did not require persuasion or prompting in order to complete it, and many added spontaneous written comments. No telephone interviews were conducted. During the first administration of the questionnaire package, an interviewer was available to answer any questions that the patient might have.

Surgical Technique

All patients underwent a standard open acromioplasty, which was performed through a deltoid-splitting approach with the patient in the beach-chair (semi-sitting) position. Following a two-step anterior acromioplasty, the subacromial bursa was excised and the distal part of the clavicle was resected, with removal of ten millimeters of bone and preservation of the coracoclavicular ligaments. We believe that degenerative changes in the acromioclavicular joint are closely related to, and may contribute to, rotator cuff impingement. Excision of the distal part of the clavicle ensures complete rotator cuff decompression, relieves pain at the site of a degenerative acromioclavicular joint, and improves exposure. The rotator cuff was inspected[35]. Forty patients had inflammation, edema, or thinning of the rotator cuff without any visible tear or defect. Thirty-one patients had a rotator cuff tear that was repaired at the time of surgery; there were ten small, twelve medium, nine large, and no massive tears[18]. All tears were debrided to healthy tissue and were repaired with use of standard mobilization and advancement techniques. Most tears were repaired into a trough in bone at the articular margin. The deltoid muscle was repaired with use of interrupted, nonabsorbable sutures that were

placed in a horizontal mattress fashion, and the subcutaneous tissue and the skin were then closed in a standard fashion.

Rehabilitation

Postoperatively, a sling was applied for comfort. Pendulum exercises were begun on the first postoperative day under the supervision of a physiotherapist. Active-assisted flexion and abduction exercises were begun two weeks postoperatively. To protect the integrity of the deltoid repair, full active exercises were restricted until the sixth postoperative week and unrestricted exercises, including resisted motion, were begun at eight weeks. The patient was allowed to return to work as early as possible, depending on the physical demands of his or her occupation, the presence or absence of a rotator cuff tear, and the progression of the rehabilitation.

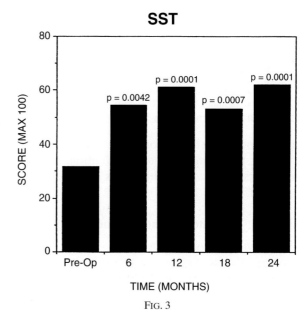

FIG. 3

Preoperative and postoperative scores for the SST (Simple Shoulder Test).

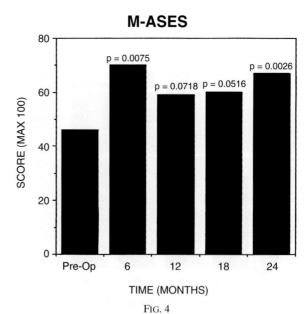

FIG. 4

Preoperative and postoperative scores for the M-ASES (Modified American Shoulder and Elbow Surgeons) Patient Self-Evaluation Form.

TABLE II
PREOPERATIVE AND POSTOPERATIVE SF-36 SCORES*

SF-36 Component	Preoperative	Postoperative			
		6 Mos.	12 Mos.	18 Mos.	24 Mos.
Physical function					
Score *(points)*	60.6	72.7	62.8	73.2	66.8
P value		0.2201	0.7504	0.0349	0.3351
Social function					
Score *(points)*	65.3	76.1	77.8	77.2	79.5
P value		0.1957	0.1034	0.0758	0.0373
Role function-physical					
Score *(points)*	20.8	42.3	50.0	54.0	42.1
P value		0.2221	0.0153	0.0028	0.0615
Role function-emotional					
Score *(points)*	39.2	51.9	37.5	55.3	54.0
P value		0.3237	0.8743	0.0829	0.1084
Mental health					
Score *(points)*	67.9	75.1	77.5	71.2	66.8
P value		0.4675	0.1065	0.5589	0.2067
Vitality					
Score *(points)*	52.3	64.6	57.8	60.5	66.8
P value		0.1019	0.4168	0.1432	0.0105
Pain					
Score *(points)*	38.6	65.8	65.3	60.3	66.1
P value		0.0011	0.0002	0.0007	0.0001
General health perception					
Score *(points)*	68.1	72.7	70.3	66.1	68.1
P value		0.7561	0.7366	0.7829	0.3200

*The p values pertain to the comparison between the postoperative score at each time-point and the preoperative score. SF-36 = Short Form-36.

Statistical Analysis

Statistical analysis was performed with use of the SAS software package (SAS Institute, Cary, North Carolina). Comparisons between preoperative and postoperative scores were performed at each time-point for each of the five limb-specific rating scales and the SF-36 questionnaire with use of a Student two-sample t test. A p value of 0.05 or less was considered significant. The normality of the data was tested with use of the Shapiro-Wilk statistic; a value of $W > 0.05$ was obtained, indicating a normal distribution of scores. The preoperative SF-36 scores for the patients in the study group were compared with normal (control) values after the calculation of z values. To assess the effect of various prognostic variables, data was subdivided and pooled in relation to each variable and evaluated in a similar fashion, with a p value of 0.05 or less considered significant.

Results

Demographic Data

Seventy-one patients (fifty of whom were men and twenty-one of whom were women) with a mean age of 56.1 years (range, thirty-two to seventy-eight years) were enrolled in the trial. The patients had had shoulder symptoms for a mean of 10.6 months (range, six to sixty-one months). All had had a failure of an adequate course of conservative care, as described previously.

Twenty-three patients (thirteen physical or manual workers, eight office or professional workers, and two full-time students) had filed a Workers' Compensation Board claim involving the shoulder. The remaining forty-eight patients (nineteen physical or manual workers, fifteen office or professional workers, ten individu-

als who were retired or unemployed, and four full-time students) had not filed such a claim. With the numbers available for study, we could detect no significant difference between the two groups with regard to the number of physical or manual workers (40 percent [nineteen] of the forty-eight patients who had not filed a claim per-

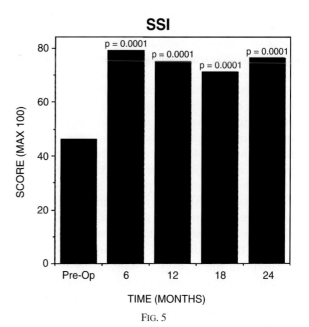

FIG. 5

Preoperative and postoperative scores for the SSI (Shoulder Severity Index).

SF-36
Role Function-Physical

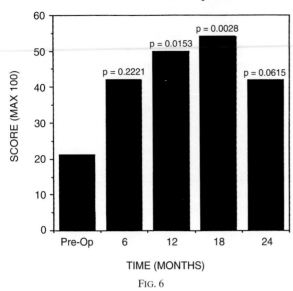

FIG. 6

Preoperative and postoperative scores for the role function-physical component of the Short Form-36 (SF-36) questionnaire.

formed physical or manual work compared with 57 percent [thirteen] of the twenty-three who had filed a claim; p = 0.18). Similarly, we could detect no significant difference between the two groups with regard to marital status (71 percent [thirty-four] of the forty-eight patients who had not filed a claim were married or had a common-law spouse compared with 70 percent [sixteen] of the twenty-three who had filed a claim; p = 0.91) or the presence of a medical comorbidity (27 percent [thirteen] of the forty-eight patients who had not filed a claim had a comorbidity compared with 22 percent [five] of the twenty-three who had filed a claim; p = 0.63). Thirty-eight percent (eighteen) of the forty-eight patients who had not filed a claim had graduated from a college or university compared with 26 percent (six) of the twenty-three who had filed a claim (p = 0.41). Data on mean household income was not available.

Four patients did not complete the study. Their demographic characteristics (age, occupation, educational level, medical comorbidity, marital status, and baseline scores) were not significantly different from those of the patients who completed the study. Two of the four patients had moved out of the country and could not be located. One of these two patients had a 14-point improvement in the SF-36 physical component summary score at twelve months, and the other had a 12-point improvement at six months; these were the last available scores for these individuals. The third patient who did not complete the study was subjectively pleased with the result of the operation but refused to complete the postoperative forms because of a pending legal claim. The fourth patient withdrew from the study because he was diagnosed with systemic lymphoma nine months postoperatively. He had a 9-point improvement in the

physical component summary score at six months, and he was subjectively satisfied with the result of the operation. Complete preoperative and postoperative data was available for the remaining sixty-seven patients (94 percent). All sixty-seven patients were followed at six-month intervals for two years after the operation.

Preoperative Scores

Preoperatively, all patients had significant impairment of upper extremity function as determined with use of the five limb-specific measures (Figs. 1 through 5 and Table I). The mean SPADI score was 34.2 (range, 21 to 75), the mean SSRS score was 47.3 (range, 33 to 87), the mean SST score was 31.6 (range, 15 to 58), the mean M-ASES score was 46.1 (range, 9 to 63), and the mean SSI score was 45.6 (range, 20 to 70). All patients also demonstrated impairment of general health status as measured with use of the SF-36 questionnaire (Figs. 6 through 9 and Table II). The mean physical component summary score was 37.0, and the mean mental component summary score was 45.6; both of these values were significantly lower than control values (p = 0.001 and p = 0.02, respectively)[14]. While the scores for pain (mean, 38.6; range, 0 to 90), role function-physical (mean, 20.8; range, 0 to 95), and physical function (mean, 60.6; range, 0 to 90) were the most severely affected (p = 0.003, p = 0.001, and p = 0.02, respectively), significant decreases also were seen in the other components of the SF-36.

Complications

Four patients (6 percent) had a postoperative complication, and two (3 percent) required a reoperation. One patient had a wound infection that necessitated

SF-36
Pain

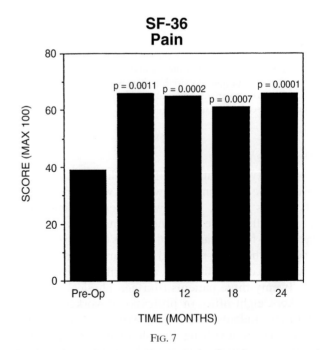

FIG. 7

Preoperative and postoperative scores for the pain component of the Short Form-36 (SF-36) questionnaire.

TABLE III
EFFECT OF ROTATOR CUFF TEAR ON LIMB-SPECIFIC AND GENERAL-HEALTH-STATUS SCORES

	Preoperative			Postoperative		
	Score *(points)*			Score *(points)*		
Outcome Measure*	Tear (N = 31)	No Tear (N = 40)	P Value	Tear (N = 30)	No Tear (N = 37)	P Value
SPADI	31.7	36.1	0.04	70.8	77.5	0.05
SF-36						
Physical component summary	36.2	37.6	0.51	42.4	44.6	0.25
Mental component summary	44.2	46.7	0.32	46.9	49.1	0.46

*SPADI = Shoulder Pain and Disability Index, and SF-36 = Short Form-36.

surgical drainage and débridement, and one patient required total shoulder arthroplasty because of rapid progression of previously minimal osteoarthritic changes. Two patients had a documented rerupture of the rotator cuff but were satisfied with the level of pain relief and declined additional surgical intervention.

Postoperative Scores

The postoperative scores were significantly higher than the preoperative scores. The limb-specific scores showed the greatest magnitude of improvement, and most were significantly improved at six, twelve, eighteen, and twenty-four months postoperatively. Scores tended to plateau by twelve to eighteen months postoperatively (Figs. 1 through 5). When the preoperative SF-36 scores were compared with the final (twenty-four-month) postoperative scores, improvement was observed in a number of categories: the physical component summary score improved from 37.0 to 43.6 (p = 0.01), the role function-physical score improved from 20.8 to 42.1 (p = 0.06), the vitality score improved from 52.3 to 66.8 (p = 0.01), and the pain score improved from 38.6 to 66.1 (p = 0.0001).

The greatest magnitudes of improvement were seen in the pain and role function-physical categories (Figs. 6 and 7 and Table II).

Prognostic Variables

We assessed the effect of a number of variables on the preoperative and postoperative scores that were determined with use of the SF-36 questionnaire and the limb-specific instruments. For the purposes of this analysis, outcome was determined by comparing the preoperative score and the final (twenty-four-month) postoperative score. We detected no relationship between outcome and the variables of age (SF-36, p = 0.55; limb-specific measures, p = 0.43 to 0.65), gender (SF-36, p = 0.87; limb-specific measures, p = 0.78 to 0.89), side of involvement (SF-36, p = 0.41; limb-specific measures, p = 0.59 to 0.75), duration of symptoms (SF-36, p = 0.23; limb-specific measures, p = 0.33 to 0.49), or type of occupation (physical or sedentary) (SF-36, p = 0.14; limb-specific measures, p = 0.23 to 0.35). Two variables were found to have a significant effect on the scores, as demonstrated in Tables III and IV (using one typical limb-

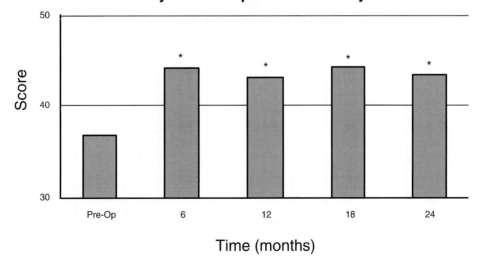

**SF-36
Physical Component Summary**

* = p < 0.05 compared to preoperative values

FIG. 8

Preoperative and postoperative scores for the physical component summary of the Short Form-36 (SF-36) questionnaire.

TABLE IV

EFFECT OF WORKERS' COMPENSATION STATUS ON LIMB-SPECIFIC AND GENERAL-HEALTH-STATUS SCORES

	Preoperative			Postoperative		
	Score *(points)*			Score *(points)*		
Outcome Measure*	No WCB Claim† (N = 48)	WCB Claim† (N = 23)	P Value	No WCB Claim† (N = 45)	WCB Claim† (N = 22)	P Value
SPADI	36.4	29.7	0.02	80.8	61.7	0.01
SF-36						
Physical component summary	38.9	32.9	0.02	45.8	38.7	0.005
Mental component summary	47.6	41.4	0.01	50.7	42.4	0.01

*SPADI = Shoulder Pain and Disability Index, and SF-36 = Short Form-36.

†WCB = Workers' Compensation Board.

specific measure [the SPADI] and the physical component summary and mental component summary of the SF-36). The presence of a rotator cuff tear had a negative effect on the limb-specific scores both preoperatively (p = 0.04) and postoperatively (p = 0.05) but did not have a significant effect on the general-health-status scores (Table III). A positive Workers' Compensation status had a negative effect on the limb-specific and general-health-status scores both preoperatively (p ≤ 0.02) and postoperatively (p ≤ 0.02) (Table IV). Although the physical component summary scores for patients who had filed a Workers' Compensation Board claim showed a similar magnitude of increase compared with the scores for patients who had not filed such a claim (p = 0.32), the mental component summary scores did not improve significantly in either group.

Discussion

Numerous reports in the orthopaedic literature have documented the effectiveness of operative treatment of rotator cuff disease that is recalcitrant to conservative care[1,2,4,5,8-10,15,17,30,35]. Those studies have been criticized because of their retrospective nature, poor follow-up rates, lack of functional outcome data, and exclusive use of limb or disease-specific outcome measures. As the evaluation of the results of medical or surgical intervention has become more sophisticated, the inadequacy of previous outcome measures that rely solely on physician assessment or on surrogate measures (such as radiographic findings) has become apparent[3,23,26-29]. As a result, investigators have developed a number of patient-oriented general-health-status measures in an effort to be more responsive to the factor that is of greatest importance — that is, the patient's perception of the impact of treatment on function and quality of life. One of the most widely used instruments has been the SF-36, which has been shown to be valid (able to measure what it is supposed to measure), reliable (able to yield consistent measurements at different times and in different settings), and responsive (able to measure a change in condition)[38,39]. The efficacy of a variety of orthopaedic interventions, including hip, shoulder, and knee arthroplasties, has been demonstrated with use of the SF-36 in a prospective fashion[12,25,28,29].

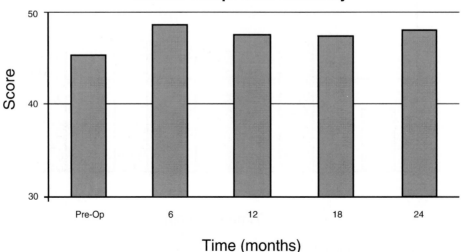

SF-36 Mental Component Summary

FIG. 9

Preoperative and postoperative scores for the mental component summary of the Short Form-36 (SF-36) questionnaire.

A number of recent studies have demonstrated that shoulder pathology has a deleterious effect on both limb-specific and general-health-status scores[13,14,25]. It is clear that shoulder pathology, including rotator cuff disease, can have a significant negative impact on quality of life and general health status and that this impact may not be limited to the so-called physical components of such outcome measures. Matsen, in a prospective study, demonstrated that total shoulder arthroplasty has a beneficial effect on osteoarthritis of the shoulder, although the follow-up period was short[29]. Similarly, Gartsman et al. documented that arthroscopic repair of rotator cuff tears has a beneficial effect on general health status as measured with the SF-36[13]. The present study provides additional information in that it focused on the effect of open surgical treatment of rotator cuff disease (defined as impingement or tearing, or both). By determining the scores at four separate postoperative intervals (ranging from six months to two years following surgery), we were able to examine the time-course of improvement following operative treatment. In most patients, improvement plateaued by twelve to eighteen months postoperatively (Figs. 1 through 9).

Preoperatively, we found a significant level of impairment as measured with use of limb-specific outcome tools (the SPADI, SSRS, SST, M-ASES, and SSI), as has been reported in previous studies[2,14,23,36]. Highly significant improvement in the scores was seen postoperatively (p = 0.0001 to 0.0026). The responsiveness of limb-specific measures to surgical intervention has been documented previously[2,12,37]. In the present study, we found that surgical intervention also had an effect on general-health-status scores, several of which showed significant improvement. While Gartsman et al. found improvements in most categories of the SF-36, including mental components such as vitality and role function-emotional[13], the improvements in the present study were limited to physical components. This may have been due to differences between the studies with regard to the indication for the operation (impingement or tearing, or both, compared with tearing only), the nature of the operative procedure (open compared with arthroscopic repair), and, most importantly, the patient population (inclusion compared with exclusion of patients who had filed a Workers' Compensation claim). The mean increase in the SF-36 pain score in the present study (27 points) was less than that in the study by Gartsman et al. (40 points).

The use of a general-health-status instrument allows for comparisons of improvement following a wide range of medical interventions. We previously reported that the SF-36 pain score improved a mean of 28 points (from 33 points preoperatively to 61 points postoperatively) in patients managed with Ilizarov reconstruction because of a posttraumatic lower-limb deformity[25]. Matsen reported a mean improvement of 26 points in the SF-36 pain score in patients managed with total shoulder arthroplasty because of glenohumeral arthritis[29]. It

seems intuitive that the magnitude of improvement after successful treatment of shoulder arthritis (26 points) or an infected tibial nonunion (28 points) would be greater than that after open (27 points) or arthroscopic (40 points) rotator cuff repair, but this was not reflected by the SF-36 pain scores. The reason for this finding is unclear, and many factors are certainly involved. It has been shown that there are significant differences between patients' and surgeons' assessments of outcome following orthopaedic procedures[23].

Compensation for work-related injuries has been associated with a poor outcome following surgical intervention and with delayed recovery leading to longer time-periods before return to work[4,11,31]. Recently, Viola et al., in a study of patients with a variety of shoulder disorders, showed that Workers' Compensation status has an effect on general health status (including mental components) prior to any surgical intervention[37]. Our results parallel those findings and demonstrate that this phenomenon is also seen postoperatively. Since the demographic characteristics of the patients who had filed a Workers' Compensation claim were similar to those of the patients who had not, we believe that any differences between these groups were related to the compensation status. While both groups had improvement in the physical component summary score, patients who were involved in a compensation claim started with a lower score and thus ended with a lower score. The mental component summary score did not improve significantly in either group. Since most surgeons are familiar with patients receiving Workers' Compensation who remain dissatisfied despite a technically successful shoulder procedure, this information is important for a number of reasons. In the future, it may help the surgeon (1) to identify individuals whose shoulder problem is only one component of their dissatisfaction, (2) to identify individuals who are less likely to have a successful result, (3) to provide a more accurate prognosis for those undergoing surgery, and (4) to focus treatment on other aspects of patient care.

It also has been well documented that a frank rotator cuff tear (as opposed to inflammation, edema, or thinning of the cuff without a tear) has a deleterious effect on function[9,10,16,18,22]. In the present study, the presence of a tear affected the limb-specific scores but did not seem to influence the general-health-status scores. This may be because general-health-status questionnaires lack the sensitivity to distinguish between these two closely related conditions.

The use of health-status questionnaires is convenient, inexpensive, and straightforward. Patients generally enjoy being asked their opinion regarding the relative success or failure of a medical intervention, and many of the patients in the present study provided additional written comments on their forms. Although health-status questionnaires may not be as responsive as limb or disease-specific instruments, they can be administered over the telephone or by mail and thus can eliminate the requirement for extensive follow-up. The information that is obtained may provide a better picture of the patient's assessment of a given medical intervention than is possible with the use of a standard history and physical examination; this information can be used both by research groups and by surgeons who wish to provide their patients with the clearest possible picture of the potential risks and benefits of a potential operation.

In summary, we found that recalcitrant rotator cuff disease had a significant effect on both limb-specific and general-health-status scores. Patients who had filed a Workers' Compensation claim had significantly lower limb-specific and general-health-status scores than those who had not, a finding that persisted postoperatively. As has been previously described in other areas of orthopaedic intervention, surgery had a beneficial effect not only on the anatomical area of interest but also on the general health status and the quality of life of the patient. Surgery for chronic rotator cuff disease reliably and significantly improves overall health status.

References

1. **Bartolozzi, A.; Andreychik, D.;** and **Ahmad, S.:** Determinants of outcome in the treatment of rotator cuff disease. *Clin. Orthop.,* 308: 90-97, 1994.
2. **Beaton, D. E.,** and **Richards, R. R.:** Measuring function of the shoulder. A cross-sectional comparison of five questionnaires. *J. Bone and Joint Surg.,* 78-A: 882-890, June 1996.
3. **Bellamy, N.; Buchanan, W. W.; Goldsmith, C. H.; Campbell, J.;** and **Stitt, L. W.:** Validation study of WOMAC: a health status instrument for measuring clinically important patient relevant outcomes following total hip or knee arthroplasty in osteoarthritis. *J. Orthop. Rheumatol.,* 1: 95-108, 1998.
4. **Bjorkenheim, J. M.; Paavolainen, P.; Ahovuo, J.;** and **Slatis, P.:** Surgical repair of the rotator cuff and surrounding tissues. Factors influencing the results. *Clin. Orthop.,* 236: 148-153, 1998.
5. **Bokor, D. J.; Hawkins, R. J.; Huckell, G. H.; Angelo, R. L.;** and **Schickendantz, M. S.:** Results of nonoperative management of full-thickness tears of the rotator cuff. *Clin. Orthop.,* 294: 103-110, 1993.
6. **Bombardier, C.; Melfi, C. A.; Paul, J.; Green, R.; Hawker, G.; Wright, J.;** and **Coyte, P.:** Comparison of a generic and a disease-specific measure of pain and physical function after knee replacement surgery. *Med. Care,* 33 (Supplement 4): AS131-AS144, 1995.
7. **Cleary, P. D.; Greenfield, S.;** and **McNeil, B. J.:** Assessing quality of life after total hip replacement. *Qual. Life Res.,* 2: 3-11, 1993.
8. **Cofield, R. H.:** Current concepts review. Rotator cuff disease of the shoulder. *J. Bone and Joint Surg.,* 67-A: 974-979, July 1985.
9. **Ellman, H.; Hanker, G.;** and **Bayer, M.:** Repair of the rotator cuff: end result study of factors influencing reconstruction. *J. Bone and Joint Surg.,* 68-A: 1136-1144, Oct. 1986.
10. **Essman, J. A.; Bell, R. H.;** and **Askew, M.:** Full-thickness rotator cuff tear. An analysis of results. *Clin. Orthop.,* 265: 170-177, 1991.
11. **Frieman, B. G.,** and **Fenlin, J. M., Jr.:** Anterior acromioplasty: effect of litigation and Workers' Compensation. *J. Shoulder and Elbow Surg.,* 4: 175-181, 1995.
12. **Gallay, S. H.; Hupel, T. M.; Beaton, D. E.; Schemitsch, E. H.;** and **McKee, M. D.:** The functional outcome of acromioclavicular joint injury in polytrauma patients. *J. Orthop. Trauma,* 12: 159-163, 1998.
13. **Gartsman, G. M.; Brinker, M. R.;** and **Khan, M.:** Early effectiveness of arthroscopic repair for full-thickness tears of the rotator cuff. *J. Bone and Joint Surg.,* 80-A: 33-40, Jan. 1998.
14. **Gartsman, G. M.; Brinker, M. R.; Khan, M.;** and **Karahan, M.:** Self-assessment of general health status in patients with five common shoulder conditions. *J. Shoulder and Elbow Surg.,* 7: 228-237, 1998.
15. **Gazielly, D. F.; Gleyze, P.;** and **Montagnon, C.:** Functional and anatomical results after rotator cuff repair. *Clin. Orthop.,* 304: 43-53, 1994.
16. **Harryman, D. T., II; Mack, L. A.; Wang, K. Y.; Jackins, S. E.; Richardson, M. L.;** and **Matsen, F. A., III:** Repairs of the rotator cuff: correlation of functional results with integrity of the cuff. *J. Bone and Joint Surg.,* 73-A: 982-989, Aug. 1991.
17. **Hawkins, R. J.; Brock, R. M.; Abrams, J. S.;** and **Hobeika, P.:** Acromioplasty for impingement with an intact rotator cuff. *J. Bone and Joint Surg.,* 70-B(5): 795-797, 1988.
18. **Iannotti, J. P.; Bernot, M. P.; Kuhlman, J. R.; Kelley, M. J.;** and **Williams, G. R.:** Postoperative assessment of shoulder function: a prospective study of full-thickness rotator cuff tears. *J. Shoulder and Elbow Surg.,* 5: 449-457, 1996.
19. **Johanson, N. A.; Charlson, M. E.; Szatrowski, T. P.;** and **Ranawat, C. S.:** A self-administered hip-rating questionnaire for the assessment of outcome after total hip replacement. *J. Bone and Joint Surg.,* 74-A: 587-597, April 1992.
20. **Kantz, M. E.; Harris, W. J.; Levitsky, K.; Ware, J. E., Jr.;** and **Davies, A. R.:** Methods for assessing condition-specific and generic functional status outcomes after total knee replacement. *Med. Care,* 30 (Supplement 5): MS240-MS252, 1992.
21. **Kohn, D.; Geyer, M.;** and **Wülker, N.:** The Subjective Shoulder Rating Scale (SSRS) — an examiner-independent scoring system. Read at the International Congress on Surgery of the Shoulder, Paris, July 12-15, 1992.
22. **Kuhlman, J. R.; Iannotti, J. P.; Kelly, M. J.; Reigler, F. X.; Gevaert, M. L.;** and **Ergin, T. M.:** Isokinetic and isometric measurement of strength of external rotation and abduction of the shoulder. *J. Bone and Joint Surg.,* 74-A: 1320-1333, Oct. 1992.
23. **Lieberman, J. R.; Dorey, F.; Shekelle, P.; Schumacher, L.; Thomas, B. J.; Kilgus, D. J.;** and **Finerman, G. A.:** Differences between patients' and physicians' evaluations of outcome after total hip arthroplasty. *J. Bone and Joint Surg.,* 78-A: 835-838, June 1996.
24. **Lippitt, S. B.; Harryman, D. T., II;** and **Matsen, F. A., III:** A practical tool for evaluating function: the Simple Shoulder Test. In *The Shoulder: A Balance of Mobility and Stability,* pp. 501-518. Edited by F. A. Matsen, III, F. H. Fu, and R. J. Hawkins. Rosemont, Illinois, American Academy of Orthopaedic Surgeons, 1993.
25. **McKee, M. D.; Yoo, D.;** and **Schemitsch, E. H.:** Health status after Ilizarov reconstruction of post-traumatic lower-limb deformity. *J. Bone and Joint Surg.,* 80-B(2): 360-364, 1998.
26. **MacKenzie, E. J.; Burgess, A. R.; McAndrew, M. P.; Swiontkowski, M. F.; Cushing, B. M.; deLateur, B. J.; Jurkovich, G. J.;** and **Morris, J. A., Jr.:** Patient-oriented functional outcome after unilateral lower extremity fracture. *J. Orthop. Trauma,* 7: 393-401, 1993.
27. **MacKenzie, E. J.; Cushing, B. M.; Jurkovich, G. J.; Morris, J. A., Jr.; Burgess, A. R.; deLateur, B. J.; McAndrew, M. P.;** and **Swiontkowski, M. F.:** Physical impairment and functional outcomes six months after severe lower extremity fractures. *J. Trauma,* 34: 528-539, 1993.

28. **Martin, D. P.; Engelberg, R.; Agel, J.;** and **Swiontkowski, M. F.:** Comparison of the Musculoskeletal Function Assessment questionnaire with the Short Form-36, the Western Ontario and McMaster Universities Osteoarthritis Index, and the Sickness Impact Profile health-status measures. *J. Bone and Joint Surg.,* 79-A: 1323-1333, Sept. 1997.

29. **Matsen, F. A., III:** Early effectiveness of shoulder arthroplasty for patients who have primary glenohumeral degenerative joint disease. *J. Bone and Joint Surg.,* 78-A: 260-264, Feb. 1996.

30. **Neer, C. S., II:** Anterior acromioplasty for the chronic impingement syndrome in the shoulder. *J. Bone and Joint Surg.,* 54-A: 41-50, Jan. 1972.

31. **Otsuka, N. Y.; McKee, M. D.; Liew, A.; Richards, R. R.; Waddell, J. P.; Powell, J. N.;** and **Schemitsch, E. H.:** The effect of comorbidity and duration of nonunion on outcome after surgical treatment for nonunion of the humerus. *J. Shoulder and Elbow Surg.,* 7: 127-133, 1998.

32. **Patte, D.:** *Directions for the Use of the Index Severity for Painful and/or Chronic Disabled Shoulders,* pp. 36-41. Paris, The First Open Congress of the European Society of Surgery of the Shoulder and Elbow, 1987.

33. **Richards, R. R.; An, K.-N.; Bigliani, L. U.; Friedman, R. J.; Gartsman, G. M.; Gristina, A. G.; Iannotti, J. P.; Mow, V. C.; Sidles, J. A.;** and **Zuckerman, J. D.:** A standardized method for the assessment of shoulder function. *J. Shoulder and Elbow Surg.,* 3: 347-352, 1994.

34. **Roach, K. E.; Budiman-Mak, E.; Songsiridej, N.;** and **Lertratanakul, Y.:** Development of a shoulder pain and disability index. *Arthrit. Care and Res.,* 4: 143-149, 1991.

35. **Rockwood, C. A., Jr.,** and **Lyons, F. R.:** Shoulder impingement syndrome: diagnosis, radiographic evaluation, and treatment with a modified Neer acromioplasty. *J. Bone and Joint Surg.,* 75-A: 409-424, March 1993.

36. **Soldatis, J. J.; Moseley, J. B.;** and **Etminan, M.:** Shoulder symptoms in healthy athletes: a comparison of outcome scoring systems. *J. Shoulder and Elbow Surg.,* 6: 265-271, 1997.

37. **Viola, R. W.; Boatright, C.; Smith, K. L.; Sidles, J. A.;** and **Matsen, F. A.:** Association of shoulder function and health status with Workers' Compensation status in twelve common disorders of the shoulder. Read at the Open Meeting of the American Shoulder and Elbow Surgeons, New Orleans, Louisiana, March 22, 1998.

38. **Ware, J. E., Jr.,** and **Sherbourne, C. D.:** The MOS 36-item short-form health survey (SF-36). I. Conceptual framework and item selection. *Med. Care,* 30: 473-483, 1992.

39. **Ware, J. E., Jr.; Snow, K.; Kosinski, M.;** and **Gandek, B.:** *SF-36 Health Survey: Manual and Interpretation Guide.* Boston, The Health Institute, New England Medical Center, 1993.

40. **Williams, A.:** Setting priorities in health care: an economist's view. *J. Bone and Joint Surg.,* 73-B(3): 365-367, 1991.

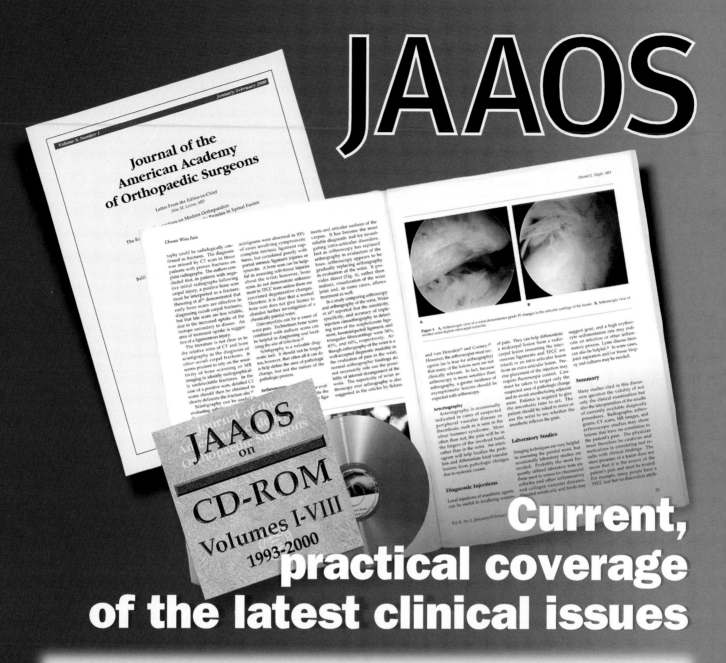

JBJS
THE JOURNAL OF BONE & JOINT SURGERY

JAAOS
JOURNAL OF THE AMERICAN ACADEMY OF ORTHOPAEDIC

section two

Basic
Research

Strength of Fixation with Transosseous Sutures in Rotator Cuff Repair*

BY GEORGE L. CALDWELL, JR., M.D.†; JON J. P. WARNER, M.D.‡; MARK D. MILLER, M.D.§; DOUGLAS BOARDMAN, M.D.‡; JEFFREY TOWERS, M.D.¶, AND RICHARD DEBSKI, M.S.‡, PITTSBURGH, PENNSYLVANIA

Investigation performed at the Department of Orthopaedic Surgery, the Musculoskeletal Research Center, University of Pittsburgh, Pittsburgh

ABSTRACT: The effect of various configurations of placement of transosseous sutures on the immediate strength of fixation was studied in forty-five fresh-frozen humeri from cadavera of older individuals (mean age at the time of death, sixty-three years). The ultimate strength (the strength to failure) was significantly greater ($p < 0.05$) when the sutures were placed at sites more distal to the tip of the greater tuberosity or when the sutures were tied over a wider bone bridge. Cortical augmentation with use of a plastic button through which the transosseous sutures were tied increased the ultimate strength approximately 1.9-fold. The increase in the ultimate strength of the transosseous repair corresponded significantly with the increasing mean thickness of the cortical bone as the sutures were placed more distally along the lateral aspect of the humerus. We concluded that the strength of the fixation of a rotator cuff repair can be increased by placing the transosseous sutures at least ten millimeters distal to the tip of the greater tuberosity and by tying them over a bone bridge that is at least ten millimeters wide. When bone is very osteoporotic, cortical augmentation with a readily available plastic button strengthens the repair.

The repair of a rotator cuff tendon generally consists of reapproximation of the torn edge to a prepared bone surface. Fixation of the tendon into a bone trough in the greater tuberosity with use of transosseous sutures — the McLaughlin technique — is considered to be the standard method for such a repair[1,2,4,10,11].

Recurrence of a tear of a tendon after operative repair is a well recognized complication, and recurrence

*No benefits in any form have been received or will be received from a commercial party related directly or indirectly to the subject of this article. No funds were received in support of this study.

†6000 North Federal Highway, Fort Lauderdale, Florida 33308.

‡The Shoulder Service, Center for Sports Medicine, University of Pittsburgh, 4601 Baum Boulevard, Pittsburgh, Pennsylvania 15213.

§Department of Orthopaedic Surgery, United States Air Force Academy Hospital, 4102 Pinion Drive, Suite 100, United States Air Force Academy, Colorado Springs, Colorado 80840-4000.

¶Department of Radiology, University of Pittsburgh Medical Center/Montifiore University Hospital, 5th Floor, 200 Lothrop Street, Pittsburgh, Pennsylvania 15213.

of large or massive tears may occur relatively frequently[8]. Failure of the fixation may be caused by rupture of the suture material, loss of the suture's so-called grasp of the tendon, or loss of the suture anchor in the bone. In most previous *in vitro* studies of rotator cuff repair, these three modes of failure could not be examined independently as testing involved loading of all three elements of the repair. The mode of failure during testing has often varied, yielding little information about the specific changes in technique that would maximize the strength of each individual component[6,9,12,13]. Gerber et al. provided valuable information on each of the three modes of failure individually. They identified stronger suture materials and improved tendon-grasping techniques but suggested that suture fixation to bone may be the weak link of a standard transosseous repair, especially in elderly individuals who have a chronic tear[7]. They concluded that, in such patients, the osteoporotic bone of the proximal part of the humerus provides poor fixation and the fixation should be augmented to improve the over-all strength of the repair.

Furthermore, the immediate strength of repair with transosseous sutures has been used as a benchmark for the adequacy of newer suture anchors[5,7,9,12] and that of different techniques to augment suture-bone fixation[6,7,13]. However, the exact anatomical placement of the transosseous sutures has not been detailed in any of these studies; thus, the so-called control values are susceptible to variability. To date, we are not aware of any investigation of the effect of different sites for placement of transosseous sutures on the immediate strength of suture fixation to bone.

Therefore, the purpose of our study was to assess how varying the site of transosseous sutures through the greater tuberosity influenced the immediate strength of the repair and to relate these observations to the thickness of the cortical bone in the proximal part of the humerus. Furthermore, we wanted to determine how augmentation of transosseous fixation with a readily available plastic button would affect the ultimate strength (the strength to failure) of the repair.

Materials and Methods

Forty-five fresh-frozen humeri were obtained from the cadavera of individuals who had been a mean of sixty-three years old (range,

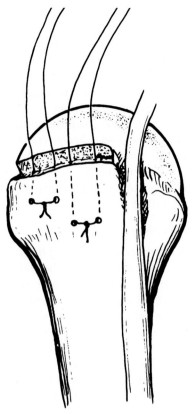

FIG. 1-A

Diagram showing two of the distances between the tip of the greater tuberosity and the placement of the sutures.

fifty-eight to seventy-one years old) at the time of death. The specimens were dissected free of all soft tissue.

Radiographic Analysis

High-quality micro-fine radiographs of thirty-five of the specimens were made, in the anteroposterior plane, before strength-testing was performed. The thickness of the cortical bone along the lateral aspect of the humerus was measured, with use of a calibrated magnifying loupe, at ten, twenty, and thirty millimeters distal to the tip of the greater tuberosity.

Fixation with Transosseous Sutures

A bone trough, four to five millimeters wide and twenty-five millimeters long, was prepared, with use of an osteotome, in the juxta-articular portion of the greater tuberosity in each specimen. Four sutures then were placed through the bone trough and were passed through four drill-holes, placed ten, twenty, or thirty millimeters distal to the tip of the greater tuberosity, in the lateral cortex of the humerus (Fig. 1-A). The four sutures were divided into pairs, and the two sutures of each pair were tied to one another over the bone bridge between the two drill-holes. The precise placement of the drill-holes permitted the pairs to be positioned in the test configurations to be described.

The bone bridge was either five or ten millimeters wide (Fig. 1-B). Because of the distal narrowing of the proximal part of the humerus, there was no ten-millimeter-wide bone bridge at a site thirty millimeters from the greater tuberosity.

A high-density polyethylene suture button (Smith and Nephew Richards, Memphis, Tennessee), with a diameter of nineteen millimeters and a thickness of 1.4 millimeters, was trimmed with a bone-cutter (Fig. 2-A). Pairs of sutures were placed ten millimeters from the tip of the tuberosity and tied over a ten-millimeter-wide bone bridge that had been reinforced with the button (Fig. 2-B). The ultimate strength of augmented fixation was compared with that of non-augmented

fixation at the same site. Seven tests were performed on both the augmented and the non-augmented repairs.

Testing Protocol

Number-five braided non-absorbable polyester sutures were used in the present study. This large suture was chosen in an attempt to eliminate the effect of suture breakage on the ultimate strength of the repair. All free ends of the suture were brought out through the bone trough and tied into a loop, ten centimeters long, over a bar in the crosshead of an Instron machine (model 4502; Canton, Massachusetts), and testing to failure was performed at an extension rate of fifty millimeters per minute. A specially designed clamp allowed the angle of pull to be adjusted to 50 degrees relative to the long axis of the humerus. Statistical comparisons of subgroups were performed with use of two-tailed Student t tests.

Results

Radiographic Analysis

The mean cortical thickness (and standard deviation) ten millimeters from the tip of the greater tuberosity (0.22 ± 0.11 millimeter; range, 0.05 to 0.55 millimeter) was significantly less ($p < 0.001$) than the thickness at the twenty-millimeter site (0.36 ± 0.13 millimeter; range, 0.15 to 0.65 millimeter), which in turn was significantly less ($p < 0.001$) than the thickness at the thirty-millimeter site (0.86 ± 0.35 millimeter; range, 0.16 to 1.50 millimeters) (Fig. 3).

Strength of the Repair

We evaluated the effect of the distance between the site of fixation and the tip of the greater tuberosity as

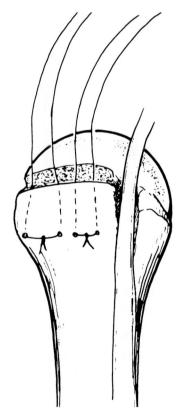

FIG. 1-B

Diagram showing the two widths of the bone bridge.

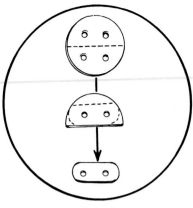

FIG. 2-A

Diagram showing the plastic button, which is divided in half and trimmed to a rectangular shape.

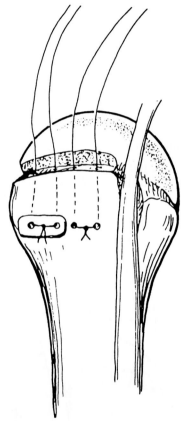

FIG. 2-B

Diagram showing the transosseous sutures tied over the augmentation device as well as the non-augmented fixation.

well as the effect of the width of the bone bridge on the ultimate strength of the repair.

Effect of the Placement of the Sutures

Five-millimeter-wide bone bridge (constant variable): When the distance between the site of fixation and the tip of the greater tuberosity increased from ten to twenty millimeters, the ultimate strength increased significantly ($p < 0.05$), from 69 ± 22 newtons to 94 ± 31 newtons. Similarly, the ultimate strength at the thirty-millimeter site (247 ± 26 newtons) was significantly greater ($p < 0.001$) than that at the twenty-millimeter site (Table I). The ultimate strength of the osseous fixation at the thirty-millimeter site exceeded that of the suture material in all specimens. This site was the only one at which the sutures broke; at the other two sites, all of the suture pulled through the bone at a force that was less than the ultimate strength of the suture material.

Ten-millimeter-wide bone bridge (constant variable): The ultimate strength was significantly greater ($p < 0.005$) at the site twenty millimeters from the tip of the greater tuberosity (165 ± 49 newtons) than at the ten-millimeter site (100 ± 26 newtons) (Table I).

Effect of the Width of the Bone Bridge

Ten millimeters distal to the tip of the greater tuberosity (constant variable): Increasing the width of the bone bridge from five to ten millimeters significantly increased ($p < 0.05$) the ultimate strength of the fixation from 69 ± 22 newtons to 100 ± 26 newtons (Table I).

Twenty millimeters distal to the tip of the greater tuberosity (constant variable): When the width of the bone bridge was increased from five to ten millimeters, the ultimate strength of the fixation significantly increased ($p < 0.05$) from 94 ± 31 newtons to 165 ± 49 newtons (Table I).

Effect of Augmentation

The mean ultimate strength of augmented fixation (183 ± 57 newtons; range, 101 to 252 newtons) was significantly greater ($p < 0.005$) than that of non-augmented fixation (96 ± 54 newtons; range, forty-two to 176 newtons).

Discussion

The fixation of a rotator cuff tendon to the proximal part of the humerus may fail in the early postoper-

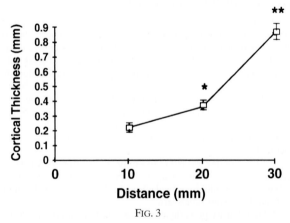

FIG. 3

Graph of the thicknesses of the cortical bone at the three sites on the lateral aspect of the greater tuberosity. The I-bars denote the standard deviation. One asterisk denotes a significant difference compared with the ten-millimeter site and two asterisks denote a significant difference compared with the twenty-millimeter site ($p < 0.001$ for both).

TABLE I
MEAN ULTIMATE STRENGTH (NEWTONS) OF FIXATION ACCORDING TO LOCATION OF SUTURES AND WIDTH OF BONE BRIDGE

Distance between Sutures and Tip of Greater Tuberosity	5-mm Bone Bridge	10-mm Bone Bridge
10 mm	69 (37-100) (n = 8)	100 (73-147) (n = 10)
20 mm	94 (67-158) (n = 7)	165 (74-250) (n = 10)
30 mm	247 (212-285) (n = 6)	—

ative period before the tendon has healed adequately. Retearing of a repaired rotator cuff has been associated with diminished functional results[8]. Furthermore, the results of operative revision of a rotator cuff repair have been less encouraging than those of primary repair[3]. Ideally, the technique for repair of a rotator cuff tendon should maximize the strength of the fixation in the immediate postoperative period. Stronger fixation may allow early rehabilitation without complete failure and may also prevent the formation of a gap at the tendon-bone interface, which may inhibit healing. In practical terms, the repair of a tendon to bone includes three separate components: the material properties of the suture, the grasping power provided by the suture technique, and the strength of the fixation to bone. The current study was designed to examine only the component of fixation to bone by negating the variables of suture material and tendon-grasping power.

Radiographic analysis demonstrated that the cortical thickness of the greater tuberosity progressively increases distally; this means that the ability of the cortex to hold transosseous sutures increases as well. Hecker et al. reported that the holding strength of suture anchors in the proximal part of the tibia was increased by more distal placement, where cortical bone was thicker. Although this concept initially may appear to be self-evident, it is surprising that previous reports[6,7,13] on rotator cuff repair have not included the details of the exact placement of the sutures relative to the greater tuberosity or of the width of the bone bridge over which the sutures were tied. Moreover, some investigators[5-7,13] have compared fixation with transosseous sutures, as a control group, with augmented fixation or fixation with use of suture anchors, as experimental groups, without stating the exact placement of the sutures. The comparisons of the techniques in those studies may be inaccurate because the investigators did not control for these variables.

We studied specimens from the cadavera of older individuals in order to obtain data relevant to a patient who has a chronic large or massive tear of the rotator cuff. We used specimens from individuals who were in the sixth, seventh, or eighth decade of life, as this is the age-group in which tears usually develop. Furthermore, in this age-group, osteopenia of the proximal part of the humerus may make it difficult to secure transosseous fixation for rotator cuff repair.

In our study, the mean strength at a single site of fixation with transosseous sutures ranged from sixty-nine to 247 newtons, depending on its exact placement. Thus, the conclusion in most previous studies[7,13], that the transosseous fixation is the so-called weak link in a rotator cuff repair, is inaccurate. Those studies did not account for the distance of the fixation from the tip of the greater tuberosity or the width of the bone bridge, both of which may affect the strength of the repair.

The purpose of the augmentation device was to increase the functional surface area of the bone bridge and to distribute the stresses of the repair effectively over a greater surface area. Several investigators have demonstrated that the strength of transosseous fixation may be improved by reinforcement of the bone along the lateral cortex of the greater tuberosity[6,7,13]. Gerber et al. noted that the ultimate strength was 2.3 times greater when fixation was augmented with an absorbable poly(L-/D-lactide) membrane, and Sward et al. demonstrated that the ultimate strength was 1.7 times greater when fixation was augmented with a polyethylene patch. Again, those studies did not include the details of the operative methods; that is, there was no information regarding the exact location of the sutures or the width of the bone bridge. Therefore, it is difficult to make direct comparisons among the different augmentation techniques. In the present study, fixation was significantly stronger when it was augmented with a modified, readily available plastic suture button; the augmented repair was approximately 1.9 times stronger than the non-augmented repair when the sutures were placed ten millimeters distal to the tip of the greater tuberosity and the bone bridge between the sutures was ten millimeters wide.

When such distal placement of sutures is not feasible or when the bone is very osteoporotic, the repair can be strengthened by tying the sutures over a bone bridge that is reinforced with a plastic button.

References

1. **Bassett, R. W.,** and **Cofield, R.H.:** Acute tears of the rotator cuff. The timing of surgical repair. *Clin. Orthop.,* 175: 18-24, 1983.
2. **Bateman, J. E.:** The diagnosis and treatment of ruptures of the rotator cuff. *Surg. Clin. North America,* 43: 1523-1530, 1963.
3. **Bigliani, L. U.; Cordasco, F. A.; McIlveen, S. J.;** and **Musso, E. S.:** Operative treatment of failed repairs of the rotator cuff. *J. Bone and Joint Surg.,* 74-A: 1505-1515, Dec. 1992.
4. **Cofield, R. H.:** Current concepts review. Rotator cuff disease of the shoulder. *J. Bone and Joint Surg.,* 67-A: 974-979, July 1985.
5. **Craft, D. V.,** and **Moseley, J. B.:** The fixation strength of rotator cuff repairs with third generation suture anchors vs the transosseous suture technique. *Orthop. Trans.,* 19: 368, 1995.

6. **France, E. P.; Paulos, L. E.; Harner, C. D.;** and **Straight, C. B.:** Biomechanical evaluation of rotator cuff fixation methods. *Am. J. Sports Med.,* 17: 176-181, 1989.

7. **Gerber, C.; Schneeberger, A. G.; Beck, M.;** and **Schlegel, U.:** Mechanical strength of repairs of the rotator cuff. *J. Bone and Joint Surg.,* 76-B(3): 371-380, 1994.

8. **Harryman, D. T., II; Mack, L. A.; Wang, K. Y.; Jackins, S. E.; Richardson, M. L.;** and **Matsen, F. A., III:** Repairs of the rotator cuff. Correlation of functional results with integrity of the cuff. *J. Bone and Joint Surg.,* 73-A: 982-989, Aug. 1991.

9. **Hecker, A. T.; Shea, M.; Hayhurst, J. O.; Myers, E. R.; Meeks, L. W.;** and **Hayes, W. C.:** Pull-out strength of suture anchors for rotator cuff and Bankart lesion repairs. *Am. J. Sports Med.,* 21: 874-879, 1993.

10. **McLaughlin, H. L.:** Lesions of the musculotendinous cuff of the shoulder. I. The exposure and treatment of tears with retraction. *J. Bone and Joint Surg.,* 26: 31-51, Jan. 1944.

11. **McLaughlin, H. L.:** Rupture of the rotator cuff. *J. Bone and Joint Surg.,* 44-A: 979-983, July 1962.

12. **Reardon, J. P.; Moseley, J. B.; Noble, P. C.; Alexander, J. W.;** and **Tullos, H. S.:** The fixation strength of suture anchors in the shoulder. *Orthop. Trans.,* 16:665, 1992-1993.

13. **Sward, L.; Hughes, J. S.; Amis, A.;** and **Wallace, W. A.:** The strength of surgical repairs of the rotator cuff. A biomechanical study on cadavers. *J. Bone and Joint Surg.,* 74-B(4): 585-588, 1992.

Experimental Rotator Cuff Repair

A PRELIMINARY STUDY*

BY CHRISTIAN GERBER, M.D.†, ALBERTO G. SCHNEEBERGER, M.D.†, STEPHAN M. PERREN, M.D.‡,
AND RICHARD W. NYFFELER, M.D., DIPL. ING ETH/FIT†, DAVOS, SWITZERLAND

Investigation performed at the Laboratory for Experimental Surgery, AO/ASIF Foundation, Davos

Abstract

Background: The repair of chronic, massive rotator cuff tears is associated with a high rate of failure. Prospective studies comparing different repair techniques are difficult to design and carry out because of the many factors that influence structural and clinical outcomes. The objective of this study was to develop a suitable animal model for evaluation of the efficacy of different repair techniques for massive rotator cuff tears and to use this model to compare a new repair technique, tested *in vitro*, with the conventional technique.

Methods: We compared two techniques of rotator cuff repair *in vivo* using the left shoulders of forty-seven sheep. With the conventional technique, simple stitches were used and both suture ends were passed transosseously and tied over the greater tuberosity of the humerus. With the other technique, the modified Mason-Allen stitch was used and both suture ends were passed transosseously and tied over a cortical-bone-augmentation device. This device consisted of a poly(L/D-lactide) plate that was fifteen millimeters long, ten millimeters wide, and two millimeters thick. Number-3 braided polyester suture material was used in all of the experiments.

Results: In pilot studies (without prevention of full weight-bearing), most repairs failed regardless of the technique that was used. The simple stitch always failed by the suture pulling through the tendon or the bone; the suture material did not break or tear. The modified Mason-Allen stitch failed in only two of seventeen shoulders. In ten shoulders, the suture material failed even though the stitches were intact. Thus, we concluded that the modified Mason-Allen stitch is a more secure method of achieving suture purchase in the tendon. In eight of sixteen shoulders, the nonaugmented double transosseous bone-fixation technique failed by the suture pulling through the bone. The cortical-bone-

augmentation technique never failed.

In definite studies, prevention of full weight-bearing was achieved by fixation of a ten-centimeter-diameter ball under the hoof of the sheep. This led to healing in eight of ten shoulders repaired with the modified Mason-Allen stitch and cortical-bone augmentation.

On histological analysis, both the simple-stitch and the modified Mason-Allen technique caused similar degrees of transient localized tissue damage. Mechanical pullout tests of repairs with the new technique showed a failure strength that was approximately 30 percent of that of an intact infraspinatus tendon at six weeks, 52 percent of that of an intact tendon at three months, and 81 percent of that of an intact tendon at six months.

Conclusions: The repair technique with a modified Mason-Allen stitch with number-3 braided polyester suture material and cortical-bone augmentation was superior to the conventional repair technique. Use of the modified Mason-Allen stitch and the cortical-bone-augmentation device transferred the weakest point of the repair to the suture material rather than to the bone or the tendon. Failure to protect the rotator cuff postoperatively was associated with an exceedingly high rate of failure, even if optimum repair technique was used.

Clinical Relevance: Different techniques for rotator cuff repair substantially influence the rate of failure. A modified Mason-Allen stitch does not cause tendon necrosis, and use of this stitch with cortical-bone augmentation yields a repair that is biologically well tolerated and stronger *in vivo* than a repair with the conventional technique. Unprotected repairs, however, have an exceedingly high rate of failure even if optimum repair technique is used. Postoperative protection from tension overload, such as with an abduction splint, may be necessary for successful healing of massive rotator cuff tears.

*No benefits in any form have been received or will be received from a commercial party related directly or indirectly to the subject of this article. Funds were received in total or partial support of the research or clinical study presented in this article. The funding source was the AO/ASIF Foundation, Davos, Switzerland.

†Department of Orthopaedics, University of Zurich, Balgrist, Forchstrasse 340, CH-8008 Zurich, Switzerland. E-mail address for Dr. Gerber: cgerber@balgrist.unizh.ch.

‡Laboratory for Experimental Surgery, AO/ASIF Foundation, Clavadelestrasse, CH-7270 Davos, Switzerland.

The repair of chronic, massive rotator cuff tears is associated with a high rate of failure[3,6,8]. The causes and mechanisms of these failures are not known. In a previous *in vitro* study, we assessed different tendon-suturing and bone-anchoring techniques in the infraspinatus tendons of sheep and the proximal ends of severely osteoporotic human humeri similar to those seen with long-standing massive rotator cuff tears[4]. A

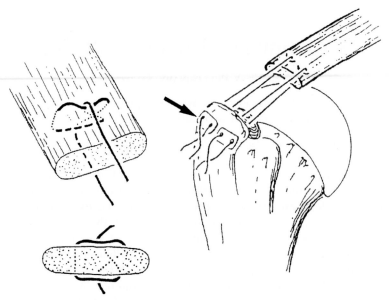

FIG. 1

Drawing showing the modified Mason-Allen stitch and cortical-bone augmentation[4] with a poly(L/D-lactide) plate (arrow). Two modified Mason-Allen stitches and two plates were used in each tendon in the experiment.

modified Mason-Allen stitch and cortical-bone augmentation with a thin, plate-like membrane of poly(L/D-lactide) (Fig. 1) yielded the most satisfactory results on mechanical testing. The goal of the present study was to examine the mechanical and biological properties of the new modified Mason-Allen stitch and bone-augmentation technique *in vivo* in sheep shoulders simulating features of long-standing rotator cuff tears and to compare it with the conventional repair technique that consists of a simple stitch and nonaugmented double transosseous bone fixation (Fig. 2).

Materials and Methods

In the absence of any established animal model suitable for *in vivo* testing of different techniques for rotator cuff repair, the shoulder of the Alpine sheep was selected for this experiment because of the similarity of its infraspinatus tendon to the human supraspinatus tendon[2,4]. The left infraspinatus tendons of forty-seven adult female Alpine sheep were used. The mean weight (and standard deviation) of the sheep was 60 ± 7 kilograms (range, forty-four to seventy-five kilograms), and the mean age was 5 ± 2 years (range, two to nine years).

Test Groups

Three test groups were compared (Table I). Group A had repair of the infraspinatus tendon with three simple stitches and the conventional double transosseous bone-fixation technique. Group B had repair with two modified Mason-Allen stitches and the conventional double transosseous bone-fixation technique. Group C had repair with two modified Mason-Allen stitches and the cortical-bone-augmentation double transosseous bone-fixation technique. Use of the conventional double transosseous bone-fixation technique in both group A and group B allowed comparison of the two different tendon-suturing techniques, whereas use of the modified Mason-Allen stitch in both group B and group C allowed comparison of the two different

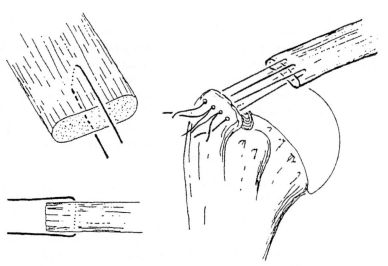

FIG. 2

Drawing showing the simple stitch and double transosseous bone fixation[4]. Three simple stitches were used in each tendon in the experiment.

TABLE I

MODIFICATION OF THE METHODS

Series	Group*	No. of Sheep	Type of Repair	Postop. Prevention of Weight-Bearing	Preload (N)	Distance of Tendon Suture from Distal End of Tendon (mm)	No. of Failures	Mode of Failure† (No. of Shoulders)
I	A	2	Delayed	None	30	10	2	Stitch in scar (2), bone fixation (2)
	B	3	Delayed	None	30	10	2	Stitch in scar (2), bone fixation (2)
	C	3	Delayed	None	30	10	3	Stitch in scar (3)
II	A	2	Delayed	None	30	20-25	2	Stitch pullout (1), bone fixation (2)
	B	2	Delayed	None	30	20-25	1	Suture rupture (1), bone fixation (1)
	C	3	Delayed	None	30	20-25	2	Suture rupture (1), stitch pullout (1)
III	A	3	Immediate	None	30	10	3	Stitch pullout (2), bone fixation (1)
	B	3	Immediate	None	30	10	3	Suture rupture (3), bone fixation (2)
	C	3	Immediate	None	30	10	2	Suture rupture (1), stitch pullout (1)
IV	A	3	Immediate	None	0	10	3	Stitch pullout (3), bone fixation (1)
	B	3	Immediate	None	0	10	2	Suture rupture (2), bone fixation (1)
	C	3	Immediate	None	0	10	2	Suture rupture (2)
V	C	10	Immediate	Partial (with ball under hoof)	0	10	2	Stitch pullout (2)

*The sheep in group A had repair of the rotator cuff with three simple stitches and double transosseous bone fixation, those in group B had repair with two modified Mason-Allen stitches and double transosseous bone fixation, and those in group C had repair with two modified Mason-Allen stitches and cortical-bone augmentation.

†Stitch in scar = failure of a stitch that had been placed into peritendinous scar tissue. Stitch pullout = the stitch pulled through the tendon but did not break.

bone-fixation techniques. The Investigational Review Board at our institution believed that a fourth test group consisting of repair with simple stitches and the cortical-bone-augmentation technique was not warranted because the first three groups would allow identification of whether the modified Mason-Allen stitch was better than the simple stitch and whether the augmented transosseous bone-fixation technique was superior to the nonaugmented transosseous bone-fixation technique.

All of the sheep were suspended in a sling postoperatively and protected from full weight-bearing. The involved limbs were started moving immediately postoperatively through an increasing range of motion. The sheep were observed to be calm postoperatively and did not visibly suffer. No analgesics or nonsteroidal anti-inflammatory drugs were used.

Development of the Sheep Model

Initially, we planned to study the delayed repair of tears of the infraspinatus tendon four to six weeks after transection of the tendon, which would have simulated features of a chronic rotator cuff tear, including retraction, atrophy, and loss of compliance of the infraspinatus muscle as well as osteoporosis of the greater tuberosity of the humerus. In addition, to simulate the condition in humans (in whom some severely retracted rotator cuff tendons can be repaired only under tension), we planned to shorten the infraspinatus tendons before the repair to create tension at the site of tendon-bone fixation. However, a variety of problems were encountered in these pilot studies. The initial protocol was therefore modified several times, and the delayed-repair model was abandoned in favor of an immediate-repair model, with the infraspinatus tendon transected and repaired during the same procedure. Nonetheless, the observations made during the course of these pilot studies have strong clinical relevance and are described in the Results section.

Characteristics of Unsutured Tears of the Infraspinatus Tendon in Sheep

To create a model of delayed repair, a tear of the infraspinatus tendon was made in the left shoulder of two sheep by releasing the tendon at its insertion. The sheep were kept partially immobilized in a hanging device for one week postoperatively to avoid excessive motion of the affected limb. The hanging device consisted of belts around the abdomen and thorax of the sheep. The belts were fixed to the ceiling of the stable with ropes. This hanging device allowed the sheep to stand and bear full weight but prevented them from walking or lying down. When sleeping, the sheep were suspended in these devices. After four to six weeks, the shoulders were removed and dissected. Scar tissue covered the tendon-bone junction. The released infraspinatus tendons were retracted by two to three centimeters, and the scar tissue filled the defects and embedded the tendon stumps. The infraspinatus musculotendinous units were completely removed from the shoulders and weighed with a balance. The volume of the units was determined by measuring the displaced volume of water in a container. Compared with the musculotendinous unit on the contralateral side, the involved musculotendinous units of the two sheep had lost 17 and 18 percent of their weight and 12 and 15 percent of their volume.

Simulation of Osteoporosis by Decortication of the Greater Tuberosity

In each of the two sheep shoulders that had the four to six-week-old iatrogenic tear of the infraspinatus, the humeral head was hard and of good bone quality. Bone-density measurements made on a computed tomography scan revealed a quantitative loss of bone of only 10 and 17 percent at the greater tuberosity compared with the contralateral side. This loss is less than that observed in the humeral heads of patients who have long-standing disease of the rotator cuff[4]. To simulate osteoporosis in humans, the cortical bone of the greater tuberosity was removed with a chisel until cancellous bone was exposed. The area of weakened bone was four centimeters by one centimeter in diameter and was located one centimeter lateral to the site of the original insertion of the infraspinatus tendon (Fig. 3). *In vitro* pullout tests of double transosseous sutures were performed on eight sheep humeral heads. The testing and loading conditions were identical to those in a previously reported *in vitro* study in which the same tests were performed on six osteoporotic humeral heads from human shoulders with a massive rotator cuff tear[4]. In our study, two Ethibond number-3 sutures pulled through the weakened sheep bones at a load of 165 ± 56 newtons, whereas they pulled through the six osteoporotic human humeral heads in the previous study[4] at a load of 146 ± 41 newtons. With the numbers available, no significant differences were found between these two values with the Mann-Whitney U test (p = 0.3).

Pilot Studies of Delayed Repair of Tears of the Infraspinatus Tendon

In the pilot studies of the delayed repair of tears of the infraspinatus tendon, the tendon was first transected at the greater tuberosity and then repaired after a delay of four to six weeks.

All procedures were performed with the sheep under general anesthesia (thiopental, halothane, and nitrous oxide).

A lateral approach was used to retract the deltoid muscle medially. This procedure widely exposed the infraspinatus tendon, which was released at its insertion. The wound was then closed in layers. Postoperatively, the sheep were kept in the hanging device until the second operation for the repair of the tendon.

For the transosseous repair of the tendon after four to six weeks, the same approach was used. The infraspinatus tendon was mobilized by releasing the peritendinous scar tissue. To simulate the intraoperative experience in humans (in whom severely retracted tendons of the rotator cuff can often be repaired only under tension), we shortened the stump of the infraspinatus tendon until an intraoperative tension of approximately thirty newtons was obtained. This level of tension was chosen arbitrarily but corresponds to a level that we have often measured during rotator cuff repairs in humans. The amount of shortening was five to ten millimeters to obtain thirty newtons of tension, which was measured with the extremity in neutral position with a spring-balance (PESOLA; Präzisionswaagen, Baar, Switzerland). Two modified Mason-Allen stitches or three simple stitches with Ethibond number-3 sutures were then placed into the tendon ten millimeters proximal to the tendon end (Fig. 3). A five-millimeter-deep bone trough was created at the site of the original insertion of the infraspinatus tendon. The bone of the greater tuberosity was weakened with decortication as described earlier, and the sutures were pulled through three two-millimeter drill-holes. Either the nonaugmented or the augmented bone-fixation technique was used. For the latter technique, the cortical bone was augmented with two two-millimeter-thick, fifteen-millimeter-long, and ten-millimeter-wide absorbable poly(L/D-lactide) plates (G. HUG, Freiburg-Umkirch, Germany).

Two metallic vascular clips were then placed into the tendon stumps and into the greater tuberosity so that the amount of gap formation between the tendon and the proximal end of the humeral head could be monitored radiographically. The wound was closed in layers. The sheep were kept in the hanging device and protected from full weight-bearing for the first postoperative week. Thereafter, no additional protection was used.

The distance between the clips was measured intraoperatively with a ruler and on radiographs immediately postoperatively; after

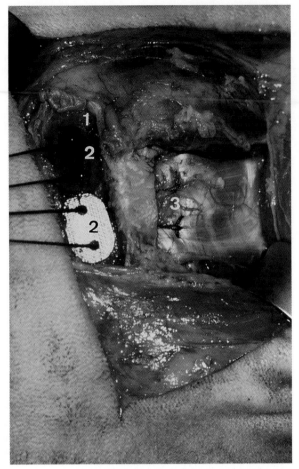

FIG. 3

Intraoperative photograph of the greater tuberosity showing (1) the weakened cortical bone, (2) the poly(L/D-lactide) plates for bone augmentation, and (3) the infraspinatus tendon sutured with the modified Mason-Allen technique and fixed into the bone trough.

one day; after two, four, six, eight, and ten weeks; and at the end of the experiment.

The sheep were killed after six weeks, three months, or six months or when a gap of fifteen millimeters or more between the two clips was discovered on the postoperative radiographs.

The shoulders were removed, and the humeral heads and the tendons were macroscopically analyzed for integrity of the repair. Eleven involved shoulders were used for mechanical pullout tests, and eight contralateral shoulders were used as a control group. For the mechanical tests, the humeral heads were freed of all soft tissues except the infraspinatus tendon and were embedded in methylmethacrylate. The infraspinatus tendon was grasped with a specially constructed clamp. The pullout tests were performed with a universal testing machine (model 4302; Instron, High Wycombe, England). No preload was used for the mechanical tests. The extension rate was five millimeters per minute. During the testing, the specimens were kept moist with saline solution.

Twenty-four specimens were analyzed histologically by one of us (R. W. N.) with the help of two board-certified pathologists. Immediately after the sheep were killed, the axillary artery was injected with a 4 percent dispersion of India ink in Ringer's lactate. The specimens were then submerged into a 4 percent formalin solution, decalcified with 15 percent formic acid, and prepared step by step with water, alcohol, and xylol. They were then embedded in methylmethacrylate and cut longitudinally in the direction of the fibers of the infraspinatus tendon vertical to its surface, in slices of six micrometers, at intervals of five millimeters.

Light microscopy with polarized and nonpolarized light was used to histologically evaluate the specimens after staining with Giemsa and van Gieson stains.

Statistical Analysis

After a discussion with our statistical consultant, we decided not to use statistical analysis to evaluate the data because strictly comparable test groups were too small after the repair methods had been modified several times.

Results

Four sheep were excluded: three had a deep wound infection, and one died of aspiration during the operation. No antibiotics were used during the experiments.

For reasons that will be described, we observed an inordinately high rate of failure in the first eight sheep treated with delayed repair in the pilot study (Table I, series I). The experiment was therefore interrupted. After analysis of the results in these sheep, the methods were modified as will be described. The next step in the experiment involved seven sheep (Table I, series II) and also led to a high rate of failure, for reasons that will be described, so the methods had to be further modified. We made a total of four modifications to the methods before we recognized that protection from full weight-bearing was absolutely essential and that it was necessary to develop an efficient method of prevention of full weight-bearing. There were thus five series: one representing the original method and four, a modification of the method. The observations made during these pilot studies are of strong clinical relevance and are therefore described.

Observations in Series I (Table I)

In series I (delayed repair), seven of the eight repairs, involving each of the three repair techniques, failed. Histological examination revealed that the stitches in the delayed repair had inadvertently been placed into peritendinous scar tissue and not into the retracted original tendon tissue. At the time of the delayed repair, this scar tissue had been indistinguishable from normal tendon. Subsequent *in vitro* pullout tests of modified Mason-Allen stitches placed into the peritendinous scar tissue of two specimens that had a failure of the repair yielded low pullout strength (sixty-four and seventy-eight newtons). This series of experiments was excluded from further analysis, and the protocol was modified as will be described.

Modification of Methods and Observations in Series II Through V (Table I)

In series II (seven sheep; delayed repair), the sutures were placed twenty to twenty-five millimeters proximal to the distal end of the tendon to ensure that the stitches were in the original tendon tissue. In these repairs, the tendon-scar stumps were sutured into the bone trough. Resection of all scar tissue at the distal end of the tendon would have caused tensions that were too high to allow repair to the bone trough. The radiographic follow-up of these sheep indicated failure of the repair in five: two in group A, one in group B, and two in group C. After the sheep were killed, histological analysis did not allow the differentiation of old scar from new scar. With this very high rate of failure, we decided to abandon the delayed repair in favor of an immediate repair of a released tendon.

In series III (nine sheep), we used a one-stage procedure with release of the infraspinatus tendon at its insertion, partial resection of the distal end of the tendon, and immediate repair under thirty newtons of preload. The musculotendinous unit was more compliant and was not retracted or atrophic. Also, direct repair of the tendon end was easily performed. The radiographic follow-up, however, revealed failure of the repair in eight of the nine sheep in this series despite the good compliance of the muscles and the ease of repair.

In series IV (nine sheep), we decided to further reduce the postoperative load. No tissue from the distal end of the tendon was resected, and the repair was performed under no tension. Seven of the nine repairs in this series failed.

At this stage of the experiment, it became clear that, regardless of technique, none of our tested repairs would withstand the loads imposed under unprotected experimental conditions. Protection from weight-bearing was essential. The hanging device still allowed full weight-bearing, and full suspension or immobilization of the limb (including the upper body) in a cast was not tolerated by the sheep. Thus, in series V (ten sheep), a hard ten-centimeter-diameter rubber ball was fixed under the hoof of the involved limb with methylmethacrylate. With this device, the sheep did not bear full weight on the limb but touched the ground, avoiding full weight-bearing and reducing rotational forces between the limb and the ground. The rubber ball was removed after five weeks.

Integrity of Repairs

In series II, III, and IV (without postoperative prevention of weight-bearing), all of the repairs in group A (simple stitch and nonaugmented bone fixation) failed with a gap of more than fifteen millimeters. The cause was pullout of all three simple stitches from the tendon in four of the eight shoulders. In two shoulders, all of the transosseous sutures were found to be pulled into the humeral head. In the remaining two shoulders, a combined failure of the tendon suture and bone fixation was observed. The suture material never broke in this group.

In the group-B sheep (modified Mason-Allen stitch and nonaugmented bone fixation) of series II, III, and IV, two of the eight repairs healed (Fig. 4). All of the modified Mason-Allen stitches were found to be intact. In two limbs both sutures ruptured, and in four limbs one suture ruptured and the other pulled through the bone.

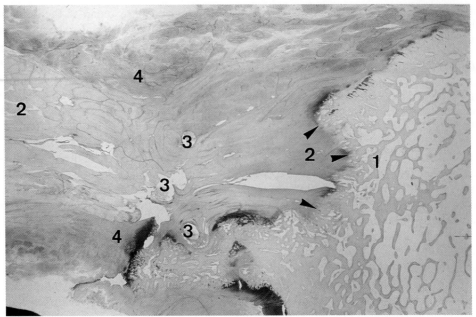

FIG. 4

Photomicrograph of a longitudinal cut through a healed infraspinatus tendon of a group-C sheep killed three months after repair with the modified Mason-Allen technique and bone augmentation (Giemsa staining). 1 = bone trough, 2 = infraspinatus tendon with collagen fibers in contact with bone trough (arrowheads), 3 = remnants of suture material, and 4 = scar tissue.

In the group-C sheep (modified Mason-Allen stitch and cortical-bone augmentation) of series II, III, and IV, three of the nine repairs healed. The modified Mason-Allen stitches slipped out of the tendon in two sheep. In four sheep, the suture material ruptured. The bone fixations were always intact.

Thus, a comparison of technique A (simple stitch) and B (modified Mason-Allen stitch), both with the non-augmented double transosseous bone fixation, revealed that the simple stitches pulled out of the tendon in six of the eight shoulders, whereas all of the modified Mason-Allen stitches of group B were intact. Comparison of techniques B (nonaugmented double transosseous bone fixation) and C (augmented double transosseous bone fixation), which both used the modified Mason-Allen stitch, revealed failure of the nonaugmented bone fixation in four shoulders, whereas the augmented fixation was always intact.

Overall, without postoperative prevention of weight-bearing, all of the repairs with use of both simple stitches and nonaugmented double transosseous bone fixation failed. The modified Mason-Allen stitches were found to be intact in fifteen of seventeen shoulders. In the two repairs that failed, the modified Mason-Allen stitches slipped out of the tendon. The bone fixation was always intact when the augmentation had been used.

Series V (with prevention of full weight-bearing) consisted only of repairs with use of the modified Mason-Allen stitch combined with the poly(L/D-lactide)-plate bone augmentation. Eight of the ten repairs healed. In the two repairs that failed, the modified Mason-Allen stitches slipped out of the tendon.

Of the twenty-two failures in series II through V, one

was identified on a radiograph immediately postoperatively; fourteen, after one week; three, after two weeks; three, after three weeks; and one, after six weeks. Thus, almost all of the failures occurred within the first three weeks after repair.

Macroscopic evaluation of the failed repairs showed that the gaps between the stump of the infraspinatus tendon and the bone trough were consistently filled with scar tissue that bridged the defect. We termed this type of rupture a failure in continuity.

Mechanical Testing of Repairs with the Modified Mason-Allen Stitch and Bone Augmentation

The eight normal infraspinatus tendons in the control group withstood a mean load (and standard deviation) of 2500 ± 286 newtons (range, 2221 to 3141 newtons). Failure at maximum load occurred by rupture of the tendon tissue at the site of the clamp, which suggests that fixation with the clamp may have weakened the tendon and that the actual strength of a normal tendon might be even higher.

Mechanical testing was performed on seven intact repairs, all of which were from group C (repair with the modified Mason-Allen suturing technique and bone augmentation). One was from series II; one, from series IV; and five, from series V (protection from weight-bearing) (Fig. 5 and Table I). In these seven successful repairs, the ultimate failure strength averaged 755 newtons (30 percent of that of normal tendon) after six weeks, 1291 newtons (52 percent) after three months, and 2030 ± 99 newtons (81 percent) after six months.

Mechanical testing was also performed on four unsuccessful repairs that had healed in continuity, with scar

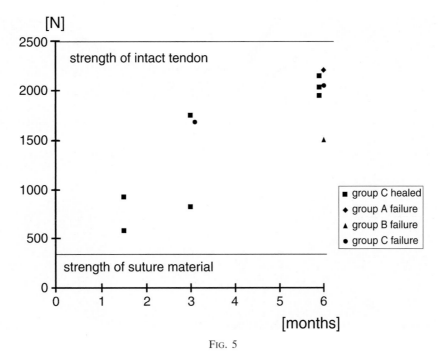

FIG. 5

Plots of the ultimate failure strengths of seven healed repairs and four failures in continuity. All healed repairs were from group C, in which the modified Mason-Allen stitch and bone augmentation were used. One sheep in group C, killed after three months, had a failure in continuity with scar tissue in the gap between the tendon stump and the bone trough. Three other sheep with a failure in continuity were killed after six months. The scar tissue was eighteen millimeters long in one specimen from group A, fifteen millimeters in one from group B, and sixteen millimeters in one from group C.

bridging the gap between the retracted end of the tendon stump and the bone trough (Fig. 5). At six months, the mechanical strength of the scar that bridged the gap between the tendon stump and the bone was approximately the same as that of a successfully healed tendon-to-bone junction (Fig. 5).

Because of the small number of samples in each group in this preliminary study, statistical analyses of the differences in the mechanical strengths of the repairs in the different groups were not carried out.

Structural Changes of the Tendons

The two types of stitches caused similar histological changes in the tendon tissue. The simple stitch caused changes as far as two millimeters around the suture material and as far as the distal tendon stump distal to it. With the modified Mason-Allen stitch, the involved tendon area was larger: there were changes within the sutured tissue, as far as two millimeters around the suture material, and distal to the stitches at the distal end of the tendon.

At one week postoperatively, these changes consisted of a reduced number of vessels and fibrocytes. The cell nuclei were pyknotic or were not stained, suggesting cell death (Fig. 6). In addition, an increased number of rounded cells were found, particularly distal to the stitches. The architecture of collagen-fiber bundles was always preserved. Between the stitches, the tendon tissue appeared normal. Around the tendon stumps, granulation tissue was found that contained vessels, fibroblasts, and longitudinally oriented collagen fibers.

At two weeks postoperatively, the tendon seemed to be edematous with a distended space between the collagen-fiber bundles and in between an increased number of vessels and fibroblasts showing numerous mitoses.

At six weeks, the tendon stumps were still edematous. Fibroblasts and vessels were present in large numbers, and inflammatory cells were observed.

Three and six months after the operation, most repairs appeared to be in continuity either by direct contact between the tendon and the bone trough or by interposition of scar tissue. The tendon stumps were less edematous but still contained numerous fibroblasts and vessels. Within the region surrounded by sutures, the number of fibroblasts was still diminished but the collagen-fiber bundles were generally intact. The scar tissue had a more mature appearance and contained dense collagen-fiber bundles that were mainly parallel and longitudinal in orientation. In some six-month specimens, it was almost impossible to distinguish the scar tissue from the edematous distal tendon stump.

Tendon-Bone Junction

In the sheep, as in humans, the insertion of a normal tendon into bone was found to consist of four layers: tendon, noncalcified fibrocartilage, calcified fibrocartilage, and bone.

At six weeks postoperatively, scar tissue consisting of fibroblasts and parallel collagen-fiber bundles filled the gap between the end of the tendon and the bone trough. Multiple osteoblasts at the border of the trough

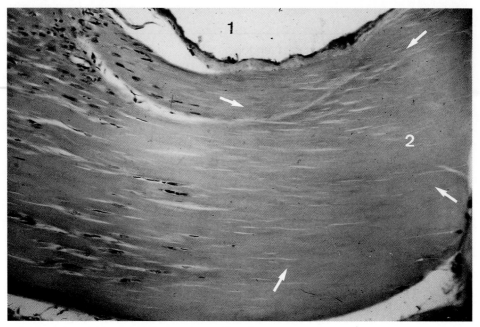

FIG. 6

Photomicrograph of a specimen of tendon sutured with the modified Mason-Allen stitch. The suture material (1) was washed out during the staining procedure. The collagen-fiber bundles (2) are intact, but there are no cell nuclei, suggesting cell death (area marked with arrows).

formed new bone, embedding these collagen-fiber bundles. Some vessels were observed to extend from the scar tissue to the bone marrow. At three months, the bone troughs were found to be completely laid out with new bone. The scar tissue was dense and parallel in orientation. At six months (Fig. 7), the scar tissue was compact and consisted mainly of collagen-fiber bundles lying tightly side by side and resembling normal tendon tissue. The fibers were packed and fixed into the adjacent bone mass, which was covered by a layer of dense,

noncalcified fibrocartilage similar to that found at a normal tendon-to-bone junction. Calcified fibrocartilage (as found in a normal tendon insertion) was not observed.

Bone Augmentation with Absorbable Poly(L/D-Lactide) Membranes

The poly(L/D-lactide) plates were covered by a thin capsule of nonreactive connective tissue with only a few inflammatory cells such as macrophages and giant cells.

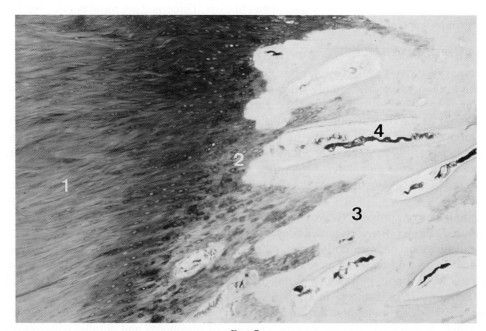

FIG. 7

Photomicrograph showing the bone trough at six months in a sheep from group C, series V, with a successful repair. 1 = mature scar tissue that resembles tendon tissue, 2 = noncalcified fibrocartilage, 3 = bone, and 4 = blood vessel filled with India ink.

After six months, the plates measured approximately 100 micrometers. All of the plates were found to be intact, but some of the membranes had a small degree of bowing, which indicated load uptake.

Discussion

More than half of the repairs of chronic, massive rotator cuff tears rupture again and fail[3,5,6]. As successful repairs that remain intact yield substantially better functional results than those that fail[3,5,6,8], obtaining healing of the repair is of crucial importance if postoperative function, rather than relief of pain alone, is a major goal. Current clinical[5,6,9] and experimental[2,4] evidence suggests that the repair technique may play an important role in the prevention of failure.

In humans, the analysis of failures of rotator cuff repairs, except those necessitating revision, is limited to imaging studies such as arthrography, ultrasonography, and magnetic resonance imaging. Even in prospective clinical series, many variables such as the size, location, and age of the tear as well as the postoperative compliance of the patients render the analysis of failures difficult. Animal experiments are necessary to define conditions for successful repairs in humans.

To our knowledge, no one has previously reported a satisfactory experimental model with which to develop techniques that lead to successful repair. After thorough study of different possibilities and in vitro experimentation with sheep shoulders[4], we developed an in vivo animal model of human rotator cuff tears. In our pilot series I and II (delayed repair), retraction and atrophy of the muscle were simulated in subacute rotator cuff tears but it was impossible to distinguish between the true tendon stump and the newly formed scar at the time of delayed repair. This problem severely compromised the experiment. Therefore, in series III, IV, and V, the tendon was detached and immediately repaired so that the experimental condition corresponded to an acute tear. Degeneration of the tendon and changes of mechanical properties of the musculotendinous unit, as encountered in long-standing tears in humans[7], were not simulated in series III, IV, and V.

Osteoporosis of the greater tuberosity is often encountered in shoulders that have a long-standing rotator cuff tear. The intraoperative finding in patients that nonaugmented transosseous suture fixation to osteoporotic humeral heads can be mechanically weak was confirmed in a previous in vitro study[4]. Other authors have also identified the greater tuberosity as a potential location for transosseous suture failure[1]. They found that the strength of transosseous suture fixation can be increased by placing the sutures at sites more distal to the tip of the greater tuberosity or by tying the sutures over a wider bone bridge. The role of osteoporosis in the failure of rotator cuff repair in human shoulders has not been studied in vivo, to our knowledge. Considering that the causes of failure of rotator cuff repairs in humans

are not known, we planned to simulate the features of rotator cuff tears that might be important factors in failures, including osteoporosis. Decortication caused weakening of the greater tuberosity of the sheep, resulting in in vitro holding strength for transosseous sutures similar to that of osteoporotic humeral heads. However, this model can only be considered an approximation of the human shoulder with a massive rotator cuff tear and consequent osteoporosis.

The potential for healing seems to be better for the sheep infraspinatus tendon than for the human supraspinatus tendon. The retracted infraspinatus tendons in failed repairs were always embedded in scar tissue that bridged the created defects, which resulted in lengthening of the tendon and shortening (retraction) of the muscle (failure in continuity). Although rotator cuff tears in humans are more likely to be characterized by a tissue defect, intraoperative observations by one of us (C. G.) led us to believe that this type of failure in continuity also exists in humans. This observation deserves further attention.

The need for protection of the shoulder after rotator cuff repair is extremely controversial. We expected that the repairs would be compatible with the limited activity of the sheep. Suspension in a sling allowed the sheep to bear full weight on all of the extremities but prevented them from walking. Inability to reach the ground was not tolerated by the sheep, and it was only in the last series of experiments that a solution was found to prevent the sheep from bearing full weight on the affected extremity. Mounting a rubber ball on the involved hoof apparently changed the proprioceptive feedback of the sheep so that they avoided weight-bearing.

The present study documented that the holding power of a modified Mason-Allen stitch was distinctly better than that of a simple stitch, as most of the simple stitches failed and only two of the modified Mason-Allen stitches failed. On histological examination, this new tendon-suturing technique was found to be biocompatible. Signs of tendon-tissue damage were identified but were limited to a small area of sutured tendon tissue. This tissue damage was found predominantly at one week postoperatively. Thereafter, the tendon had mostly recovered. The simple stitch was less strangulating. Nevertheless, the same local tendon damage was found in a small area surrounding the stitches. The increased area of tendon damage with the modified Mason-Allen stitch was temporary and had no apparent clinical effect.

The failure modes in this study also documented that fixation over augmented cortical bone was distinctly more reliable than that over nonaugmented cortical bone. The repairs with augmented fixation never failed at their knot or over the plate; the in vivo results with bone augmentation therefore confirmed those of the corresponding in vitro study[4]. The absorbable poly(L/D-lactide) membranes were well tolerated by the sheep, but advanced degradation of the membranes had not yet taken place; a longer duration of follow-up is necessary for analysis of tolerance of this type of implant. In clinical practice, a titanium plate is currently used and has not yet been associated with complications. A repair with a modified Mason-Allen stitch and cortical-bone augmentation transformed the suture into the weakest link in the chain.

Regardless of the repair technique, the suture material was not able to withstand the loads that were imposed on the repair if the sheep were not prevented from weight-bearing. However, without weight-bearing, the loads imposed on the repairs performed with the modified Mason-Allen stitch and cortical-bone augmentation could be managed successfully and the repairs healed.

Poor-quality tendon tissue may be another cause of failure of rotator cuff repairs. It was not possible to address this question in the present study. However, placing the stitches into peritendinous scar tissue resulted in disruption of the repair. The four to six-week-old scar tissue felt hard when the suture needle was passed through it, but mechanical tests showed that this immature scar tissue was weak. We therefore try never to put stitches into tendon-like tissue that is hard or stiff or appears myxomatous, and we usually debride such tissue, during rotator cuff repair in patients.

The model in the present study certainly cannot be accepted as fully simulating rotator cuff repair in humans. Nonetheless, the study documented that a modified tendon-suturing technique was associated with fewer failures than a simple stitch, without causing strangulation and tendon necrosis. It confirmed that non-augmented fixation in the greater tuberosity could fail, whereas augmented bone fixation did not, and that the use of such a repair technique did not cause any apparent complications. Most of all, the study documented that, regardless of the technique, no repair was able to withstand the high loads imposed by weight-bearing. Given that the clinical results of successful repairs are superior to those of failed repairs[3,5,6,8], the use of an optimum repair technique and adequate protection of the repair until healing appear warranted.

NOTE: The authors wish to acknowledge the enormous technical support of Roland Würgler, mechanical engineer, throughout the study. Thanks are also due to Jiangming Xu, M.D., Werner Wüst, M.D., and Hubert Laeng, M.D., for their contributions to the histological evaluation; to Iris Keller, Elena Rampoldi, Petra Romer, Katrin Kampf, and Margret Hostettler for the preparation of the histological specimens and operative assistance; and to Urban Lanker for the care of the sheep. The support of Prof. Berton Rahn, M.D., throughout this study is especially and gratefully acknowledged.

References

1. **Caldwell, G. L., Jr.; Warner, J. J. P.; Miller, M. D.; Boardman, D.; Towers, J.; and Debski, R.:** Strength of fixation with transosseous sutures in rotator cuff repair. *J. Bone and Joint Surg.,* 79-A: 1064-1068, July 1997.

2. **France, E. P.; Paulos, L. E.; Harner, C. D.; and Straight, C. B.:** Biomechanical evaluation of rotator cuff fixation methods. *Am. J. Sports Med.,* 17: 176-181, 1989.

3. **Gazielly, D. F.; Gleyze, P.; and Montagnon, C.:** Functional and anatomical results after rotator cuff repair. *Clin. Orthop.,* 304: 43-53, 1994.

4. **Gerber, C.; Schneeberger, A. G.; Beck, M.; and Schlegel, U.:** Mechanical strength of repairs of the rotator cuff. *J. Bone and Joint Surg.,* 76-B(3): 371-380, 1994.

5. **Gerber, C.; Fuchs, B.; and Hodler, J.:** The clinical and structural results of direct repair of massive tears of the rotator cuff. Read at the Annual Meeting of the American Shoulder and Elbow Surgeons, New Orleans, Louisiana, March 22, 1998.

6. **Harryman, D. T., II; Mack, L. A.; Wang, K. Y.; Jackins, S. E.; Richardson, M. L.; and Matsen, F. A., III:** Repairs of the rotator cuff. Correlation of functional results with integrity of the cuff. *J. Bone and Joint Surg.,* 73-A: 982-989, Aug. 1991.

7. **Hersche, O., and Gerber, C.:** Passive tension in the supraspinatus musculotendinous unit after long-standing rupture of its tendon. A preliminary report. *J. Shoulder and Elbow Surg.,* 7: 393-396, 1998.

8. **Postel, J. M.; Goutallier, D.; Lavau, L.; and Bernageau, J.:** Anatomical results of rotator cuff repairs. Study of 57 cases controlled by arthrography [abstract]. *J. Shoulder and Elbow Surg.,* 3: 20, 1994.

9. **Thomazeau, H.; Boukobza, E.; Morcet, N.; Chaperon, J.; and Langlais, F.:** Prediction of rotator cuff repair results by magnetic resonance imaging. *Clin. Orthop.,* 344: 275-283, 1997.

Thermal Modification of Connective Tissues: Basic Science Considerations and Clinical Implications

Steven P. Arnoczky, DVM, and Alptekin Aksan, MS

Abstract

Thermal modification (shrinkage) of capsular connective tissue has gained increasing popularity as an adjunctive or even a primary procedure in the arthroscopic treatment of shoulder instability. Although the physical effects of heat on collagenous tissues are well known, the long-term biologic fate of these shrunken tissues is still a matter of debate. The temperatures required to alter the molecular bonding of collagen and thus cause tissue shrinkage (65°C to 70°C) are also known to destroy cellular viability. Therefore, thermally modified tissues are devitalized and must undergo a biologic remodeling process. During this remodeling, the mechanical properties of the treated tissues are altered (decreased stiffness) and can be at risk for elongation if the postoperative rehabilitation regimen is too aggressive. Although anecdotal reports suggest that thermal capsular shrinkage does have a beneficial effect, the exact mechanism responsible for this clinical improvement has yet to be fully defined. The reported improvement could be due to the maintenance of initial capsular shrinkage, secondary fibroplasia and resultant thickening of the joint capsule, a loss of afferent sensory stimulation due to the destruction of sensory receptors, or a combination of all three. The clinical role for thermal modification of connective tissues has not yet been defined, but it appears that it may prove most useful as a stimulant for inducing a biologic repair response.

J Am Acad Orthop Surg 2000;8:305-313

The application of heat as a therapeutic modality has evolved from the ancient use of fire to sterilize wounds and control bleeding to the modern-day use of hyperthermia to treat various forms of cancer. This evolution arose from a better understanding of the tissue biology associated with the application of thermal energy and an improved ability to control the amount of heat delivered, as well as the precision of its application. Although the use of boiling oils, heated metals, and magnified sunlight in medicine has been replaced by modern electrocautery and laser energy, the major therapeutic uses of these sources of heat in surgery remain essentially the same: hemostasis and tissue ablation.

Recently, the use of thermal energy has been proposed as a means of shrinking redundant or lax connective tissues through the well-established mechanism of collagen denaturation.[1-18] Although numerous in vitro[4,7,8,10-12,15,16,19] and in vivo[6,9,17,20,21] experimental studies have investigated the biology and biomechanics of thermally modified tissues, there is still no unanimity of opinion regarding the optimal therapeutic algorithm (e.g., the degree of tissue shrinkage required and the optimal postoperative regimen), the ultimate mechanism of the reported clinical improvements, or the long-term fate of the thermally modified tissues. There is, however, agreement on the basic science of the thermal modification of connective tissues, as well as on some of the potential clinical implications associated with its use.

Mechanism of Thermal Shrinkage of Collagen

Ligaments and joint capsule are composed primarily of type I collagen. The type I collagen molecule is made up of three polypeptide chains, which are stabilized in a triple-helix arrangement by intramolecular cross-links. These molecules are, in turn, aggregated into a parallel pattern to form collagen

Dr. Arnoczky is Director, Laboratory for Comparative Orthopaedic Research, College of Veterinary Medicine, Michigan State University, East Lansing. Mr. Aksan is a doctoral student, Department of Mechanical Engineering, College of Engineering, Michigan State University.

Reprint requests: Dr. Arnoczky, Laboratory for Comparative Orthopaedic Research, College of Veterinary Medicine, Michigan State University, East Lansing, MI 48824.

fibrils. This fibrillar arrangement is maintained by intermolecular cross-links and provides the tissue with its tensile properties. The intramolecular cross-links are reducible covalent aldehyde bonds, which are progressively replaced by irreducible multivalent cross-links as the tissue ages.

When collagen is heated, the heat-labile intramolecular cross-links are broken, and the protein undergoes a transition from a highly organized crystalline structure to a random, gel-like state (denaturation) (Fig. 1).[22] Collagen shrinkage occurs through the cumulative effect of the "unwinding" of the triple helix, due to the destruction of the heat-labile intramolecular cross-links, and the residual tension of the heat-stable intermolecular cross-links (Fig. 2).[22,23]

Collagen denaturation typically occurs at approximately 65°C. The precise heat-induced behavior of connective tissues (and the extent of tissue shrinkage) are dependent on several factors, including the maximum temperature reached and exposure time[23] and the mechanical stress applied to the tissue during heating.[19] The thermal properties of

a tissue can also vary with species, age, the pH and electrolyte concentration of the surrounding environment, the concentration and orientation of the collagen fibers, and the hydration level of the tissue.[24,25]

Increased collagen content, directionality of fiber orientation, and increased tensile load have been shown to increase the temperature necessary for shrinkage of connective tissue.[24] Aging has also been shown to increase this temperature, probably due to the age-related increased ratio of heat-stable to heat-labile cross-links.[24,25] In addition, increased pH of the surrounding medium and dehydration of the tissues are known to increase the shrinkage temperature.

On the macroscopic level, the effect of heat on dense, regularly oriented connective tissues (e.g., ligaments and tendons) may be summarized as shrinkage along an axis parallel to the dominant direction of fiber orientation accompanied by swelling on the transverse axis. In dense, irregularly oriented connective tissues (e.g., joint capsule), shrinkage still occurs along the long axis of the collagen fibers. However, because the fiber orienta-

tion is multidirectional in these tissues, the extent and principal axis of shrinkage are less predictable.

Experimental Studies

Since the initial clinical application of thermal shrinkage in the shoulder joint, there have been numerous in vitro and in vivo studies that characterize the biomechanical and biologic effect of thermal modification on tendons, ligaments, and the joint capsule.

In Vitro Studies

Examination and quantification of the thermal response characteristics of collagenous tissues are difficult due to the diversity of species and the compositional variance among tissues. In the past four decades, researchers have performed various experiments with tendon, ligament, skin, joint capsule, and corneal tissue specimens harvested from different species (cow, dog, rat, rabbit, sheep, and human).[7,8,10,21]

It has been established that when collagenous tissues are exposed to high temperatures (in the range of 65°C to 85°C for most tissue types

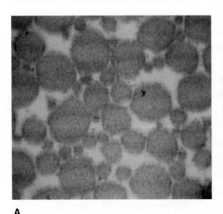 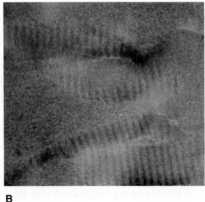 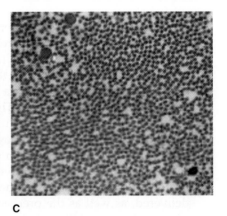

A B C

Figure 1 **A,** Electron-photomicrograph of a cross section of a normal rabbit patellar tendon. Note the normal bimodal pattern of large- and small-diameter collagen fibers and the longitudinal orientation of all fibers (original magnification ×34,000). **B,** Cross section of rabbit patellar tendon immediately after thermal shrinkage. Note the random orientation of the collagen fibers (original magnification ×34,000). **C,** Cross section of a rabbit patellar tendon 8 weeks after thermal modification shows remodeling with small-diameter collagen fibers, indicative of scar tissue (original magnification ×34,000).

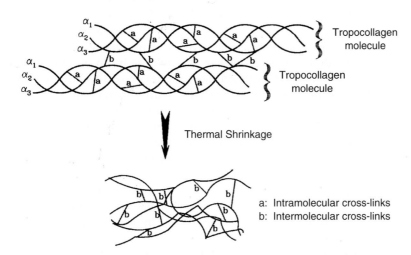

Figure 2 Molecular mechanism of collagen shrinkage. The intramolecular cross-links within the tropocollagen molecules are denatured, but the intermolecular cross-links between the tropocollagen molecules are maintained.

and species), they undergo rapid denaturation.[22] The resultant effect of the microscopic phenomenon of collagen denaturation is tissue shrinkage.[23] At a constant temperature, shrinkage increases with increased exposure until it reaches a plateau value beyond which no additional shrinkage is observed. This ultimate value of shrinkage changes with the treatment temperature[23] and the mechanical load applied to the tissue during heating.[19] Heating to excessive temperatures for extended periods of time results in hyalinization, extensive thermal damage, and necrosis of the tissue.[26]

Hydrothermal heating experiments performed on specimens taken from different regions of cadaver glenohumeral joint capsules point to a correlation between the maximum temperature reached and the amount of tissue shrinkage.[8] Exposure to heating at 65°C for 10 minutes results in 10% shrinkage, whereas 60% shrinkage occurs after only 1.5 minutes at 80°C. These results support the axiom that the higher the maximum temperature reached during heating, the greater

the shrinkage. It is also evident from the same data that the time required to reach the same amount of shrinkage decreases with increasing temperature. A similar experiment with the use of radio-frequency heating of specimens harvested from sheep glenohumeral joint capsules demonstrated less than 4% shrinkage at temperatures below 65°C, but reached a peak value of 14% shrinkage at 80°C.[11]

Discrepancies among these results may have resulted from the interspecies differences in tissue composition and the possible nonthermal effects of the two heating modalities.[3] The variability of the amount of shrinkage of similar tissues from different species under identical heating conditions is well established in the literature.[19,21] It has also been shown that these variations correlate well with the differences in the physiologic body-core temperatures of the species. Another factor is that laser heating causes local dehydration of the tissues due to evaporation of fluids in the target volume, whereas this is not a problem with hydrothermal heating. It has also been postulated that laser

energy enhances healing by stimulating collagen synthesis; however, as yet no study has compared the nonthermal effects of the various healing modalities.

There are other differences among heating modalities. In hydrothermal heating, the tissue sample is immersed in a constant-temperature bath, and the tissue rapidly comes into thermal equilibrium with its surroundings. Therefore, a homogeneous temperature distribution can be obtained within the tissue. In laser or radio-frequency heating, the temperature distribution created within the tissue is a function of the probe-sweep velocity, the distance between the target tissue and the probe, and the heat-penetration depth. The combination of these factors may easily cause nonhomogeneous heating. Differences between the thermal histories of regions within the same tissue volume may cause significant changes in ultrastructure and overall behavior, resulting in nonuniform shrinkage.

Researchers realize that hydrothermal and laser heating cause differences in the resultant collagenous tissue ultrastructure,[8] but these variations have not been specifically attributed to either nonthermal effects or differences between applications. In addition, after heating, if the collagenous tissue is cooled to room temperature, some collagen molecules regain their triple-helix structure (renaturation). This may be accompanied by relaxation of 5% to 10% of the total amount of shrinkage obtained.[19]

The effect of mechanical stress on the shrinkage and postheating relaxation characteristics of bovine chordae tendineae has been investigated. In one study,[19] a fivefold increase in the applied stress caused about a 15% decrease in the final plateau value of shrinkage and delayed the renaturation process. The authors suggested that there is a time-temperature-load equivalency in the heat-induced shrinkage of collagenous tissues. That is, these variables are to an extent interchangeable (they have similar effects on gross tissue behavior), and a change in any of them affects the shrinkage process. This hypothesis may have very important clinical applications, in that the same amount of tissue shrinkage may be obtained at a lower temperature, minimizing the risk of excessive loss of stiffness and thermal damage to the surrounding tissues.

Research performed on cadaver glenohumeral capsular tissues suggests that the stiffness of heated collagenous tissue decreases while viscoelastic properties remain unaltered.[4,8] Stiffness values down to 90% of normal have been measured after aggressive laser heating.[4,8] Similar to the shrinkage response, the decrease in stiffness is also dose-related.[16] The higher the heating (and thus the greater the shrinkage), the greater the loss of stiffness. It has been suggested that the loss of stiffness is of concern because it may make the tissues more vulnerable to postoperative mechanical loading.[5,21]

In Vivo Studies

There have been only a limited number of studies of the in vivo effects of thermal modification on connective tissue biology and biomechanics.[6,8,17,20,21] However, most researchers agree that after thermal modification and the accompanying local cell death, modified tissues undergo a repair response characterized by fibroplasia, neovascularization, and fibrovascular scar formation. In studies on sheep[8] and rabbits,[6] tissue has been shown to begin to regenerate only 7 days after treatment, as evidenced by hyperplasia and increased fibroblastic activity. Vascularization of the scar region and migration of more fibroblasts to the treated site accompany the long-term healing response of the tissue. After 1 month, newly

synthesized collagen molecules and small-diameter fibrils are present in the scar area.[6,8]

Subphysiologic loads are known to accelerate healing. However, it has been observed that when thermally modified tissue is subjected to physiologic loads in the immediately postoperative period, it can elongate to its preoperative length within 4 weeks.[21] Although the initial shrinkage values obtained in rabbit patellar tendons with laser treatment in both in vivo and in vitro experiments were the same, the in vivo study showed relaxation back to the original length by 4 weeks and beyond the original length by 8 weeks.[21]

A recent study has suggested that it may take as long as 12 weeks for thermally modified tissues to regain normal strength.[20] However, another study has shown that during that same period of time the tissue has an increased susceptibility to creep.[17] There is no unanimity of opinion as to the time at which thermally modified tissues regain their normal material and biologic properties. Anecdotal reports have described a total absence of capsular tissues at surgery in patients who had previously failed laser-assisted capsular shrinkage for shoulder stabilization. However, the mechanisms potentially responsible for this loss of tissue (e.g., overzealous shrinkage, extensive heat) have yet to be identified. These findings point to the need for further research on the response of thermally modified tissues in the postoperative period and the effects of various rehabilitation regimens (e.g., immobilization).

Delivery of Thermal Energy

Clinically, two types of energy systems have been used to thermally modify connective tissues: laser energy and radio-frequency energy.[11,27]

Laser Energy

The laser is an electro-optical device capable of efficiently transmitting energy in the form of an intense beam of light. The radiant energy of the laser beam can be transformed into heat energy through its interaction with tissues. This interaction is dependent on the wavelength of the laser and the properties of the tissue. Laser light is absorbed by water, and, as most biologic tissues are composed mainly of water, the tissues are heated.

In addition to the nature of the interaction with the tissue, the extent of the thermal effect of a laser is also controlled by the power density, the spot size, and the duration of application. The total power output of a laser is measured in watts, and the power density (measured in watts per square centimeter) is directly correlated with the thermal effect produced in the tissue. The spot size (the tissue area on which the laser light is concentrated) is an important factor in determining power density. Power density can be increased by increasing power output or by decreasing spot size (i.e., power density varies as the inverse of the area). The time of laser application can also affect the amount of energy delivered to the tissue and the resultant thermal effect. Pulsing the laser beam (rapidly alternating the beam off and on) creates a cooling effect between pulses in a fluid medium and can limit heat transfer to adjacent tissues. This helps limit the depth of penetration and tissue damage.

The holmium–yttrium-aluminum-garnet (Ho:YAG) laser was the first system used clinically for the thermal modification of connective tissues. No one therapeutic algorithm has yet been rigorously tested. Because of the noncontact nature of the Ho:YAG laser probe, there is no specific mechanism for temperature feedback; temperature control and ultimate thermal effect are determined by the surgeon through the control of spot size and the duration of laser application to a specific area. It has been suggested that the laser be set to a low power setting (10 to 15 W) and the beam defocused (by holding the tip of the probe 2 mm from the surface of the tissue). Once visible tissue shrinkage occurs, the laser beam is advanced to another area. However, it should be remembered that simply decreasing the spot size (focusing the laser beam by bringing the tip of the probe closer to the tissue) and/or keeping the beam focused too long on the same spot can result in tissue ablation.

Radio-frequency Energy

Radio-frequency energy is a form of electromagnetic energy. When applied to tissues, rapidly oscillating electromagnetic fields cause movement of charged particles within the tissue, and the resultant molecular motion generates heat.[3] Electromagnetic energy can be applied between two points on the tip of a probe (bipolar) or between a single electrode tip and a grounding plate (monopolar). In monopolar devices, the molecular friction created within the tissues adjacent to the probe produces heat. Thus, the actual source of heat is the frictional resistance of the tissues rather than the probe itself. With bipolar probes, the electromagnetic energy follows a much shorter path through a conductive irrigating solution (electrolytes) or through the tissues between the tips of the probe. Less current is required with a bipolar device than with a monopolar device to achieve the same effect, because the current passes through a much smaller volume of tissue. In addition, the depth of tissue damage relative to the probe tip may be less with a bipolar device.

Similar to laser energy, the thermal effect of radio-frequency energy in tissues is determined by the level of energy (related power and impedance), duration of treatment, and nature of the tissues. In addition, the electrode type (monopolar or bipolar), size, and shape all have an effect.

Some radio-frequency devices are capable of monitoring and/or controlling the temperature at the tip of the probe. Although this is thought to provide the highest margin of safety and efficacy, no data (clinical or experimental) have been published to support this claim. Indeed, as with the laser, the extent of thermal modification with radio-frequency devices is operator-dependent and relies on the visual observation of the tissue response. Because the tissue response is both time- and heat-dependent, the longer a probe (laser or radio-frequency) is left in one place, the greater the resultant tissue damage. In addition, the biologic variables of age and the thickness, hydration status, and quality of the tissue all affect the thermal response. Thus, application of a uniform amount of thermal modification with either class of devices appears, at best, subjective.

Although radio-frequency devices and lasers differ fundamentally in the way they generate heat within a tissue, both classes of devices are capable of producing temperatures within the critical temperature range (65°C to 75°C) for collagen denaturation and subsequent tissue shrinkage. Both types of devices have advantages and disadvantages (e.g., price, temperature monitoring). It must also be remembered that when it comes to cell viability and tissue response, heat is heat. Once critical temperatures are reached, cells will die, (45°C)[2] and collagen will become denatured (65°C)[22,23] no matter what the source of thermal energy. Therefore, claims of a better or different type of heat have little bearing on the biologic response of the tissue. Indeed, histologic, ultrastructural, and biomaterial alterations induced by laser and radio-frequency energy have been shown to be similar.[3]

Clinical Implications

Although the effect of heat energy on collagen molecules has been well established, the reason for the reported efficacy of this mode of therapy in the treatment of lax or redundant collagenous tissues is less clear. It has not yet been established what is really responsible for the clinical improvement after thermal capsular shrinkage—whether it is the initial connective tissue shrinkage, which appears to tighten and thus stabilize the joint; the fibroplasia, capsular thickening, and secondary cicatrix formation that occur in response to the traumatic insult; the loss of afferent sensory stimulation due to destruction of sensory receptors; or perhaps a combination of those three possible explanations.[1,2,13]

Although this fundamental question remains unanswered, certain clinical implications are clear. The initial degree of tissue shrinkage (and ultimate tissue damage) is directly related to the amount and rate of thermal energy applied. It has also been shown that the amount of tissue shrinkage is directly related to the loss of tissue stiffness.[4,16,21] Thus, the surgeon is faced with the dilemma of trying to minimize tissue damage while at the same time trying to achieve sufficient tissue shrinkage. Once shrunken (and devitalized), the tissues must be revitalized; during that period of repair, they are susceptible to elongation if left unprotected, due to compromise of their material properties.

Maintenance of Initial Capsular Shrinkage

Experimental studies have shown that immediately after thermal shrinkage, connective tissues demonstrate a significant ($P<0.05$) loss of stiffness.[4,16,17,21] This loss of stiffness has also been shown to be a significant important covariant of shrinkage (more shrinkage results in a greater loss of stiffness). Thus, tightening a lax joint by inducing thermal shrinkage in the joint capsule and/or ligaments makes these tissues weaker and more compliant, putting them at risk postoperatively.

It is also important to note that since most experimental studies have been performed on normal, healthy tissues, the heat response of abnormal tissues is unknown. It is possible that normal and abnormal tissues respond differently to thermal modification. One study has demonstrated an increased prevalence of reducible cross-links in joint capsules from joints demonstrating pathologic changes irrespective of the age of the patient.[28] This suggests that collagen from such joints may be more susceptible to thermal modification and could put them at even greater risk in the immediately postoperative period.

If the degree of tissue shrinkage is directly related to the loss of tissue stiffness in the immediately postoperative period, it is logical to assume that the degree of postoperative tissue repair is directly related to the extent of tissue damage. However, the application of thermal energy and the visual confirmation of the tissue response are both subjective. Indeed, in describing the technique, one author instructs that the probe should be swept slowly back and forth along the capsule "while the surgeon visually inspects for the capsular response."[2] With this in mind, it should be remembered that while it takes a temperature of at least 65°C to shrink connective tissues, a temperature of 45°C is lethal to most cells.[26] This suggests that after thermal application, at minimum, a significant portion of all visibly shrunken tissue has been

killed. In addition, it is possible that adjacent nonshrunken tissue has been subjected to lethal temperatures. Thus, the extent of actual tissue injury may not be accurately reflected by the visual impression of the amount of shrinkage.

All traumatized or devitalized tissues induce an inflammatory response leading to repair and/or removal and replacement of the injured tissue. This process is more protracted after thermal injury than after traumatic incisional injury.[26] Numerous experimental studies have documented that thermally modified tissues undergo a repair and remodeling process characterized by fibroplasia (Fig. 3), increased collagen deposition, and a remodeling phase in which the collagen-diameter profile changes from a bimodal (large- and small-diameter) fiber pattern to a unimodal (small-diameter) fiber pattern indicative of scar tissue (Fig. 1, C).[6,17,20,21] These morphologic changes are associated with a decrease in tensile stiffness, making the tissue susceptible to elongation due to tissue creep.[17,21] Studies have suggested that at least 3 months is required before thermally modified tissue can fully recover its biomechanical properties.[19] Restric-

tion of activity during this time is a recommended consideration for the postoperative regimen. Thus, it appears that the maintenance of initial tissue shrinkage is directly dependent on controlling the postoperative stresses exerted on the tissue and is indirectly dependent on the amount of shrinkage induced at the time of surgery.

Posttreatment Capsular Thickening and Cicatrix Formation

Inherent to all wound repair is a period of fibroplasia and collagen deposition that, in most cases, is directly related to the extent of tissue damage (caused by either the initial injury or the surgical treatment). Although extensive fibroplasia and subsequent tissue thickening are unwelcome sequelae of most surgical procedures, the creation of a hypertrophied joint capsule after thermal modification may actually contribute to the ultimate stability of the joint.

This method of shoulder stabilization has historical precedent. Hippocrates treated recurrent shoulder dislocations with insertion of a red-hot iron into the axillary region.

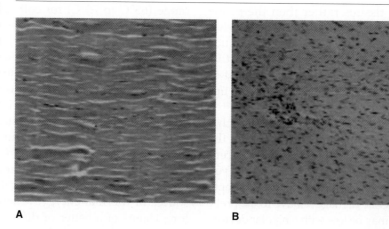

A   **B**

Figure 3   Photomicrographs of a longitudinal section of a normal rabbit patellar tendon before **(A)** and 8 weeks after **(B)** thermal modification (hematoxylin-eosin, original magnification ×100). Note the marked fibroblastic response still present within the tissue at 8 weeks.

In the 1950s, Hackett[29] developed a treatment for the correction of lax ligaments and tendons by means of a minimally invasive technique involving the injection of various irritant solutions in an effort to incite a fibroblastic response. Focal injections of a dextrose solution were used to stimulate a generalized inflammatory reaction, which, in turn, led to the deposition of new collagen, making the thickened structure stronger and stiffer. Hackett termed this treatment "prolotherapy" (derived from the Latin root of "proliferate") and defined it as "the rehabilitation of an incompetent structure by the generation of new cellular tissue." He reported a gradual return of joint stability, but cautioned against the early mobilization of these joints, which he felt could result in disruption of the healing process and stretching of the tissue.

Some currently utilized open procedures for shoulder stabilization rely on tightening and reinforcement of the joint capsule to provide stability. It is logical to assume that the exposure and surgical trauma associated with these procedures could also result in postoperative fibroplasia and thickening of the joint capsule, which may contribute to the ultimate stability of the shoulder. Therefore, the inability of arthroscopic shoulder stabilizations to equal the results of open stabilization procedures may be due, in part, to the decrease in tissue trauma (and attendant fibroplastic response of the joint capsule) associated with this minimally invasive technique. The use of thermal energy to incite an inflammatory cascade in the joint capsule and produce a fibroplastic response may induce the secondary capsular thickening seen in open stabilizations (Fig. 4).

A possible consequence of the creation of such a proliferative response is that excessive fibroplasia due to extensive tissue trauma may cause problems in the joint (e.g., arthrofibrosis, adhesive capsulitis). Appropriate stresses are required to remodel these healing tissues. This is especially true in the shoulder, where the portions of the capsule contributing to joint stability vary according to arm position. As with healing in all connective tissues, rehabilitation regimens must be developed to coincide with the various phases of repair in order to permit functional remodeling of the maturing tissues (Fig. 5). As yet unresolved is the question of which is the best postoperative protocol for modulation of scar formation and remodeling after thermal modification.

Loss of Afferent Sensory Stimulation

The joint capsule of the shoulder is a richly innervated structure containing a variety of sensory receptors.[30] It seems logical to assume that temperatures that denature and shrink collagen (>65°C) can also destroy these receptors and alter, if not completely disrupt, the afferent sensory pathway of the shoulder. It has been suggested that in some arthroscopic surgical procedures on the shoulder, destruction (excision) of neural elements may decrease painful stimuli and thus allow more joint movement, strength, and function.[30] Therefore, thermal modification of the shoulder joint capsule could result in local or regional anesthesia of the joint capsule, providing symptomatic relief. In addition, the loss of neurosensory input secondary to thermal modification could make the shoulder more susceptible to future injury due to the

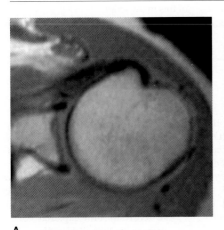 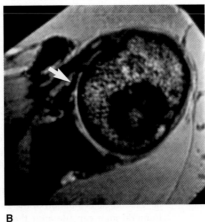 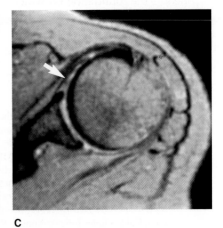

A　　　　　　　　　　**B**　　　　　　　　　　**C**

Figure 4 **A,** Magnetic resonance image of a normal shoulder joint. The anterior joint capsule is indistinct. **B,** Image of a shoulder of another subject 1 year after open stabilization. Note the increased thickness of the anterior joint capsule (arrow). **C,** Image of a shoulder of yet another subject 1 year after arthroscopic thermal modification of the anterior joint capsule. Note the thickening of the capsule (arrow).

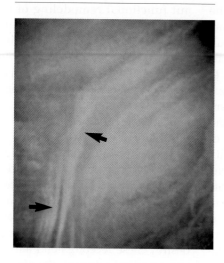

Figure 5 Arthroscopic view of the anterior capsule of a shoulder joint 1 year after arthroscopic thermal capsular shrinkage. Note that the bands of fibrous tissue that have formed (arrows) are oriented at right angles to the normal course of the inferior glenohumeral ligament.

loss of reflex-protective muscle activity. However, this theory has yet to be proved.

Summary

Wound healing is a natural and well-orchestrated biologic event. Indeed, the ability of wounds to heal is the foundation on which the practice of surgery is predicated. The successful surgeon maintains a delicate alliance with Mother Nature, balancing the magnitude of the surgical insult against the capacity of the tissue for repair. Thermal injury is one of the most traumatic insults a tissue can sustain, and the high degree of cell death and matrix alteration associated with thermal burns has been shown to result in a protracted healing time. Thus, the use of thermal energy as a stimulant for tissue shrinkage must be tempered with an appreciation of the biologic events that accompany this phenomenon. Furthermore, it must be realized that the initial degree of capsular shrinkage observed after the application of thermal energy may have little bearing on the long-term biologic and biomechanical status of the joint capsule. Therefore, the desire to see a redundant capsule shrink and become taut at surgery should be weighed very carefully against the level of damage imparted to the tissue to achieve this result. In the words of Hackett, the simple initiation of the healing response may be, in itself, sufficient "to rehabilitate an incompetent structure through the generation of new cellular tissue."[29]

It is probable that no one mechanism is totally responsible for the reported clinical improvement after thermal modification of the joint capsule. Indeed, it is entirely possible that all three of the mechanisms discussed—initial shrinkage, postoperative capsular thickening, and loss of regional afferent sensory input—may be involved in the ultimate postoperative improvement reported by some clinicians. Careful, long-term follow-up of these patients is needed to provide some insight into which factors have the greatest impact on functional outcome after thermal modification of connective tissues.

Although the ultimate applications of thermal modification of connective tissues have yet to be completely defined, its ultimate role may be as a low-level stimulant for inducing a biologic repair response, rather than as a highly aggressive mechanism for primary tissue shrinkage. As with all procedures, long-term, prospective clinical studies are required to define the precise indications and the appropriate therapeutic algorithm for this treatment modality.

Acknowledgments: The authors thank Charles Ho, MD, and Jonathan B. Ticker, MD, for their assistance in the preparation of this manuscript.

References

1. Fanton GS: Arthroscopic electrothermal surgery of the shoulder. *Operative Techniques Sports Med* 1998;6:139-146.
2. Fanton GS, Wall MS, Markel MD: Electrothermally-assisted capsule shift (ETAC) procedure for shoulder instability, in *The Science and Applications of ElectroThermal Arthroscopy*. Menlo Park, Calif: Oratec Interventions, 1998.
3. Hayashi K, Markel MD: Thermal modification of joint capsule and ligamentous tissues: The use of thermal energy in sports medicine. *Operative Techniques Sports Med* 1998;6:120-125.
4. Hayashi K, Markel MD, Thabit G III, Bogdanske JJ, Thielke RJ: The effect of nonablative laser energy on joint capsular properties: An *in vitro* mechanical study using a rabbit model. *Am J Sports Med* 1995;23:482-487.
5. Hayashi K, Massa KL, Thabit G III, et al: Histologic evaluation of the glenohumeral joint capsule after the laser-assisted capsular shift procedure for glenohumeral instability. *Am J Sports Med* 1999;27:162-167.
6. Hayashi K, Nieckarz JA, Thabit G III, Bogdanske JJ, Cooley AJ, Markel MD: Effect of nonablative laser energy on the joint capsule: An *in vivo* rabbit study using a holmium:YAG laser. *Lasers Surg Med* 1997;20:164-171.
7. Hayashi K, Thabit G III, Bogdanske JJ, Mascio LN, Markel MD: The effect of nonablative laser energy on the ultrastructure of joint capsular collagen. *Arthroscopy* 1996;12:474-481.
8. Hayashi K, Thabit G III, Massa KL, et al: The effect of thermal heating on the length and histologic properties of the glenohumeral joint capsule. *Am J Sports Med* 1997;25:107-112.

9. Hecht P, Hayashi K, Cooley AJ, et al: The thermal effect of monopolar radiofrequency energy on the properties of joint capsule: An *in vivo* histologic study using a sheep model. *Am J Sports Med* 1998;26:808-814.

10. Naseef GS III, Foster TE, Trauner K, Solhpour S, Anderson RR, Zarins B: The thermal properties of bovine joint capsule: The basic science of laser- and radiofrequency-induced capsular shrinkage. *Am J Sports Med* 1997;25:670-674.

11. Obrzut SL, Hecht P, Hayashi K, Fanton GS, Thabit G III, Markel MD: The effect of radiofrequency energy on the length and temperature properties of the glenohumeral joint capsule. *Arthroscopy* 1998;14:395-400.

12. Selecky MT, Vangsness CT Jr, Liao WL, Saadat V, Hedman TP: The effects of laser-induced collagen shortening on the biomechanical properties of the inferior glenohumeral ligament complex. *Am J Sports Med* 1999;27:168-172.

13. Thabit G: The arthroscopically assisted holmium:YAG laser surgery in the shoulder. *Operative Techniques Sports Med* 1998;6:131-138.

14. Thabit G: The arthroscopic monopolar radiofrequency treatment of chronic anterior cruciate ligament instability. *Operative Techniques Sports Med* 1998;6:157-160.

15. Tibone JE, McMahon PJ, Shrader TA, Sandusky MD, Lee TQ: Glenohumeral joint translation after arthroscopic, non-ablative, thermal capsuloplasty with a laser. *Am J Sports Med* 1998;26:495-498.

16. Vangsness CT Jr, Mitchell W III, Nimni M, Erlich M, Saadat V, Schmotzer H: Collagen shortening: An experimental approach with heat. *Clin Orthop* 1997;337:267-271.

17. Wallace AL, Sutherland CA, Marchuk LL, et al: Early *in vivo* effects of electrothermal shrinkage on viscoelastic properties and cellular responses in a model of ligament laxity. *Trans Orthop Res Soc* 1999;24:309.

18. Lopez MJ, Hayashi K, Fanton GS, Thabit G, Markel MD: The effect of radiofrequency energy on the ultrastructure of joint capsular collagen. *Arthroscopy* 1998;14:495-501.

19. Chen SS, Wright NT, Humphrey JD: Heat-induced changes in the mechanics of a collagenous tissue: Isothermal, isotonic shrinkage. *J Biomech Eng* 1998;120:382-388.

20. Sandusky MD, Schulz MM, McMahon PJ, Tibone JE, Lee TQ: The effects of laser on joint capsular tissue: An *in vivo* rabbit study. *Trans Orthop Res Soc* 1999;24:366.

21. Schaefer SL, Ciarelli MJ, Arnoczky SP, Ross HE: Tissue shrinkage with the holmium:yttrium aluminum garnet laser: A postoperative assessment of tissue length, stiffness, and structure. *Am J Sports Med* 1997;25:841-848.

22. Flory PJ, Garrett RR: Phase transitions in collagen and gelatin systems. *J Am Chem Soc* 1958;80:4836-4845.

23. Allain JC, Le Lous M, Cohen-Solal L, Bazin S, Maroteaux P: Isometric tensions developed during the hydrothermal swelling of rat skin. *Connect Tissue Res* 1980;7:127-133.

24. Chvapil M, Jensovsky L: The shrinkage temperature of collagen fibres isolated from the tail tendons of rats of various ages and from different places of the same tendon. *Gerontologia* 1963;1:18-29.

25. Le Lous M, Cohen-Solal L, Allain JC, Bonaventure J, Maroteaux P: Age related evolution of stable collagen reticulation in human skin. *Connect Tissue Res* 1985;13:145-155.

26. Boykin JV Jr, Molnar JA: Burn scar and skin equivalents, in Cohen IK, Diegelmann RF, Lindblad WJ (eds): *Wound Healing: Biochemical and Clinical Aspects.* Philadelphia: WB Saunders, 1992, pp 523-540.

27. Shaffer B: The holmium:YAG laser in knee arthroscopy. *Operative Techniques Sports Med* 1998;6:139-146.

28. Herbert CM, Jayson MIV, Bailey AJ: Joint capsule collagen in osteoarthrosis. *Ann Rheum Dis* 1973;32:510-514.

29. Hackett GS: *Ligament and Tendon Relaxation (Skeletal Disability) Treated by Prolotherapy (Fibro-osseous Proliferation),* 3rd ed. Springfield, Ill: Charles C Thomas, 1958.

30. Vangsness CT Jr, Ennis M, Taylor JG, Atkinson R: Neural anatomy of the glenohumeral ligaments, labrum, and subacromial bursa. *Arthroscopy* 1995;11:180-184.

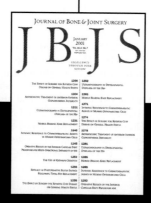

JBJS
THE JOURNAL OF BONE & JOINT SURGERY

JAAOS
JOURNAL OF THE AMERICAN ACADEMY OF ORTHOPAEDIC

section three

Evaluation and Treatment

Partial-Thickness Tears of the Rotator Cuff: Evaluation and Management

Owen R. McConville, MD, and Joseph P. Iannotti, MD, PhD

Abstract

The approach to management of a partial-thickness rotator cuff tear is best made with the understanding that this is not a singular condition. Rather, partial tears represent the common outcome of a variety of insults to the rotator cuff. Degenerative changes due to aging, anatomic impingement, and trauma may all be etiologic agents. Overhead athletes may develop tears due to repetitive microtrauma or internal impingement. Outlet radiographs and magnetic resonance imaging are recommended for routine preoperative evaluation. A nonoperative treatment program for rotator cuff strengthening and stretching is appropriate as initial treatment; modification of activities and anti-inflammatory medication are often used as well. Operative management may be considered when nonoperative treatment fails. Arthroscopic evaluation is required to determine the true extent of the cuff lesion. Arthroscopic subacromial decompression is recommended when outlet impingement is present. Rotator cuff debridement or formal cuff repair is dependent on the size of the cuff defect and the age and activity level of the patient. The importance of recognizing the different causes of partial-thickness rotator cuff tears is emphasized in this review of pathogenesis, clinical diagnosis, imaging, and treatment.

J Am Acad Orthop Surg 1999;7:32-43

Partial-thickness rotator cuff tears (PTRCTs) have long been recognized as an often asymptomatic consequence of the aging process as well as a potential source of shoulder dysfunction. Other possible etiologic factors include anatomic impingement and trauma (including repetitive microtrauma). In the past, the difficulty in accurately diagnosing and characterizing the elements contributing to PTRCTs has compromised the ability to understand the natural history of this condition. More recently, magnetic resonance (MR) imaging and arthroscopic assessment have allowed more precise characterization of PTRCTs. Nevertheless, the optimal clinical approach to this entity has not yet been completely defined.

Natural History

Partial cuff tears may involve either the articular surface or the bursal surface or may be confined entirely within the tendon substance. Tears on the articular surface are two to three times more common than bursal-surface tears in most reports.[1-7] Throwing athletes may show a predilection for articular-surface tears.[8,9] Most tears affect the supraspinatus tendon. The infraspinatus, subscapularis, and teres minor tendons are much less commonly involved.[4,10]

Intratendinous tears are characterized as having no communication to either cuff surface,[11] and their relationship to symptomatology is uncertain. Cadaveric studies have demonstrated a higher incidence of intratendinous tears than clinical studies,[12] because arthroscopic techniques allow inspection of only the tendon surfaces of the rotator cuff. Current techniques of MR imaging have the ability to demonstrate intrasubstance tears and tendon degeneration[13] (Fig. 1). The abnormal signal changes seen within the tendon on MR imaging correlate with pathologic changes seen on histologic examination.

In studies involving cadaveric specimens, the incidence of partial tears has ranged from 13% to

Dr. McConville is Assistant Clinical Professor, Department of Orthopedics, Tufts University School of Medicine, Boston; and is in private practice with South Shore Orthopaedic Specialists, South Weymouth, Mass. Dr. Iannotti is Professor, Department of Orthopaedic Surgery, University of Pennsylvania School of Medicine, Philadelphia; and Chief, Shoulder and Elbow Service, University of Pennsylvania Health System, Philadelphia.

Reprint requests: Dr. Iannotti, Penn Musculoskeletal Institute, Department of Orthopaedic Surgery, 39th and Market Street, 1 Cupp Pavilion, Presbyterian Medical Center, Philadelphia, PA 19104-2699.

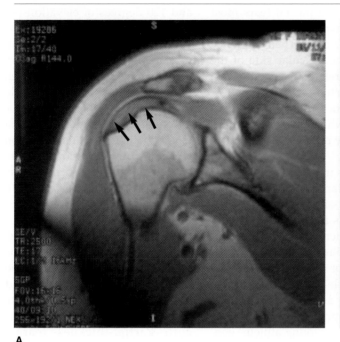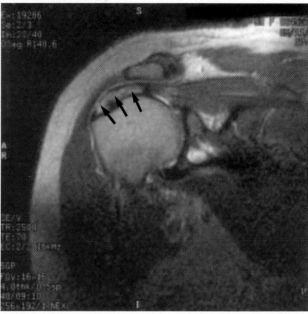

A   **B**

Fig. 1 Proton-density **(A)** and T2-weighted **(B)** coronal oblique MR images show tendon thickening and extensive intrasubstance tendon degeneration (arrows), indicated by hyperintensity of the signal in the tendon.

37%.[12] Most clinical and cadaveric reports have demonstrated that partial tears are more common than full-thickness rotator cuff tears (FTRCTs).[12,14] In part, this finding is age-dependent, as the peak incidence of PTRCTs occurs in the fifth and sixth decades, whereas FTRCTs occur with greater frequency in the later decades of life.

The natural history of PTRCT has never been completely documented. Codman suggested that spontaneous healing of PTRCTs might occur, although he provided little evidence to support his contention. Fukuda et al[11] examined histologic sections of PTRCTs and found no evidence of active tissue repair. The earlier peak incidence of PTRCTs relative to FTRCTs demonstrated by epidemiologic data[15] and imaging studies[16] suggests that progression may occur. However, it is not clear whether this progression in

cuff tear size correlates with clinical symptoms.

Serial arthrography has been used in an attempt to define the progression of symptomatic articular-surface PTRCTs when treated nonoperatively.[17] In a study of 40 shoulders, 11 tears (28%) progressed to being FTRCTs in just over 1 year. Four PTRCTs (10%) were thought to have healed completely. The authors concluded that although some small posttraumatic articular-surface PTRCTs in young patients may have the potential for healing, most tears continue to enlarge with time.

The role of operative treatment in modifying the natural history of PTRCT is poorly defined. There is no evidence that debridement of a partially torn cuff stimulates a healing response.[1,6] Intuitively, subacromial decompression might delay the progression of cuff disruption in cases of PTRCT caused by subacromial outlet narrowing.

Rehabilitation to restore normal joint mechanics and strengthen the rotator cuff musculature might itself influence progression of cuff disease, particularly in cases of dynamic impingement.

Anatomy

The suprascapular artery is the primary vascular supply to the supraspinatus tendon.[18] Selective injection studies have shown that the articular surface of the cuff is relatively hypovascular compared with the bursal cuff surface.[18] This finding has been suggested as a factor in the tendency for partial tears to occur more frequently on the articular surface of the cuff.

Histologic studies of cadaveric[19] and clinical[20] specimens have defined the rotator cuff microstructure. Collagen bundles located near the articular surface of the cuff are thinner and less uniform than the thick parallel bundles found closer to the bursal surface. The articular surface of the cuff has an ultimate failing stress only half as high as the bursal surface.[20] This relative weakness may be another contributing factor accounting for the observed predilection of cuff injuries to occur on the articular surface.

Pathogenesis

Factors related to the development of PTRCTs may be classified as intrinsic, extrinsic, or traumatic. Intrinsic tendinopathy, related to changes in cuff vascularity or other metabolic phenomena associated with the aging process, may lead to degenerative tears. Extrinsic impingement due to supraspinatus outlet narrowing caused by coracoacromial arch abnormalities can result in cuff irritation and is thought to play a major role in many partial cuff tears. Tensile overload of the cuff, due to either a single violent traumatic injury or repetitive microtrauma, may also cause partial cuff injury. On occasion, more than one etiologic factor may be involved.

The location of the cuff tear on either the articular or the bursal surface may offer a clue to the cause of the tear. Histologic changes have been found on the undersurface of cadaveric acromion specimens with bursal-surface tears but not in those with articular-surface tears.[15] This suggests that bursal-surface tears may be more likely to be related to abrasion of the cuff by the acromion.

Some authors feel that extrinsic impingement due to coracoacromial arch narrowing can lead to partial tears on the articular as well as the bursal surface of the cuff.[10] Differential shear stress affecting the layered anatomy of the cuff has been proposed as one mechanism involved in the production of articular-surface tears.

Degenerative partial tears most commonly involve the deep surface of the rotator cuff. Their tendency to involve the articular side of the cuff may be related to tenuous vascularity, particularly with senescence. Degenerative tears are often associated with extensive lamination and may remain entirely intratendinous.

Trauma is more often associated with articular-surface tears than with bursal-surface tears.[3] This association is also seen in cases of repetitive microtrauma. Glenohumeral instability and traction stress on the rotator cuff in the throwing athlete can lead to undersurface tears in the absence of extrinsic anatomic impingement. Articular-surface tears in young athletes generally occur in otherwise healthy tissue, in contrast to the degenerative tears seen in older individuals.

Recently, Walch et al[21] and Jobe[22] described a subset of articular-surface PTRCTs that develop secondary to "internal impingement." Throwers and other overhead athletes may experience posterior shoulder pain when repetitive contact occurs between the undersurface of the supraspinatus and the posterosuperior glenoid during the late cocking phase of the throwing motion. Fatigue of the dynamic stabilizers and excessive external rotation secondary to overstretching of the anterior capsule may predispose individuals to development of internal impingement.

Clinical Presentation

The frequent occurrence of PTRCTs in both cadaveric studies and MR imaging studies of asymptomatic individuals suggests that such tears are not always symptomatic.[16] The symptoms of PTRCT are nonspecific, with pain being predominant. A painful arc of motion between 60

and 120 degrees of elevation (seen in many patients with subacromial pain of various causes) is present in most symptomatic patients.[3] Partial tears may be associated with glenohumeral joint contracture and loss of motion,[11] which manifests as posterior capsular tightness and resultant restriction of internal rotation.[10] Obligate anterosuperior translation of the humeral head may result from posterior capsular contracture and may serve to potentiate impingement symptoms.

Strength is generally preserved on clinical examination. However, pain inhibition may result in both apparent loss of strength and a decrease in active range of motion in patients with a partially intact cuff. Partial-thickness tears are often associated with pain on testing for the classic Jobe sign (active resistance to shoulder abduction with the shoulder positioned in 90 degrees of abduction).

The lag signs described by Hertel et al[23] may be helpful in separating PTRCTs from FTRCTs. The external-rotation lag sign is nearly always negative with PTRCTs and, in many cases, is positive with complete tears (particularly with larger tears). Discernible weakness (unrelated to discomfort) and atrophy of cuff musculature indicate a high likelihood of full-thickness involvement. The impingement signs described by Neer (pain with forced passive forward elevation) and Hawkins (pain with passive internal rotation of the arm placed in 90 degrees of forward elevation) are positive in nearly all patients with symptomatic PTRCTs.[10] These maneuvers may be repeated after injection of 10 mL of 1% lidocaine into the subacromial space (impingement test). Diminution of pain on repeat testing after subacromial injection is indicative of a subacromial lesion.

Throwing athletes warrant particular attention to the shoulder laxity examination. Increased anterior translation has been proposed as the instability pattern likely to generate rotator cuff lesions. Subtle degrees of anterior subluxation may be difficult to discern on physical examination with the standard means of manually evaluating glenohumeral translation. To better define the presence of instability, apprehension is assessed with the shoulder placed in 90 degrees of abduction and external rotation in the supine patient. The expression of apprehension in this position is highly suggestive of underlying anterior instability. Augmentation with an anteriorly directed force on the proximal humerus increases diagnostic yield. A posteriorly directed force that reduces apprehension lends further support to the diagnosis of anterior instability. The presence of pain alone with testing in this fashion is nonspecific and an unreliable indicator of anterior instability. Pain produced with external rotation of the abducted shoulder may be related to a variety of conditions, including glenohumeral instability, rotator cuff disease, and degenerative joint disease or internal glenoid impingement.

In the overhead athlete, external rotation in abduction is characteristically increased in the dominant shoulder, with a concomitant loss of internal rotation. Pain at the posterior joint line with maximal external rotation of the abducted shoulder in these individuals may be related to internal impingement. Posterior translation of the humeral head (the Jobe relocation maneuver) characteristically relieves this pain. It is a matter of debate whether rotator cuff injury observed in individuals with internal impingement develops as a result of pathologic anterior glenohumeral subluxation or whether it occurs as a result of repetitive cuff abrasion in an otherwise stable shoulder.

The clinical course of patients with PTRCTs is often indistinguishable from that of patients with impingement syndrome without cuff failure or with small FTRCTs.[24] Most patients improve with conservative measures over 6 months, and some continue to improve up to 18 months from initiation of treatment.

Because of the considerable overlap in clinical presentation, symptoms caused by PTRCTs may be difficult to differentiate from those due to other conditions, such as subacromial bursitis, bicipital tendinitis, and mild cases of frozen shoulder. Furthermore, associated shoulder lesions are common in patients with surgically diagnosed PTRCT. These associated conditions may contribute to the symptoms experienced by individuals with PTRCTs. Biceps tendon fraying or rupture may accompany a PTRCT.[2,25] Labral degeneration or tearing occurs in as many as a third of patients even if those with symptomatic instability are excluded.[2,26] Posterosuperior labral lesions or osteochondral lesions of the humeral head are occasionally present in throwing athletes with articular-surface PTRCTs.[21]

Imaging

Arthrography, ultrasonography, and MR imaging are all used to evaluate rotator cuff disorders. These studies are particularly accurate in the diagnosis of full-thickness tears, but have generally been found to be less accurate in the assessment of partial-thickness tears. These studies do have value, however, in ruling out FTRCT and other non-cuff-related disorders.

Radiographic Evaluation

While conventional x-ray films are helpful in the general evaluation of a painful shoulder, there is no specific plain-radiographic diag-

nostic feature of PTRCT. Indirect evidence of an advanced rotator cuff disorder, such as greater tuberosity or acromial sclerosis or anterior acromial spurring, may be present on plain films. Larger chronic FTRCTs may have a decreased acromiohumeral interval. However, most patients with a PTRCT do not have these radiographic abnormalities, especially younger patients and those in whom trauma or instability is the cause of the tear. Nevertheless, plain radiographs are helpful in ruling out other causes of shoulder pain, such as acromioclavicular lesions or glenohumeral arthritis.

Standard x-ray views include an anteroposterior view of the shoulder, an axillary lateral view, and a supraspinatus outlet view. The supraspinatus outlet view best demonstrates curved or hooked acromial morphology, which is seen in some individuals with PTRCTs due to supraspinatus outlet narrowing. Os acromiale, which can cause impingement symptoms, can be seen on an axillary lateral film. Degenerative changes of the acromioclavicular joint are seen with a 15-degree cephalic-tilt anteroposterior (Zanca) view. An apical oblique (Garth) or West Point axillary view may be added if glenohumeral instability is suspected.

Arthrography and Bursography

Arthrography of the glenohumeral joint allows evaluation of the integrity of the undersurface of the rotator cuff. Proponents of arthrography report accuracy of better than 80% in the diagnosis of PTRCT.[3] However, other clinical studies have found arthrography less valuable.[11,27] Gartsman and Milne[10] reported that arthrography detected only 7 of 46 arthroscopically proven articular-surface PTRCTs. Walch et al[21] reported positive arthrograms in only 8 of 17 surgically proven articular-surface

PTRCTs. The use of fluoroscopy in conjunction with arthrography has been suggested to improve detection of PTRCTs.

Bursography may be performed as an adjunct to arthrography to aid in detection of bursal-surface PTRCTs that are inaccessible to the arthrographic dye. However, subacromial inflammation and adhesions limit the value of this technique. The accuracy of bursography in detecting surgically proven bursal-surface PTRCTs has been reported to range from 25% to 67%.[3,11,12]

Arthrography may have value in the diagnosis of FTRCT. It has the advantages of relatively low cost and ready availability. However, its role in the evaluation of PTRCT is limited. A negative arthrogram obtained for evaluation of a painful shoulder cannot reliably rule out the presence of a PTRCT. Further advanced imaging (i.e., MR imaging) or arthroscopic evaluation should be considered in this situation if clinically indicated.

Ultrasound

Sonographic evaluation of rotator cuff integrity has been shown to be accurate for the diagnosis of FTRCT.[28] A PTRCT may be somewhat more difficult to detect. Fluid within the substance of the rotator cuff produces a focal hypoechoic area. Thus, a focal hypoechoic area at one of the cuff surfaces or within the cuff substance signifies a PTRCT. Linear echogenicity within the cuff substance with or without thinning of the cuff may also represent a partial-thickness tear.

Wiener and Seitz[28] reported a sensitivity of 94% and a specificity of 93% in a series of 69 PTRCTs diagnosed by ultrasound. The authors suggest ultrasound as a reliable, quick, and cost-effective means of evaluating the rotator cuff.

Despite the high degree of accuracy in some reports, the clinical utility of ultrasonography for diagnosis of rotator cuff disorders may be limited by the availability of personnel experienced in the performance and interpretation of the study. These limitations may be particularly applicable in the somewhat more subtle ultrasonographic diagnosis of PTRCT.

Magnetic Resonance Imaging

Magnetic resonance imaging has become an established technique for diagnosis of FTRCT. Recently, techniques have been developed to more accurately characterize subtle cuff lesions, such as PTRCTs. Diagnosis of PTRCT is suggested by increased signal in the rotator cuff without evidence of tendon discontinuity on T1-weighted imaging. A PTRCT is depicted as further signal increase on T2-weighted images with a focal defect that is intratendinous or limited to one surface and does not extend through the entire tendon (Fig. 2). Rotator cuff tendinitis may produce increased signal and loss of anatomic definition of the cuff on T1-weighted and proton-density images, similar to the appearance of a PTRCT. Tendinitis is distinguished from PTRCT

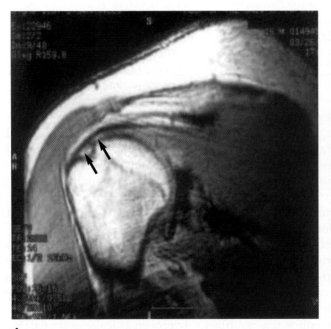 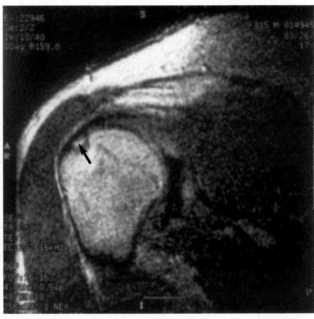

A　　　　　　　　　　　　　　　　　　**B**

Fig. 2 Proton-density **(A)** and T2-weighted **(B)** coronal oblique MR images demonstrate an articular-surface partial-thickness tear (arrows).

by the finding of only moderate or decreased signal on T2-weighted images.

With the use of standard MR imaging techniques, the detection of PTRCT has been unreliable.[29] Most series have reported that standard techniques are relatively insensitive in the detection of partial cuff tears. Traughber and Goodwin[29] reported a sensitivity of 56% to 72% and a specificity of 83% to 85% for arthroscopically proven PTRCTs. Gartsman and Milne[10] reported an 83% rate of false-negative MR studies of 12 arthroscopically proven articular-surface PTRCTs. Wright and Cofield[27] found only 6 definite PTRCTs on preoperative MR studies in a series of 18 patients.

Fat-suppression techniques accentuate fluid signal contrast on T2-weighted images and have been suggested as a means of increasing sensitivity of PTRCT detection. Clinical studies, however, have not consistently demonstrated improved reliability with this technique. In a study of 11 arthroscopically proven PTRCTs, fat-suppressed MR imaging had a sensitivity of 82%, a specificity of 99%, and an accuracy of 85%.[30] Other studies have yielded less impressive results. Reinus et al[31] compared fat-suppressed MR imaging with conventional T2-weighted imaging in the diagnosis of cuff lesions in a series of 20 arthroscopically proven PTRCTs. Although fat-saturated images improved the rate of detection of PTRCT, overall results were poor; 35% of PTRCTs were identified with fat-saturation technique, compared with only 15% with conventional MR imaging.

Magnetic resonance arthrography has also been suggested as a means of better evaluating cuff integrity.[32] Although it appears to improve sensitivity, MR arthrography still has a fairly high false-negative rate. Hodler et al[32] found that 5 of 13 partial tears found at the time of arthroscopy had been missed on preoperative MR arthrography.

The clinical utility of MR findings is further limited by the frequent occurrence of abnormal rotator cuff signal in asymptomatic individuals.[16] The MR findings consistent with PTRCT or FTRCT are uncommon in asymptomatic adults less than 40 years old. However, both tear types become more common when older individuals are evaluated. In the study by Sher et al,[16] PTRCTs were the predominant cuff lesion (24%) in asymptomatic shoulders of those between 40 and 60 years of age; in patients over 60 years old, FTRCT and PTRCT were nearly equally prevalent (28% and 26%, respectively). Thus, a substantial proportion of the population over the age of 40 may have abnormal findings on MR evaluation of the rotator cuff in the absence of clinical complaints. The possibility that MR evidence of a PTRCT could be an incidental finding should be considered when evaluating symptomatic patients, especially those over 40 years old.

Further developments in MR technology may improve its accuracy. At the present time, MR findings suggestive of PTRCT should be interpreted cautiously and used only as an adjunct to clinical evaluation when determining a treatment strategy.

Classification

Neer's classification[33] described three stages of rotator cuff disease: stage I, characterized by hemorrhage and cuff edema; stage II, cuff fibrosis; and stage III, cuff tear. Partial tears were not categorized separately. They have been considered advanced stage II lesions by some authors and early stage III lesions by others.

Ellman[5] pointed out the difficulty of classifying partial tears in Neer's scheme. He proposed a more detailed classification scheme that included specific consideration of the site and extent of partial cuff tears. The location (articular surface, bursal surface, or intratendinous) was recorded. Tear grade was defined in terms of depth. Grade I tears had a depth of less than 3 mm; grade II, a depth of 3 to 6 mm; and grade III, involvement of more than half of the cuff thickness (average cuff thickness, 9 to 12 mm).

Many authors have suggested that tears involving more than half of the tendon thickness are a significant threat to cuff integrity. Thus, the presence of a grade III PTRCT is often considered a relative indication for surgical repair in the symptomatic patient. Clinical data, although limited, seem to support this contention and suggest that it is a reasonable management guideline.

The etiology of PTRCT is not considered in most classification schemes. However, it may be important in terms of both prognosis and treatment selection. Gartsman and Milne[10] and Morrison[34] have emphasized the need to accurately define etiology in order to determine the most appropriate treatment plan.

In summary, classification of PTRCT should be descriptive in terms of the location (both the tendon involved and the surface affected), the size (depth) of the tear, and the cause.

Treatment

There is no simple treatment algorithm that can adequately address the management of PTRCT. In most cases, treatment of a symptomatic shoulder with a PTRCT is directed toward a primary diagnosis (such as impingement syndrome or instability), with treatment of the PTRCT often considered secondarily.

Thus, treatment selection is often dependent on defining the cause of the PTRCT. Because PTRCTs are frequently present in asymptomatic shoulders, the contribution of a PTRCT to symptoms in a painful shoulder is difficult, if not impossible, to establish in most cases. Therefore, careful identification and treatment of any associated condition is prudent.

Nonoperative Management

Individuals with a suspected PTRCT due to extrinsic outlet impingement or intrinsic tendinopathy are initially treated in the standard manner for patients with impingement syndrome. Subacromial bursal inflammation is controlled with activity modification, nonsteroidal medication, and the judicious use of injectable corticosteroids. Physical therapy is advanced as inflammation diminishes and pain subsides. Therapy should be first directed at eliminating capsular contractures and regaining full motion. Posterior capsular contracture is addressed by progressive stretching in adduction and internal rotation. Horizontal (cross-body) adduction exercises also serve to stretch the posterior capsule.

As pain decreases and motion improves, attention is focused on strengthening the rotator cuff and periscapular musculature. The function of the rotator cuff in dynamic stabilization of the glenohumeral joint is maximized through a program emphasizing progressive resistive exercises involving the use of elastic tubing or free weights. Rehabilitation of the periscapular musculature may serve to restore normal scapulothoracic mechanics and minimize dynamic impingement secondary to scapulothoracic dyskinesis.

Patients with PTRCTs thought to be due to instability are likewise treated initially with control of inflammation and pain. Particular attention is paid to rehabilitation of the rotator cuff and periscapular muscle groups. Restoration of proper shoulder mechanics is especially important in overhead athletes.

Operative Management

The timing of surgical intervention when conservative treatment fails has not been well defined. For tears considered to be related to extrinsic outlet impingement, 6 months of nonoperative treatment is generally considered appropriate. Patient factors, especially activity level, may influence the duration of the nonoperative program. In some cases, longer or shorter conservative treatment periods may be indicated.

The surgical treatment of PTRCTs has generally involved one of three approaches: tear debridement, acromioplasty along with tear debridement, or cuff repair in addition to acromioplasty. Surgery may be open, arthroscopically assisted, or entirely arthroscopic.

Arthroscopic Technique

Arthroscopic examination allows visualization of the articular surface of the cuff (Fig. 3), which is a distinct advantage over open surgery. The frequent association of glenohumeral lesions with PTRCTs suggests that a glenohumeral inspection should be performed at the time of every arthroscopic subacromial decompression. Hill-Sachs lesions, labral lesions, and other markers of anterior instability should be sought during glenohumeral arthroscopy.

The diagnosis of PTRCT is often not made with certainty until the rotator cuff is examined arthroscopically. Partial tears have been found unexpectedly in as many as 15% to 33% of patients undergoing arthroscopic treatment of impingement syndrome.[5,25] The preferred treatment of some of these unsuspected tears may be open surgical repair. Therefore, the possibility of encountering a PTRCT and the need to convert to an open procedure should be anticipated and discussed with the patient before shoulder arthroscopy.

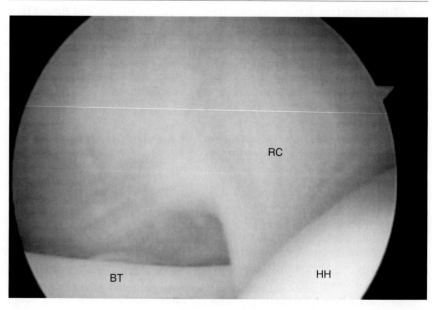

Fig. 3   Intact rotator cuff insertion site viewed from the posterior portal. BT represents the long head of the biceps tendon; HH, humeral head; RC, rotator cuff.

Arthroscopy may be performed with the patient in the beach-chair or lateral decubitus position. With the beach-chair position, the undersurface of the rotator cuff is best viewed by rotating the arthroscope in the standard posterior portal to look laterally while abducting the shoulder 30 degrees and externally rotating it 30 to 45 degrees in a position of slight forward flexion (Fig. 3). By sweeping the scope along the cuff insertion, one is generally afforded an excellent view of the biceps, supraspinatus, infraspinatus, and teres minor attachment sites. Placing the shoulder in maximum external rotation with 90 degrees of abduction allows direct assessment of internal impingement lesions.

Gentle debridement of undersurface tears is sometimes neces-sary to determine the true extent of the tear and may allow better estimation of tear depth (Fig. 4). Probing through an anterior portal allows assessment of cuff integrity in cases in which tear depth is difficult to discern. A probe introduced into the subacromial space is often helpful, allowing palpation of the cuff from above while viewing from the glenohumeral joint. A marker suture may be placed to localize the tear so that it may be more easily evaluated later when viewing from the subacromial space. An 18-gauge spinal needle is introduced from the lateral aspect of the shoulder and passed through the site of the cuff lesion. A No. 0 absorbable monofilament suture is passed through the spinal needle, and the needle is then removed, leaving the suture in place.

Bursal-surface tears are sometimes more difficult to evaluate, as hypertrophic bursitis can obscure the cuff surface. Occasionally, partial disruption of the bursal surface of the cuff is apparent on initial viewing of the subacromial space. In this situation, there is often an accompanying subacromial spur or prominent coracoacromial ligament. A complete inspection of the bursal side of the cuff should be performed, particularly if preoperative imaging studies indicate a cuff lesion. After debridement of hypertrophic bursal tissue, the shoulder is carried through a range of motion while viewing from the posterior portal. The shoulder is slightly abducted and rotated both internal-

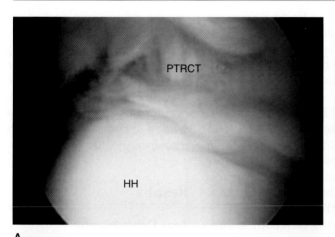

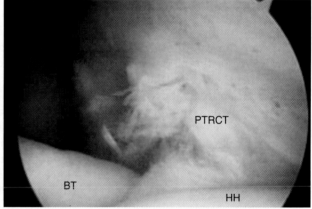

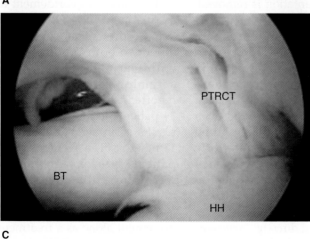

Fig. 4 Arthroscopic views of grade I (**A**), grade II (**B**), and grade III (**C**) articular-surface PTRCTs, as classified in Ellman's scheme.[5] In that system, both the site and the extent of partial cuff tears are considered. Tear grade is defined in terms of depth. Grade I tears have a depth of less than 3 mm, and grade II tears have a depth of 3 to 6 mm. In grade III tears, there is involvement of more than half of the cuff thickness.

ly and externally to best visualize the supraspinatus insertion, which is the common site of bursal-surface PTRCTs (Fig. 5). Complete cuff visualization may be achieved by moving the arthroscope to the lateral or anterior subacromial portal. After debridement of frayed fibers, tear depth and extent can be assessed. Bursal-surface tears with associated articular-surface cuff lesions should be inspected carefully, as very often these represent full-thickness tears even if they do not appear so on initial inspection.

Arthroscopy affords no substantial advantage in the evaluation and treatment of intratendinous tears. Generally, these tears cannot be identified arthroscopically. Digital palpation and tissue appearance during open surgery have been used by some to identify and localize these lesions.

Open Technique

Open surgical approaches to the subacromial space offer excellent exposure of the bursal surface of the rotator cuff. Furthermore, inspection and palpation of the cuff may allow detection of intratendinous tears. However, articular-surface PTRCTs and other intra-articular lesions may be missed if the cuff is not incised.

"The color test," an intraoperative cuff-staining technique described by Fukuda et al,[14] can be used to more accurately diagnose and localize articular-surface tears during open surgery. Indigo carmine or methylene blue (3 mL) mixed with normal saline (17 mL) is injected into the glenohumeral joint. The shoulder is then put through a range of motion. Torn cuff tissue is preferentially stained by the dye. The biceps tendon sheath (long head) and rotator interval normally demonstrate uptake of the dye. Fukuda et al reported that the staining test detected articular surface tears in 65% of cases. The color test

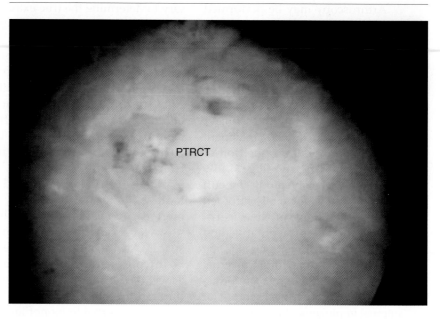

Fig. 5 Bursal-surface PTRCT viewed from a posterolateral bursoscopy portal.

is more likely to be positive when more than half of the tendon thickness is involved. Laminated tears may take up dye along intratendinous extensions.

"Mini-open" Technique

A combined arthroscopic and open surgical approach is useful in many situations. Arthroscopic glenohumeral examination is followed by arthroscopic subacromial decompression. If a PTRCT is deemed worthy of repair, arthroscopic instrumentation is removed, and a "mini-open" repair is performed. This is done through a deltoid-splitting approach, often incorporating the lateral portal in the incision. Adequate exposure is usually achieved without the need for detachment of the deltoid from the acromion. A deltoid-splitting incision placed too far anteriorly may increase the risk of avulsion of the deltoid from its attachment to the anterior acromion by overzealous retraction. Bursal-surface tears can be visualized directly. Articular-surface tears may be localized dur-

ing the arthroscopic portion of the procedure with a marker suture.[26]

Entirely arthroscopic techniques have been described and may be applicable in some instances. These include side-to-side repair of certain bursal-surface tears and tendon-to-bone fixation of tears at the supraspinatus insertion site.

Results

Tear Debridement

The value of debridement alone as treatment for PTRCT is uncertain. Andrews et al[9] and Snyder et al[26] have both reported success with tear debridement without acromioplasty. Andrews et al[9] reported that debridement alone in 34 patients led to 85% satisfactory results at an average follow-up of 13 months. The average age of the patients was 22 years, and most were competitive overhead athletes.

Snyder et al[26] proposed debridement alone as a treatment for articular-surface PTRCTs. They reported 94% satisfactory results in a mixed series of articular- and bursal-surface tears. Articular-surface tears were treated by debridement alone. Arthroscopic subacromial decompression was added for bursal-surface tears. The authors suggested that acromioplasty be performed selectively on the basis of clinical presentation and arthroscopic findings. Tear debridement was thought to provide pain relief in patients with articular-surface PTRCTs not due to primary impingement syndrome.

Success with debridement has not been uniform, however. Ogilvie-Harris and Wiley[35] reported their results with arthroscopic debridement of 57 PTRCTs without subacromial decompression. Satisfactory outcomes were achieved in only approximately 50%. Walch et al[21] reported suboptimal results for arthroscopic debridement of PTRCTs secondary to "internal impingement" with only transitory relief of pain.

Arthroscopic Subacromial Decompression

Most authors perform subacromial decompression (with or without debridement) either selectively or routinely as part of treatment of PTRCTs. Satisfactory results have been reported in 75% to 83% of cases treated by tear debridement and subacromial decompression.[4,5,36] Success with arthroscopic subacromial decompression in patients with partial tears has been equal to that in patients with intact cuffs in most series.[36,37]

The location of the partial tear may be an important determinant of the success of subacromial decompression. At an average follow-up of 23 months (minimum, 1 year), Ryu[2] reported 86% satisfactory results in the treatment of 35 PTRCTs by arthroscopic subacromial decompression. Of note, only one of the four patients with an isolated articular-surface tear had a satisfactory result. Patients with bursal-surface lesions had 94% satisfactory results. Exclusion of patients with instability likely led to a lower incidence of isolated articular-surface tears (4/35 [11%]) than in other reports. This suggests that arthroscopic subacromial decompression is particularly effective in patients with bursal-surface PTRCTs, at least in the short term.

Selective Repair

Because of concerns about cuff integrity and tear progression, repair of more extensive PTRCTs has been suggested.[6,8,10] Miller and Lewis[8] used the thickness of the cuff tear as the criterion for determining the need for open repair in 55 patients. In the patients in whom less than 50% of the tendon thickness was involved, arthroscopic subacromial decompression and cuff debridement alone was performed. In the 24 patients with more extensive tears (more than 50% involvement), a mini-open or arthroscopic cuff repair was added (20 and 4 patients, respectively). When this treatment guideline was used, 52 of 55 patients (95%) had satisfactory results, as evaluated with the UCLA scoring system at short-term follow-up (minimum, 1 year). The authors concluded that cuff repair should be considered for active patients with dominant-arm involvement and extensive tears (more than 50% of the cuff thickness) as determined arthroscopically. However, this study lacked a control group, which would have allowed comparison of the results of the more extensive repair with those of decompression alone.

Weber[6] included a control group when he compared the results in 55 patients with grade III PTRCTs (those with involvement of more than half of the tendon thickness) treated by arthroscopic debridement and subacromial decompression with the results in a group of similar patients treated with mini-open cuff repair in addition to decompression. Significantly better ($P<0.05$) results were obtained in those treated with open repair; a reoperation rate of 19% was reported for the arthroscopic group, but no reoperations were required in the mini-open group.

Open Treatment

Open treatment of PTRCT may be compromised somewhat by inability to directly visualize the articular surface of the cuff. However, repair of bursal-surface tears and subacromial decompression are readily performed with open techniques. Fukuda et al[11] have advocated open anterior acromioplasty as well as excision of the partially torn cuff segment with repair. They reported 92% satisfactory results at an average 34-month follow-up.

Itoi and Tabata[3] reviewed the results of treatment of 38 partial-thickness tears by complete excision of the involved tissue followed by repair. Open acromioplasty was used selectively. Follow-up averaged 4.9 years. The results were satisfactory in 31 of the 38 tears (82%), as evaluated with the UCLA scoring system.

Treatment Recommendations

The approach to treatment of PTRCTs must take into account the heterogeneous nature of the condition. Etiology, tear location, tear depth, and patient age and activity level should be considered in selecting treatment. Acromial morphology should influence the decision to perform subacromial decompression, but treatment should be tailored to the individual patient. Bursal-surface tears are often the result of mechanical outlet impingement. For this reason, acromioplasty should generally accompany debridement or repair of bursal-surface tears. Acromioplasty should also be given strong consideration when degenerative articular surface tears are seen in older individuals. Subacromial decompression without acromioplasty (i.e., bursectomy or coracoacromial ligament release) may be appropriate for selected patients with hypertrophic bursal tissue and flat acromial morphology.

The decision to proceed to cuff repair is based primarily on the extent of the tear. Most authors use tear depth alone as an indicator of the need for repair, with no mention of tear size in terms of area. Tears involving less than half of the tendon thickness should be treated by debridement. Tears involving more than half of the tendon thickness may benefit from repair.[6] Patients with higher activity levels may be more readily considered for cuff repair. However, caution should be exercised when dealing with the elite throwing athlete, in whom cuff debridement alone may be the most appropriate initial surgical intervention.

Articular-surface tears in young athletic individuals should be approached with a suspicion of occult instability.[25] These undersurface tears of the supraspinatus may be the result of acute eccentric loading or repetitive stress with microinstability. The hypermobility associated with the dominant shoulders of throwing athletes may subject the cuff to abnormal stress. Internal impingement may play a role in some of these tears. Anterior capsulorrhaphy might reduce symptoms in cases of anterior capsular redundancy and instability by limiting external rotation but would be expected to decrease function in the overhead athlete. In the absence of evidence of instability, rotator cuff debridement alone may provide symptomatic relief. Acromioplasty is rarely indicated for the young athlete.

Surgical treatment may be effectively performed with the use of either open or arthroscopic techniques. Glenohumeral arthroscopy offers the advantage of direct viewing of the cuff undersurface. Repair of a high-grade PTRCT is generally performed with an open deltoid-splitting approach. Some tears may be amenable to arthroscopic repair techniques, but only limited data are currently available to demonstrate the efficacy of this approach. Purely arthroscopic repair as well as mini-open techniques do not require deltoid detachment and its attendant postoperative concerns. However, rehabilitation is not accelerated because healing of the rotator cuff remains the limiting factor.

Summary

Partial-thickness tearing of the rotator cuff is a relatively common condition. However, the natural history of partial cuff tears and their contribution to clinical symptoms remain poorly characterized. Imaging modalities can be helpful but do not reliably depict partial tears.

Partial cuff tears can result from a variety of factors. These possible causes must be considered when designing a treatment plan. Extensive tears in individuals with high activity levels should be given particular consideration for repair.

References

1. Gartsman GM: Arthroscopic treatment of rotator cuff disease. *J Shoulder Elbow Surg* 1995;4:228-241.
2. Ryu RKN: Arthroscopic subacromial decompression: A clinical review. *Arthroscopy* 1992;8:141-147.
3. Itoi E, Tabata S: Incomplete rotator cuff tears: Results of operative treatment. *Clin Orthop* 1992;284:128-135.
4. Gartsman GM: Arthroscopic acromioplasty for lesions of the rotator cuff. *J Bone Joint Surg Am* 1990;72:169-180.
5. Ellman H: Diagnosis and treatment of incomplete rotator cuff tears. *Clin Orthop* 1990;254:64-74.
6. Weber SC: Arthroscopic debridement and acromioplasty versus mini-open repair in the management of significant partial-thickness tears of the rotator cuff. *Orthop Clin North Am* 1997; 28:79-82.
7. Olsewski JM, Depew AD: Arthroscopic subacromial decompression and rotator cuff debridement for stage II and stage III impingement. *Arthroscopy* 1994;10:61-68.
8. Miller DV, Lewis JM: Surgical management of partial rotator cuff tears. Presented at the Second Annual Meeting of the American Orthopaedic Society for Sports Medicine, Lake Buena Vista, Fla, June 1996.
9. Andrews JR, Broussard TS, Carson WG: Arthroscopy of the shoulder in the management of partial tears of the rotator cuff: A preliminary report. *Arthroscopy* 1985;1:117-122.
10. Gartsman GM, Milne JC: Articular surface partial-thickness rotator cuff tears. *J Shoulder Elbow Surg* 1995;4: 409-415.
11. Fukuda H, Craig EV, Yamanaka K, Hamada K: Partial-thickness cuff tears, in Burkhead WZ Jr (ed): *Rotator Cuff Disorders*. Baltimore: Williams & Wilkins, 1996, pp 174-181.
12. Fukuda H, Mikasa M, Yamanaka K: Incomplete thickness rotator cuff tears diagnosed by subacromial bursography. *Clin Orthop* 1987;223:51-58.
13. Williams GR Jr, Iannotti JP, Rosenthal A, Kneeland JB, Dalinka M, Schwaam H: Anatomic, histologic, and magnetic resonance imaging abnormalities of the shoulder. *Clin Orthop* 1996;330:66-74.
14. Fukuda H, Mikasa M, Ogawa K, Yamanaka K, Hamada K: "The color

test": An intraoperative staining test for joint-side rotator cuff tearing and its extension. *J Shoulder Elbow Surg* 1992;1:86-90.

15. Ozaki J, Fujimoto S, Nakagawa Y, Masuhara K, Tamai S: Tears of the rotator cuff of the shoulder associated with pathological changes in the acromion: A study in cadavera. *J Bone Joint Surg Am* 1988;70:1224-1230.

16. Sher JS, Uribe JW, Posada A, Murphy BJ, Zlatkin MB: Abnormal findings on magnetic resonance images of asymptomatic shoulders. *J Bone Joint Surg Am* 1995;77:10-15.

17. Yamanaka K, Matsumoto T: The joint side tear of the rotator cuff: A followup study by arthrography. *Clin Orthop* 1994;304:68-73.

18. Lohr JF, Uhthoff HK: The microvascular pattern of the supraspinatus tendon. *Clin Orthop* 1990;254:35-38.

19. Clark JM, Harryman DT II: Tendons, ligaments, and capsule of the rotator cuff: Gross and microscopic anatomy. *J Bone Joint Surg Am* 1992;74:713-725.

20. Nakajima T, Rokuuma N, Hamada K, Tomatsu T, Fukuda H: Histologic and biomechanical characteristics of the supraspinatus tendon: Reference to rotator cuff tearing. *J Shoulder Elbow Surg* 1994;3:79-87.

21. Walch G, Boileau P, Noel E, Donell ST: Impingement of the deep surface of the supraspinatus tendon on the posterosuperior glenoid rim: An arthroscopic study. *J Shoulder Elbow Surg* 1992;1:238-245.

22. Jobe CM: Superior glenoid impingement. *Orthop Clin North Am* 1997;28:137-143.

23. Hertel R, Ballmer FT, Lambert SM, Gerber C: Lag signs in the diagnosis of rotator cuff rupture. *J Shoulder Elbow Surg* 1996;5:307-313.

24. Bartolozzi A, Andreychik D, Ahmad S: Determinants of outcome in the treatment of rotator cuff disease. *Clin Orthop* 1994;308:90-97.

25. Paulos LE, Franklin JL: Arthroscopic shoulder decompression development and application: A five year experience. *Am J Sports Med* 1990;18:180-189.

26. Snyder SJ, Pachelli AF, Del Pizzo W, Friedman MJ, Ferkel RD, Pattee G: Partial thickness rotator cuff tears: Results of arthroscopic treatment. *Arthroscopy* 1991;7:1-7.

27. Wright SA, Cofield RH: Management of partial-thickness rotator cuff tears. *J Shoulder Elbow Surg* 1996;5:458-466.

28. Wiener SN, Seitz WH Jr: Sonography of the shoulder in patients with tears of the rotator cuff: Accuracy and value for selecting surgical options. *AJR Am J Roentgenol* 1993;160:103-107.

29. Traughber PD, Goodwin TE: Shoulder MRI: Arthroscopic correlation with emphasis on partial tears. *J Comput Assist Tomogr* 1992;16:129-133.

30. Quinn SF, Sheley RC, Demlow TA, Szumowski J: Rotator cuff tendon tears: Evaluation with fat-suppressed MR imaging with arthroscopic correlation in 100 patients. *Radiology* 1995;195:497-500.

31. Reinus WR, Shady KL, Mirowitz SA, Totty WG: MR diagnosis of rotator cuff tears of the shoulder: Value of using T2-weighted fat-saturated images. *AJR Am J Roentgenol* 1995;164:1451-1455.

32. Hodler J, Kursunoglu-Brahme S, Snyder SJ, et al: Rotator cuff disease: Assessment with MR arthrography versus standard MR imaging in 36 patients with arthroscopic confirmation. *Radiology* 1992;182:431-436.

33. Neer CS II: Impingement lesions. *Clin Orthop* 1983;173:70-77.

34. Morrison DS: Conservative management of partial-thickness rotator cuff lesions, in Burkhead WZ Jr (ed): *Rotator Cuff Disorders*. Baltimore: Williams & Wilkins, 1996, pp 249-257.

35. Ogilvie-Harris DJ, Wiley AM: Arthroscopic surgery of the shoulder: A general appraisal. *J Bone Joint Surg Br* 1986;68:201-207.

36. Esch JC, Ozerkis LR, Helgager JA, Kane N, Lilliott N: Arthroscopic subacromial decompression: Results according to the degree of rotator cuff tear. *Arthroscopy* 1988;4:241-249.

37. Altchek DW, Warren RF, Wickiewicz TL, Skyhar MJ, Ortiz G, Schwartz E: Arthroscopic acromioplasty: Technique and results. *J Bone Joint Surg Am* 1990;72:1198-1207.

Now a powerful web-based reference tool

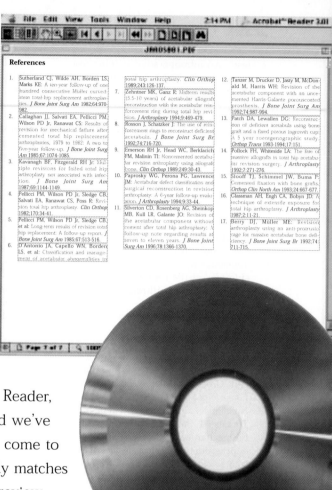

This year, *JAAOS on CD-ROM* is integrated with the World Wide Web. Point and click on links in the reference list of any article, and your web browser will display the abstract of the referenced article in *Index Medicus* on your screen. In addition, *JAAOS on CD-ROM* uses a more powerful version of Adobe's popular Acrobat Reader, with an updated toolbar that's even easier to use. And we've retained all the features of *JAAOS on CD-ROM* you've come to rely on: easy searchability, a familiar layout that exactly matches the printed version, and, of course, the finest clinical review articles in the orthopaedic specialty—now updated through 2000.

Using the CD-ROM

The articles on *JAAOS on CD-ROM* are written in Adobe's Portable Document Format (.pdf) and may only be viewed with the Adobe Acrobat Reader. You may run Acrobat directly from the CD or, for enhanced performance, install it to your system first. Windows users running an older release of Acrobat (prior to version 4.05), are strongly encouraged to erase it entirely before installing the new version, as system conflicts may occur otherwise. For detailed installation and operating instructions, open the file "ReadMe" on the disk.

To run Acrobat from the CD-ROM:
Open (double-click) the "Start Here" file on the CD. A Welcome screen will appear with two buttons. Click the button labeled "Open JAAOS on CD" to open the CD's Home page, which will lead you to the next screen. Click the other button, "Exit," to quit.

Installing Acrobat on a Windows-based PC:
The Acrobat 4.05 installer is located here: D:\Acrobat Reader 4.0\rs405eng.exe. (If your CD drive letter is not D: please substitute the appropriate letter.) If you have an older version of Acrobat on your system, uninstall it (see the ReadMe file for detailed instructions).

Exit any running applications and disable any virus protection software.

Run (double-click) the installer program. When the installation is complete, you may need to restart your system.

Installing Acrobat on a Macintosh:
The Acrobat 4.05 installer is located here: JAAOSCD:Acrobat Reader 4.0:Reader+Search 4.05 Installer. If you have an older version of Acrobat on your system, you may uninstall it by dragging it to the Trash.

Exit any running applications and disable any virus protection software.

Run (double-click) the installer program. When the installation is complete, you may need to restart your system.

JAAOS on CD-ROM is distributed as a benefit of membership to Fellows, Candidate Members, International Affiliate and Honorary Members of the American Academy of Orthopaedic Surgeons®. To purchase, contact AAOS Customer Service: phone: 800-626-6726, fax ++847-823-8033, e-mail: custserv@aaos.org.

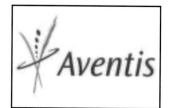

Production and distribution of *JAAOS on CD-ROM* is underwritten by an unrestricted educational grant from Aventis Pharmaceuticals Products, Inc.

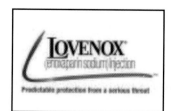

Current Concepts Review

Débridement of Partial-Thickness Tears of the Rotator Cuff without Acromioplasty

LONG-TERM FOLLOW-UP AND REVIEW OF THE LITERATURE*

BY JEFFREY E. BUDOFF, M.D.†, ROBERT P. NIRSCHL, M.D.‡, AND ERIC J. GUIDI, M.D.‡, ARLINGTON, VIRGINIA

Investigation performed at Nirschl Orthopedic and Sportsmedicine Clinic, Arlington

The rotator cuff, a musculotendinous unit that acts in combination with the deltoid to allow elevation of the shoulder, is a frequent source of pain and disability. In addition, the rotator cuff maintains the humeral head centered on the glenoid and opposes the superior translatory and shearing force of the deltoid by compressing the humeral head in the glenoid concavity as well as by imparting an inferiorly directed force vector to the proximal aspect of the humerus.

The term impingement syndrome has been used to describe symptoms related to the rotator cuff in the absence of a full-thickness tear of the cuff. The abnormality of the rotator cuff may range in severity from an acute strain or tendinitis to frank tearing. In all but the most acute situations, the lesion is one of chronic tendinopathy or angiofibroblastic hyperplasia rather than tendinitis. We recommend the use of the term tendinosis in lieu of the histologically inaccurate term tendinitis, since histopathological studies as well as analyses of cadaveric specimens have repeatedly shown that inflammatory cells are not part of the abnormality. Disorders of the rotator cuff may be due to an intrinsic factor, such as intrasubstance degenerative tearing or tendinosis caused by avascularity, aging, or overuse. Alternatively, they may be due to an extrinsic factor, such as outlet stenosis or glenohumeral instability[19].

The most commonly performed procedure to treat symptoms of impingement in the absence of a full-thickness tear of the rotator cuff is acromioplasty. This treatment is based on the theory that primary abnormal acromial morphology (an extrinsic cause), popularized by Neer[36] in 1972, is the initiating factor leading to dysfunction of the rotator cuff and eventual tearing. Therefore, subacromial decompression, which is now often performed arthroscopically, is done in an attempt to alter presumed aberrant acromial morphology, thereby eliminating a theorized impingement on the rotator cuff.

However, newer evidence suggests that, in most patients who have an abnormality of the rotator cuff, the primary problem is intrinsic. The supraspinatus, a small and relatively weak muscle, is in a key position and is therefore susceptible to overuse and injury. When eccentric tensile overload occurs at a rate that is greater than the ability of the rotator cuff to repair itself, injury occurs, resulting in weakness of the musculotendinous rotator-cuff unit. Trauma to the shoulder may initiate the same process, and a weak, fatigued, or injured rotator cuff is unable to oppose the superior pull of the deltoid effectively and to keep the humeral head centered on the glenoid during elevation of the arm. This leads to inappropriate superior migration of the humeral head with active elevation of the arm, which functionally narrows the subacromial space. Continued dysfunction of the rotator cuff and further superior migration of the humeral head cause the greater tuberosity and the rotator cuff to abut against the undersurface of the acromion and the coracoacromial ligament, leading to signs of secondary impingement.

The secondary impingement between the greater tuberosity and the acromion may lead to reactive and degenerative osseous changes, such as osteophytic spurring of these structures. The already injured and weakened rotator cuff is then damaged further by this process of secondary impingement, especially by osteophytes on the undersurface of the acromion. Subacromial impingement does occur, therefore, but in most circumstances it is a secondary, rather than a primary, phenomenon. Superimposed trauma may then cause the weakened cuff to rupture. Thus, in most instances impingement is a dynamic process secondary to intrinsic failure of the tendon that, with time, results in reactive osseous changes, causing the classic radiographic changes seen with impingement syndrome. Erosion or exostosis of the greater tuberosity has been reported to occur in nineteen (20 per cent) of ninety-six cases, probably as a result of the same mechanism[40].

*No benefits in any form have been received or will be received from a commercial party related directly or indirectly to the subject of this article. No funds were received in support of this study.

†Palm Beach Orthopaedic Associates, 603 Village Boulevard, Suite 300, West Palm Beach, Florida 33409.

‡Nirschl Orthopedic and Sportsmedicine Clinic, 1715 North George Mason Drive, Suite 504, Arlington, Virginia 22205.

The coracoacromial ligament, which stabilizes the rotator cuff to prevent uncontrolled superior migration of the humeral head[40], may also undergo degenerative changes within its substance[56] or a traction spur may form at its insertion into the anteromedial corner of the acromion, or both phenomena may occur. The traction spur, first described by Neer[36] in 1972, may easily be mistaken for an abnormal acromial hook, or type-3 acromion[6], on a radiograph of the supraspinatus outlet. This reactive spur has often been thought, erroneously we believe, to be the initiating factor in dysfunction of the rotator cuff. This etiological theory of primary extrinsic impingement led to the currently popular operative approach of subacromial decompression, which we also believe is erroneous.

We recommend that decisions involving operative treatment be based on demonstrated pathoanatomy, not theoretical concepts. Because the coracoacromial ligament and the undersurface of the acromion both function as important passive stabilizers against superior migration of the humeral head, we believe that these structures should not be sacrificed without evidence of pathological changes. Both of these structures are usually normal. Neer, in his original series of partial-thickness tears[36], found reactive acromial changes in only eight of nineteen patients, a prevalence similar to that which we found in our patients (twenty of seventy-nine shoulders). Neer did not mention any changes in the twenty patients who had a full-thickness tear. Although spurs may result in secondary damage to the cuff in only a few patients, acromioplasty was recomended by Neer 100 per cent of the time.

Acromioplasty fails to address the primary problem, which is intratendinous degeneration or tendinosis, in most symptomatic rotator cuffs. This was demonstrated by Gerber[11], who found that an injection into the subacromial space does not relieve pain caused by resisted abduction in patients who have a partial-thickness tear. It is our contention that at least some of the pain in a patient who has a partial tear is due to the damaged supraspinatus tendon. Failure of operative treatment, such as acromioplasty, likely occurs when the pathoanatomy of the tendinosis is not addressed. In addition, acromioplasty disrupts the periosteum and cortical bone of the acromion, exposing a large surface of raw cancellous bone that may predispose to extensive scar formation. Subsequent fibrosis of the coracoacromial arch may result in decreased motion of the shoulder.

Since 1988, the senior one of us (R. P. N.) has based his treatment of symptoms of impingement on demonstrated pathoanatomy[38,39]. The degenerative tissue of the rotator cuff is identified and arthroscopically debrided, thus removing the primary pathoanatomy[40,51]. Clearly identified excrescences underneath the acromion are also resected; however, such excrescences are the exception rather than the rule. A complete acromioplasty is not performed and the coracoacromial ligament is not resected, although small (less than 25 per cent) segments may be removed when occasional osseous subacromial excrescences are addressed.

Review of the Literature

We believe that 90 to 95 per cent of abnormalities of the rotator cuff are secondary to tension overload, overuse, and traumatic injury. There is no objective evidence that primary extrinsic factors are involved in most disorders of the rotator cuff[39], as changes within the rotator cuff often occur without accompanying changes on the acromion[19,42]. Ozaki et al.[42] examined 200 cadaveric shoulders and found that, while a lesion on the anterior one-third of the undersurface of the acromion was always associated with a tear of the cuff, the reverse was not always true. In fact, in all specimens that had a partial-thickness tear on the articular side, the undersurface of the acromion was intact. Ozaki et al., like one of us (R. P. N.)[38,40], concluded that "the pathogenesis of most tears of the rotator cuff is a degenerative process" that predates the formation of osteophytes and that the acromial changes, when present, are reactive osseous changes secondary to impingement from superior humeral migration rather than primary acromial variants. Ozaki et al. also noted that the severity of the pathological changes on the undersurface of the acromion were commensurate with the severity of the damage to the rotator cuff and that a cycle subsequently develops, with the irregularity of the undersurface of the acromion abrading the cuff and vice versa. The prevalence of incomplete tears increased with increasing age.

Gerber[10] stated that if a repair of the rotator cuff and an acromioplasty are performed together and the repair fails, a type-3 acromion will recur. The change in the morphology of the acromion following an acromioplasty cannot cause the rupture, but the rupture causes new deformation of the acromion[10].

Neer[36], in 1972, and Bigliani et al.[6], in 1986, popularized the theory of extrinsic subacromial impingement. However, it cannot be concluded from either the clinical series described by Neer or the cadaver series described by Bigliani et al. that acromial variations are primary (due to heredity) as opposed to secondary changes. Neer frequently noted, in 100 dissected scapulae, a characteristic ridge of proliferative spurs and excrescences on the undersurface of the anterior process of the acromion that were apparently caused by repeated impingement of the rotator cuff on the humeral head, with traction of the coracoacromial ligament. He also noted that many radiographs showed corresponding areas of proliferation at the anterior edge of the acromion. One of us (R. P. N.)[38-40] observed similar findings and concluded that Neer misinterpreted the etiology of these pathoanatomical abnormalities.

Morrison[10] has stated that the basis of rotator-cuff disorders is a muscle imbalance between the elevators and depressors of the humeral head — that is, between the rotator cuff and the deltoid. As a natural part of the aging process, the deltoid retains its strength longer than the relatively diminutive rotator cuff, resulting in a loss of the depressor effect of the rotator cuff on the humeral head during elevation and leading to subsequent impingement. Morrison also thought that acromial morphology is not the cause of tears of the rotator cuff, although he believed that acromial variants may predispose some people to tears of the rotator cuff once muscle imbalance occurs.

Deutsch et al.[15], in a radiographic study, noted that patients who had stage-II or III impingement, with or without a full-thickness tear, had superior migration of the humeral head with elevation of the arm. The humeral head stayed centered within the glenoid cavity in normal volunteers under normal conditions. However, when the volunteers were fatigued, they also had migration of the humeral head. This may explain the belief that occupational and athletic activities may play a greater role in degeneration of the tendon than does age[11]. Young patients frequently overload the rotator cuff during intense athletic activities, specifically swimming, racquet sports, or throwing sports, or because of occupational demands. This hypothesis may also explain the beneficial effects of rest and rehabilitative exercises in restoring strength to the rotator cuff. According to Gerber[10], "the main problem is degeneration and weakness in the musculotendinous unit and the tendinous insertion on the bone."

Uhthoff[10] believed that most changes on the acromion result from intrinsic tendinopathies. Tears of the cuff, if they are caused by attrition or impingement, should originate at the bursal aspect of the cuff[10]; however, autopsy evaluations[42,56] as well as clinical observations have revealed a higher prevalence of partial tears on the articular side than on the bursal side. Gerber[10] concurred, reporting that iatrogenic impingement exclusively caused lesions on the superior surface of the cuff in rats. He believed that the confusion regarding the etiology of dysfunction of the rotator cuff stems from the fact that the pain experienced by the patient is at least partly caused by secondary impingement.

Burkhead[11] found that the hook of a type-3 acromion represents spurring on the medial aspect of the acromion. We agree that this hook, when present, is a traction spur of the coracoacromial ligament rather than a radiographically misinterpreted primary acromial variant.

Uhthoff et al.[56] confirmed the presence of degenerative changes in the coracoacromial ligament in patients who had impingement syndrome. We believe that this degeneration is probably the result of repetitive overloading of the ligament as it works to function as a secondary, passive superior stabilizer of the humeral head once the rotator cuff is too weak or dysfunctional to dynamically maintain the humeral head centered in the glenoid cavity.

Osteoarthrosis of the acromioclavicular joint is present in association with many symptomatic problems of the rotator cuff that necessitate operative intervention. While inferior acromioclavicular osteophytes may contribute to subacromial stenosis and subsequent impingement and may need to be removed, osteoarthrosis of the acromioclavicular joint itself appears to be independent of injury of the rotator cuff[40].

Ozaki et al.[42] found that, in contrast to partial-thickness tears on the articular side, each partial-thickness tear on the bursal side was associated with an attritional lesion on the coracoacromial ligament as well as on the anterior one-third of the undersurface of the acromion. Those authors observed the same kind of attritional changes in each specimen that had a full-thickness tear.

One of us (R. P. N.)[40,51] also noted attritional subacromial changes in association with full-thickness tears, but only in 46 per cent (forty-four) of ninety-six tears.

Several mechanisms may be responsible for partial-thickness tears on either the articular side or the bursal side. If the articular side degenerates simultaneously with weakening of the cuff, a tear occurs on the articular side and secondary impingement may then lead to a partial-thickness tear on the bursal side, as well as to osteophytes on the underside of the acromion. If weakness occurs without a tear on the articular side, an isolated partial-thickness tear occurs on the bursal side. In either case, further damage from continued overload, overuse, secondary impingement, or traumatic injury may then lead to a full-thickness tear. We believe that a primarily intrinsic etiology is responsible for most tears on the bursal side, but a few tears may be due to extrinsic causes, such as acromial variants.

Pathophysiology

Both Uhthoff et al.[56] and Ozaki et al.[42] performed anatomical studies on cadaveric shoulders and found that most partial-thickness tears were on the articular side. Payne et al.[44] found that 91 per cent of the partial-thickness tears in forty-three young athletes were on the articular side. Ellman[17] noted that, when partial-thickness tears were openly explored, "a surprising degree of lamination can be encountered, with the most inferior [articular surface] fibers demonstrating the greatest degree of retraction." Loehr and Uhthoff[34] studied 306 cadaveric rotator cuffs and concluded that most degenerative tears originated on the articular side of the supraspinatus tendon, near the insertion, and that such tears are primarily intrinsic tendinopathies and are not secondary to anatomical variations or wear and tear resulting from contiguous structures. This finding may be due to the poor blood supply of the articular side of the supraspinatus insertion. Lohr and Uhthoff[35] confirmed the presence of the hypovascular critical zone just proximal to the insertion of the supraspinatus tendon that had first been noted by Codman[12] in 1934. Lohr and

Uhthoff[35] reported that the articular side of the supraspinatus insertion had only a sparse vascular supply, with almost no vessels. However, the bursal side of the supraspinatus insertion was well vascularized. Those authors also noted that this critical zone of ischemia on the articular side seemed to correspond well with the common site of rupture of the tendon. The relative ischemia of this area may be one reason why the cuff is unable to repair itself, leading to degeneration and weakness.

Rothman and Parke[47] noted that areas of hypovascularity coincided with the common sites of degeneration in the supraspinatus and infraspinatus tendons. Those authors concluded that this strongly suggests that a poor blood supply may be important in the pathogenesis of degeneration of the rotator cuff. They found no effect of aging on this vasculature. We also noted that the area of degenerative tendinosis occurs most often in the hypovascular zone of the articular side of the supraspinatus insertion and the anterior infraspinatus insertion. This area corresponds well with the crescent described by Burkhart[8,10]. In fact, just outside this well defined area of degeneration one can often see the cable originally described by Burkhart[8]. We have never found this cable to be degenerated, and all attempts to debride it with a motorized shaver have been futile; this further proves that the tissue is intrinsically healthy. We agree with Burkhart[8] that loss of the hypovascular crescentic area of rotator cuff tissue within the cable may be a normal part of aging, similar to hair loss. Elevation of the arm is still possible because of stress transmission through the cable. This may explain why approximately 72 per cent of all tears of the rotator cuff are asymptomatic[11]: they are a normal part of aging. The approximately 28 per cent of tears that cause pain may do so because they involve more than just the crescentic area of the insertion or are associated with increased tendinopathy.

This degenerative tissue, identified histologically as angiofibroblastic hyperplasia[39,40], appears to be painful in and of itself, although we do not know why this is so. Goldie[25] noted free nerve endings in this tissue, but we have been unable to duplicate his findings. We suggest that it is painful because it is ischemic or chemically irritated. If degeneration of the crescentic area is a normal part of aging, however, then it should be painless. This is probably true in most people, in whom the tissue degenerates at a rate at which the body can absorb it, leaving an asymptomatic non-retracted full-thickness tear of the rotator cuff with the cable intact. Symptoms may develop when the rate of tissue breakdown, or the formation of tendinosis, exceeds the body's ability to absorb the tissue, as may occur with overuse or traumatic injury even in the absence of a full-thickness tear.

Because of the high prevalence of asymptomatic shoulders with a full-thickness tear of the rotator cuff as well as the high prevalence of very painful shoulders without a full-thickness tear, we do not routinely perform preoperative magnetic resonance imaging or arthrography. Once a diagnosis of tendinosis and dysfunction of the rotator cuff is made on the basis of history, physical examination, and routine radiographs and after appropriate non-operative treatment has failed, decisions regarding operative treatment are made on the basis of the symptoms and wishes of the patient, not the presence or absence of a hole in the cuff. Once diagnostic arthroscopy is performed, it becomes clear whether the tear is full thickness.

Arthroscopic Subacromial Decompression

Most reports regarding arthroscopic treatment of abnormalities of the rotator cuff have presented only short-term results and have focused on arthroscopic subacromial decompression. While this procedure has been performed since 1985, no long-term results (after a minimum of five years of follow-up) have been published, to our knowledge. Our objections to subacromial decompression and the destruction of the normal static superior stabilizers of the humeral head concern the long-term effects of iatrogenic removal of the coracoacromial arch. Long-term follow-up is essential in the evaluation of any procedure. Many procedures that had good short-term results have now been condemned on the basis of the long-term data. The orthopaedic experience with total medial meniscectomy and various total joint arthroplasty techniques and prostheses has borne this out.

The rate of short-term (average, 25.9 months; range, 16.7 to 48.0 months) success after arthroscopic subacromial decompression has been reported to be between 46 per cent[29] (forty-six of 100) and 100 per cent[58] (fifty of fifty)[1,3,16-18,21,22,24,30,33,43,44,48-50,53,57]. These so-called successes probably occur because subacromial decompression relieves the pain caused by secondary impingement, which, even though it is a secondary manifestation of primary dysfunction of the rotator cuff, is the cause of the clinical symptoms. This situation is analogous to the subtle anterior instability and resultant dysfunction of the rotator cuff in a thrower; the primary pathoanatomy (glenohumeral instability) is subtle and is easily missed if one focuses exclusively on the immediate source of pain. Harryman[10] stated: "Before focusing on the coracoacromial arch and the shape of the acromion, we must understand why fiber failure occurs." Gerber[10] agreed that acromioplasty is effective in relieving pain, but he did not think that impingement causes the tear of the cuff. Ryu[49] reviewed the literature and concluded that the improvement noted after subacromial decompression in patients who have a partial-thickness tear on the articular side of the rotator cuff may be a result of postoperative rest rather than an intrinsic benefit of the operation itself. Another potential source of pain relief could be the denervation of subacromial soft tissue.

We are concerned that, with the passage of time after an acromioplasty, the lack of the passive stabilizing influence of the coracoacromial arch in the presence of a marginally functional rotator cuff may compromise the ability to elevate the arm. This point is best illustrated by patients who have a full-thickness tear of the rotator cuff with marginal function that is dependent on an intact coracoacromial arch. Acromioplasty may cause a torn rotator cuff that is functional to become completely non-functional, with the patient no longer able to elevate the arm secondary to uncontrolled superior humeral migration[11]. Since it is impossible to predict which torn rotator cuffs may become marginally functional in the distant future, prudence suggests retaining the secondary stabilizers if at all possible.

Ozaki et al.[42], in support of this point of view, stated that "histological evidence . . . suggests that the anterior one-third of the undersurface of the acromion plays a major role in the mechanism of movement of the shoulder, because it works as a subacromial joint." Paulos and Franklin[43] believed that excessive resection of acromial bone or removal of the coracoacromial ligament may not be advisable in patients who have a massive irreparable full-thickness tear of the rotator cuff because these structures provide restraint to anterior and anterosuperior migration of the humeral head. Harryman[11] believed that the function of the shoulder may become fully dependent on the deltoid if the rotator cuff fails and remains irreparable. In such instances, the coracoacromial arch functions as a secondary constraint to provide humeroscapular stability. When a major portion of the acromion is resected, resection of the coracoacromial ligament should be avoided or severe anterosuperior instability may occur; if such instability does occur, no reconstruction will be satisfactory[11]. Harryman also thought that the shoulder may eventually become dependent on the arch for functional stability. Williams[11] agreed, stating that patients who have a marginally functional torn cuff need the coracoacromial arch. If the arch is removed, the cuff may become completely non-functional. In fact, Williams stated that he was "appalled to find that some patients have a shoulder that is no longer functional following what was considered to be reasonable surgery." He also noted that a marginally functional torn rotator cuff can be difficult to identify preoperatively.

We believe that acromioplasty is infrequently indicated for disorders of the rotator cuff. Primary aberrant acromial morphology is probably the cause of less than 5 to 10 per cent of impingement syndromes. In addition, Burkhart[9] described congenital subacromial stenosis, which also may warrant a traditional acromioplasty. However, both of these conditions are uncommon.

Adolfsson and Lysholm[1] reported an overall 67 per cent rate of satisfactory results, according to a modification of the system described by Neer, following seventy-nine arthroscopic subacromial decompressions performed for various stages of impingement, including full-thickness tears. Of the twenty-nine patients who had a partial-thickness tear, 90 per cent had a satisfactory result; however, of the eleven patients who had clinical signs of impingement alone without tendinosis or a tear, only 19 per cent had a satisfactory result. The average duration of follow-up was seventeen months (range, nine to twenty-four months).

Altchek et al.[3] reported a 73 per cent rate of good and excellent results at an average of seventeen months (range, one to three years) after forty arthroscopic subacromial decompressions performed for various stages of impingement. The twenty-four patients who did not have a partial or full-thickness tear had the highest rate of success (83 per cent). Seventy-six per cent of the thirty-three patients who had participated in sports activity had returned to sports activity at the time of the most recent follow-up.

In a series described by Ellman[16], 88 per cent of forty-nine arthroscopic subacromial decompressions performed for various stages of impingement yielded a good or excellent result. The rate of success for the thirty-nine patients who did not have a full-thickness tear was 90 per cent. The average duration of follow-up was seventeen months (range, twelve to thirty-six months). In a later study[17], Ellman reported a satisfactory short-term result in fifteen (75 per cent) of twenty patients who had been managed with arthroscopic subacromial decompression for a partial-thickness tear.

Esch et al.[18] reported a 78 per cent rate of good and excellent results, according to the rating scale of the University of California at Los Angeles, after seventy-one arthroscopic subacromial decompressions performed for impingement syndrome and partial-thickness tears. The average duration of follow-up was nineteen months (range, twelve to thirty-six months).

Gartsman[21] noted improvement, at an average of twenty-eight months, in eighty-one (88 per cent) of ninety-two patients who had had arthroscopic subacromial decompression for stage-II impingement. In another report, Gartsman[22] reported that seventy-eight (88 per cent) of eighty-nine shoulders that had been treated with arthroscopic subacromial decompression for stage-II impingement without a partial-thickness tear had a satisfactory result at an average of thirty-one months (minimum, two years). In addition, thirty-three (83 per cent) of forty shoulders had a satisfactory result at an average of twenty-nine months after arthroscopic subacromial decompression combined with débridement of the frayed edges of a partial-thickness tear. Gartsman and Milne[24] later reported an 88 per cent rate of subjective satisfaction after arthroscopic subacromial decompression, combined with débridement of the rotator cuff when appropriate, in 111 shoulders with a partial-thickness tear on the articular side of the rotator cuff. The average duration of follow-up was thirty-two months (range, twenty-six to eighty-four months). Objective scoring systems were not used to rate the outcome of the operation.

In the study by Hawkins et al.[30], there was a satisfactory result (indicating no or minimum pain, normal use, within 20 degrees of a full range of motion, normal strength, and a negative impingement sign) after 46 per cent (fifty-one) of 110 arthroscopic subacromial decompressions performed for stage-II impingement. When patients who were involved in a Workers' Compensation claim were excluded, the rate was 56 per cent (thirty-seven of sixty-six shoulders). The minimum duration of follow-up was two years (maximum, fifty-two months).

Van Holsbeeck et al.[57], in a study of fifty-three arthroscopic subacromial decompressions performed for advanced stage-II or early stage-III disease (full-thickness tears of less than one centimeter), reported an 83 per cent rate of good and excellent results, according to the rating scale of the University of California at Los Angeles. The average duration of follow-up was twenty months (range, twelve to twenty-six months).

Lazarus et al.[33] reported a good or excellent result (on the basis of the University of Pennsylvania score) after 57 per cent of forty-six arthroscopic subacromial decompressions performed for impingement syndrome without a full-thickness tear. The average duration of follow-up was twenty-five months (minimum, twelve months). Those authors stated that patients who had a more hooked acromion postoperatively did better. Patients who had made a Workers' Compensation claim had the worst results. The results following twenty-four open subacromial decompressions were comparable.

In a study of forty-two arthroscopic subacromial decompressions and twenty-four so-called simple decompressions, which involved resection of the bursa and the coracoacromial ligament without acromioplasty, Paulos and Franklin[43] noted improvement after 85 per cent of the arthroscopic subacromial decompressions, no change after 10 per cent, and worsening after 5 per cent. They also noted improvement after 83 per cent of the simple decompressions and no change after 17 per cent. The average duration of follow-up was thirty-two months (range, twelve to fifty-four months). Patients who did not have an acromioplasty did slightly better, especially with regard to pain at night and persistence of the impingement sign. These patients also tended to be younger, which could mean that they had less extensive disease but probably also meant that they had higher functional demands.

Payne et al.[44] reported a satisfactory result, as determined with the rating system of the American Shoulder and Elbow Surgeons, for 72 per cent of forty-three athletes who had a partial-thickness tear treated with arthroscopic subacromial decompression or débridement; 51 per cent of the athletes returned to sports. However, the results of the two procedures were not compared. The duration of follow-up averaged forty-eight months (range, twenty-four to 120 months). Patients who had subtle instability had the worst results.

Roye et al.[48] reported a good or excellent result, according to the rating scale of the University of California at Los Angeles, after 94 per cent of ninety arthroscopic subacromial decompressions performed for various stages of impingement, including full-thickness tears of less than one centimeter. Sixty-one per cent (thirty-four) of the fifty-six athletes overall and 53 per cent (eighteen) of the thirty-four who participated in a sport that required throwing returned to sports activity. Only 79 per cent of the thirty-four athletes whose sport involved throwing and eight of the twelve competitive baseball or softball pitchers had a satisfactory result. The average duration of follow-up was forty-one months (range, twenty-four to eighty-two months).

At an average of twenty-three months (range, twelve to fifty months) after fifty-three arthroscopic subacromial decompressions performed for various stages of impingement, Ryu[49] reported an 81 per cent rate of good and excellent results, according to the rating scale of the University of California at Los Angeles. The result was good or excellent after 86 per cent of the thirty-five procedures that were performed for a partial-thickness tear.

Sampson et al.[50] reported a good or excellent result, according to the rating scale of the University of California at Los Angeles, after 90 per cent of ninety-one arthroscopic subacromial decompressions. The minimum duration of follow-up was one year; the average duration was not reported.

In a study of twenty-five arthroscopic subacromial decompressions performed for impingement without a full-thickness tear, Speer et al.[53] reported an 88 per cent rate of good and excellent results, on the basis of the rating scale of the University of California at Los Angeles. The patients were able to return to sports after 76 per cent of the procedures. The average duration of follow-up was twenty months (range, fourteen to thirty-two months). Only four of the twelve patients who were involved in a sport that required throwing were able to return to the sport without discomfort, even though examination under anesthesia was negative for glenohumeral instability.

Warner et al.[58] reported a successful result after 94 per cent of seventy arthroscopic subacromial decompressions at an average of twenty-four months (range, twenty-two to twenty-eight months) postoperatively. The modified technique that was used by those authors led to complete resolution of the symptoms at an average of twenty-two months (range, eighteen to twenty-four months) postoperatively in all fifty patients who had impingement syndrome. No objective measures were used to evaluate the success of the procedure.

Bigliani et al.[7] reported an 81 per cent rate of good and excellent results following twenty-six arthroscopic subacromial decompressions performed on patients who were less than forty years old. The average duration of follow-up was thirty-three months (range, twelve to eighty months). Seven of the ten patients who had been recreational athletes were able to return to their recreational activities.

Open Subcromial Decompression

Hawkins et al.[29] reported a satisfactory result (no or minimum pain, normal use, within 20 degrees of a full range of motion, normal strength, and a negative impingement sign) for 87 per cent of 108 patients who had been managed with an open subacromial decompression because of impingement without a full-thickness tear. When the thirty-five patients who had made a Workers' Compensation claim were excluded, the rate of satisfactory results was 92 per cent. The long-term follow-up evaluation was performed at an average of 5.2 years (range, 2.6 to 8.1 years).

Van Holsbeeck et al.[57] reported a good or excellent result, on the basis of the rating scale of the University of California at Los Angeles, after 81 per cent of fifty-three open subacromial decompressions performed for stage-II and early stage-III disease. The average duration of follow-up was twenty-seven months (range, twelve to forty-seven months).

In a study by Neer[36], the result was satisfactory for fifteen of sixteen shoulders at an average of two and a half years after an open subacromial decompression.

Neviaser et al.[37] reported that all patients had a subjective decrease in pain, compared with the preoperative status, following a four-in-one arthroplasty (subacromial decompression, excision of the lateral end of the clavicle and the coracoacromial ligament, and biceps tenodesis). The average duration of follow-up was four years (range, two to eight years). Many authors[11,40] currently condemn this so-called shotgun operative approach, and it should be noted that Neviaser et al. did not document any objective criteria for success.

In a study of seventy-two open subacromial decompressions performed for impingement syndrome without a full-thickness tear, Post and Cohen[46] reported an 80 per cent rate of good and excellent results at an average of twenty-three months (range, five to forty-eight months) postoperatively.

Stuart et al.[54] reported a successful result after 73 per cent of forty open subacromial decompressions without resection of the lateral end of the clavicle. The average duration of follow-up was eight years (range, three to thirteen years).

In the series described by Thorling et al.[55], the result was good or excellent for twenty-six (65 per cent) of forty patients at an average of twenty-one months (range, six to forty-two months) after an open subacromial decompression performed for impingement without a full-thickness tear.

Open Division of the Coracoacromial Ligament

The short-term results of open division of the coracoacromial ligament without subacromial decom-

pression are at least as good as, if not better than, those of open or arthroscopic subacromial decompression.

Nineteen (90 per cent) of twenty-one patients in a study by Ha'eri and Wiley[27] reported that they were satisfied after an open resection of the coracoacromial ligament, which was combined with open subacromial decompression (four patients) and open resection of the lateral end of the clavicle (six patients) when appropriate. The minimum duration of follow-up was one year, but no average was noted.

Johansson and Barrington[32] reported a 95 per cent rate of satisfactory results at an average of thirty-six months (range, eight to seventy-six months) after forty-one open resections of the coracoacromial ligament in the absence of substantial acromial osteophytes.

In the study by Penny and Welsh[45], twelve of fourteen patients who had signs of impingement without a full-thickness tear of the rotator cuff returned to sports activity. There was no difference in the results between ten patients who had a simple excision of a one-to-two-centimeter segment of the coracoacromial ligament and ten who had a complete open subacromial decompression. The average duration of follow-up was three and a half years (minimum, six months).

Débridement of the Rotator Cuff

The reported results of open or arthroscopic débridement of the rotator cuff have been good; however, in many series, the procedure was combined with a subacromial decompression. Fu et al.[19] stated that "the emphasis of treatment is shifting from that of decompression to restoring the health of the rotator cuff."

Altchek and Carson[2] reported an 80 per cent rate of favorable results after arthroscopic débridement of a symptomatic rotator cuff in fifty athletes who engaged in a sport that required throwing. Five of the fifty also had an arthroscopic subacromial decompression for a narrowed subacromial space that had been noted either on radiographs or intraoperatively. Those authors believed that the 20 per cent rate of failure was due to excessive capsular laxity that could not be controlled by strengthening of the shoulder.

Andrews et al.[4] reported a good or excellent result for 85 per cent of thirty-four young athletes (average age, twenty-two years) who had an arthroscopic débridement of the rotator cuff; 64 per cent of the patients were pitchers. The average duration of follow-up was thirteen months.

In a study of thirty-nine open subacromial decompressions combined with open débridement of the rotator cuff performed for partial-thickness tears, Fukuda et al.[20] found a 92 per cent rate of satisfactory results; no objective criteria were given. The average duration of follow-up was thirty-four months; no range was reported.

Snyder et al.[52] reported a good or excellent result, on the basis of the rating scale of the University of

California at Los Angeles, for 93 per cent of thirty-one shoulders in which a partial-thickness tear was treated with débridement; eighteen of the shoulders were also treated with an arthroscopic subacromial decompression. The average duration of follow-up was twenty-three months (range, ten to forty-three months).

Ogilvie-Harris and Wiley[41] reported a successful result for approximately two-thirds of twenty patients who had an arthroscopic débridement of the rotator cuff for tendinitis and for approximately 50 per cent of sixty-five patients who had that procedure for a partial-thickness tear. The minimum duration of follow-up was one year.

Analysis of the Present Study

Materials and Methods

Ninety-eight shoulders (ninety-five patients) were treated with arthroscopic débridement because of tendinosis of the rotator cuff in the absence of a full-thickness tear. Seventy-nine of these shoulders (seventy-six patients) were available for follow-up. Forty-two shoulders were examined by one of us (J. E. B.), and thirty-seven were evaluated with use of a telephone interview. Fifty shoulders were in male patients, and twenty-nine were in female patients. Fifty-three of the shoulders were dominant, and twenty-six were non-dominant. Sixty-five of the shoulders were in patients who were involved in athletic activity on at least a recreational level. The average age of the patients was forty-five years (range, seventeen to seventy-seven years). Fifty-two shoulders were in patients who were forty years old or more, and twenty-seven shoulders were in patients who were less than forty years old.

The overall duration of follow-up was fifty-three months (range, twenty-five to ninety-three months). Two subgroups were examined: thirty-two shoulders (thirty-one patients) that were followed for five years or more (average, seventy-five months; range, sixty to ninety-three months) and forty-seven shoulders (forty-five patients) that were followed for two to less than five years (average, thirty-nine months; range, twenty-five to fifty-six months).

The main preoperative symptom was pain in all patients. In addition, forty-five patients had weakness and thirty-eight had stiffness or loss of functional motion. The average duration of the preoperative symptoms was thirty-four months (range, two months to twenty-three years).

The preoperative diagnosis of impingement syndrome or abnormality of the rotator cuff was made on the basis of the history and the physical examination; radiographs were made for all patients. All of the patients had failed to respond to non-operative therapy that included an intensive program of rehabilitative exercises designed to restore strength, flexibility, and endurance to the rotator cuff, deltoid, scapulothoracic stabilizers, and thoracic muscles. All of the rehabilita-

TABLE I

RATING SCALE OF THE
UNIVERSITY OF CALIFORNIA AT LOS ANGELES[16]*

	No. of Points
Pain	
Present always and unbearable; strong medication needed frequently	1
Present always but bearable; strong medication needed occasionally	2
None or little at rest; present during light activities; salicylates needed frequently	4
Present during heavy or particular activities only; salicylates needed occasionally	6
Occasional and slight	8
None	10
Function	
Unable to use limb	1
Only light activities possible	2
Able to do light housework and most activities of daily living	4
Most housework, shopping, and driving possible; able to brush hair and to dress and undress, including fastening of brassiere	6
Slight restriction only; able to work above shoulder level	8
Normal activities	10
Active flexion	
>150 degrees	5
121-150 degrees	4
91-120 degrees	3
46-90 degrees	2
30-45 degrees	1
<30 degrees	0
Strength of flexion (on manual muscle-testing)	
Grade 5	5
Grade 4	4
Grade 3	3
Grade 2	2
Grade 1	1
Grade 0	0
Satisfaction of patient	
Satisfied and better	5
Not satisfied and worse	0

*The maximum score is 35 points. A score of 34 or 35 points is considered excellent; 28 to 33 points, good; 21 to 27 points, fair; and 0 to 20 points, poor. A satisfactory result is indicated by a score of 28 points or more, and a failure is indicated by a score of 27 points or less.

tion programs were supervised by a physical therapist.

A substantial number of other patients had arthroscopic procedures during this time-period, but they were excluded from the present study because they had a full-thickness tear of the rotator cuff, glenohumeral instability (noted on examination under anesthesia or on glenohumeral arthroscopy, or both), glenohumeral chondromalacia that was grade III (fissuring to bone) or grade IV (subchondral bone exposed), osteoarthrosis of the acromioclavicular joint that necessitated full resection of the lateral end of the clavicle, arthroscopically confirmed adhesive capsulitis, previous repair of the rotator cuff, previous subacromial decompression, rheumatic disease, calcific tendinitis, or osteochondromatosis. In addition, one patient had concomitant chronic neck pain with radiculopathy and could not distinguish that pain from the pain in the shoulder.

Preoperative and postoperative pain was assessed according to whether it occurred at night (that is, whether it was present while the patient was trying to fall asleep or it awoke the patient), at rest, with activities of daily living, or during athletic activities.

Operative Technique

The procedure was performed with the patient under general anesthesia, and antibiotic prophylaxis was provided. If needed, the shoulder was manipulated to regain a full passive range of motion. The patient was placed in the lateral decubitus position with ten to fifteen pounds (4.5 to 6.8 kilograms) of traction placed on the arm. Marcaine (bupivacaine hydrochloride) with epinephrine was injected into the subacromial space to aid in hemostasis of the coracoacromial arch. An arthroscopic pump (Davol, Cranston, Rhode Island) was utilized for the operative interventions in both the glenohumeral joint and the coracoacromial arch. A standard posterior arthroscopic portal was made. The rotator interval between the biceps tendon and the leading edge of the subscapularis was identified, and an anterior portal was established in this space through an inside-out technique with use of a Wissinger rod. Diagnostic arthroscopy was then performed in the glenohumeral joint.

Areas of labral degeneration were debrided with a motorized shaver. SLAP lesions (lesions of the superior portion of the labrum, anterior and posterior, or a bucket-handle tear of the labrum) were repaired or debrided as appropriate. The superior aspect of the glenoid as well as the underside of the labrum were burred to enhance biological healing. The biceps tendon was debrided if it was degenerated. The supraspinatus and infraspinatus tendons were evaluated for any degenerative tendinotic changes, which were usually identified by a change in appearance. (A normal rotator-cuff tendon appears firm, taut, shiny, and yellow-white, whereas tendinosis gives the tendon a softened texture and it appears gray, dull, sometimes edematous, and frayed.)

The degenerative portions of the affected tendons are arthroscopically debrided with straight or curved motorized shavers moved in a sweeping motion across the involved area. This is the arthroscopic equivalent of the Nirschl scratch test developed for open débridement of degenerative tendinosis about the elbow. Healthy tendon tissue is not substantially affected by a motorized shaver that is operated without undue force. However, analogous to peeling paint, friable, degenerative intratendinous tissue is readily removed, without harming healthy tissue. The abnormal tissue was most frequently located in the critical zone of the supraspinatus tendon, especially in its insertions, and in the more anterior aspect of the infraspinatus. If the abnormality extended inferiorly into the infraspinatus, the portals

TABLE II
FUNCTIONAL SCORE OF CONSTANT AND MURLEY[13]

	No. of Points
Subjective symptoms	35
Pain	
Severe	0
Moderate	5
Mild	10
None	15
Activities of daily living	
Handicap affecting work	0 to 4*
Handicap affecting recreation	0 to 4*
Sleep affected	0
Sleep not affected	2
Level of use of hand	
Waist	2
Xiphoid	4
Neck	6
Top of head	8
About head	10
Objective findings	65
Active range of motion, seated	
Flexion	
<30 degrees	0
30-60 degrees	2
60-90 degrees	4
90-120 degrees	6
120-150 degrees	8
>150 degrees	10
Abduction	
<30 degrees	0
30-60 degrees	2
60-90 degrees	4
90-120 degrees	6
120-150 degrees	8
>150 degrees	10
Internal rotation (dorsum of hand to)	
Thigh	0
Buttock	2
Sacrum	4
L3	6
T12	8
T7	10
External rotation	
Hand behind head with elbow held forward	2
Hand behind head with elbow held back	2
Hand on top of head with elbow held forward	2
Hand on top of head with elbow held back	2
Full elevation from on top of head	2
Strength	
Grade 0	0
Grade 1	5
Grade 2	10
Grade 3	15
Grade 4	20
Grade 5	25

*0 = severe handicap and 4 = full function.

were reversed to debride the abnormal areas through the posterior portal.

We believe that many partial-thickness tears of the rotator cuff are missed by both experienced and inexperienced shoulder surgeons because the synovial tissue covering the articular side of the rotator cuff gives it a deceptively normal appearance. The underside of the

TABLE III

SHOULDER-RATING SCORE (IN POINTS) FOR ABNORMALITY OF THE ROTATOR CUFF
AND THE ACROMIOCLAVICULAR JOINT, ACCORDING TO NIRSCHL AND BUDOFF*

Pain
- None — 30
- Phase I: pain <48 hours *after* exercise — 25
- Phase II: pain >48 hours *after* exercise — 22
- Phase III: pain *with* exercise; no change in activity — 20
- Phase IV: pain *with* exercise causes change in activity — 12
- Phase V: pain *with* heavy activities of daily living (e.g., housework) — 9
- Phase VI: pain with light activities of daily living (e.g., grooming) — 6
- Phase VII: pain at rest — 3
- Phase VIII: pain disturbs sleep without pressure on shoulder — 0

Overall function
- Able to perform all normal functions as well as exercise activities — 25
- Able to perform normal activities of daily living; mild restrictions in exercise; able to work above shoulder level — 20
- Major restrictions in exercise; mild restrictions in activities of daily living — 15
- Moderate restrictions in activities of daily living; able to dress, groom, and drive — 10
- Major restrictions in activities of daily living but independent; limitations in ability to dress and drive — 5
- Dependent on others for activities of daily living — 0

Active motion with patient standing
Flexion
- Normal — 5
- >150 degrees — 4
- 121-150 degrees — 3
- 91-120 degrees — 2
- 45-90 degrees — 1
- <45 degrees or scapulothoracic motion only — 0
Abduction
- Normal — 5
- >150 degrees — 4
- 121-150 degrees — 3
- 91-120 degrees — 2
- 45-90 degrees — 1
- <45 degrees or scapulothoracic motion only — 0

Internal rotation
- Normal — 5
- Thumb cephalad to T12 — 4
- Thumb to T12-L3 — 3
- Thumb to L3-L5 — 2
- Thumb to buttock — 1
- Thumb distal to buttock — 0

Passive motion with patient supine
Flexion
- Normal — 3
- >150 degrees — 2
- 120-150 degrees — 1
- <120 degrees — 0
Abduction
- Normal — 3
- >150 degrees — 2
- 120-150 degrees — 1
- <120 degrees — 0
Total rotation (external and internal rotation) at 90 degrees of abduction
- Normal — 2
- ≤20-degree loss — 1
- >20-degree loss — 0
External rotation with upper extremity at side
- Within 10 degrees of normal or other side — 2
- 11-to-20-degree loss — 1
- >20-degree loss — 0

Strength
Abduction with upper extremity at 90 degrees
- Grade 5 — 10
- Grade 4 — 7
- Grade 3 — 4
- Grade 2 — 2
- Grade 1 or 0 — 0
External rotation with upper extremity at side (eccentric)
- Grade 5 — 10
- Grade 4 (minor-to-moderate loss of strength) — 5
- Grade 3 or less (major loss of strength) — 0

*The maximum total score is 100 points. A score of 90 to 100 points is considered excellent; 80 to 89 points, good; 70 to 79 points, fair; and 0 to 69 points, poor.

rotator cuff is therefore routinely tested with a motorized shaver. If the diagnosis is correct, a cuff that had a normal appearance will be found to be abnormal and to have a partial-thickness lesion. On the basis of our findings, we believe that most patients who are diagnosed as having an impingement syndrome have, instead, a partial-thickness intrasubstance tear of the rotator cuff or tendinosis.

The same anterior and posterior skin portals were used to enter the subacromial space, which was first explored with use of a blunt trocar to disrupt any adhesions and to feel the undersurface of the acromion and the lateral aspect of the clavicle for any inferior osteophytes.

A bursectomy was performed as needed to visualize the rotator cuff, especially at its insertion onto the greater tuberosity. The bursal side of the rotator cuff

was tested with a motorized shaver, and tendinotic changes were identified and debrided in the same manner as the intrasubstance changes on the articular side. Any thickened bursa or subacromial or subclavicular osteophytes contributing to stenosis of the coracoacromial arch were arthroscopically debrided with motorized instruments. No formal acromioplasties were performed, and the coracoacromial ligament was preserved in all shoulders.

Early in the study, one patient had an open bursectomy and débridement of osteophytes because technical difficulties were encountered during subacromial arthroscopy.

The two portals were routinely closed. Postoperative rehabilitation was begun as soon as tolerated, usually within two days. The patients progressed with active and active-assisted exercise as tolerated. All of the patients followed a postoperative program of active therapeutic exercise that was similar to the preoperative program.

Assessment of the Patients

The subjective result was rated satisfactory when the patient thought that the result was good or excellent and that he or she would have the same procedure performed again under similar circumstances. Otherwise, the rating was unsatisfactory.

Three objective scoring systems were used: the rating scale of the University of California at Los Angeles[16] (Table I), the functional rating score of Constant and Murley[13] (Table II), and a new rotator-cuff score designed by two of us (R. P. N. and J. E. B.) (Table III). Only the rating scale of the University of California at Los Angeles, which has a maximum possible score of 35 points, was used to determine the objective result. A score of 34 or 35 points was considered excellent; a score of 28 to 33 points, good; a score of 21 to 27 points, fair; and a score of 0 to 20 points, poor. A good or excellent result was considered objectively satisfactory, and a fair or poor result was considered a failure. Any patient who had a second procedure on the shoulder was considered to have had an objective failure of the index operation, regardless of the score.

Statistical Analysis

Statistical analysis was performed with the chi-square test of independence with the Yates correction. We analyzed the objective result with respect to the age of the patient, side of involvement, tendons involved, performance of exostectomy, duration of follow-up, and presence of a Workers' Compensation claim.

Results

Sixty-one (77 per cent) of the seventy-nine shoulders had a labral abnormality. Eleven shoulders had a SLAP-type lesion (a lesion of the superior portion of the labrum, anterior and posterior, or a bucket-handle tear of the labrum that necessitated excision of the loose fragment). Also, most of the shoulders had labral degeneration in addition to a partial-thickness tear, often in more than one location: fifty-four had degeneration of the anterosuperior portion of the labrum; twenty-five, of the posterosuperior portion; five, of the superior portion; two, of the mid-posterior portion; and two, of the anteroinferior portion.

Grade-I (softening of the cartilage) or grade-II (fibrillation) chondromalacia (excluding the normal spot of chondromalacia often found in the center of the glenoid) was noted in nineteen glenoids and seven humeral heads. Subacromial bursitis or thickening was noted in fifty-four shoulders (68 per cent). Seven shoulders (9 per cent) had degeneration of the coracoacromial ligament, and eleven (14 per cent) had thickening of the ligament.

The partial-thickness tear of the rotator cuff was on the articular surface in fifty-one shoulders, on the bursal surface in one, and on both surfaces in twenty-seven. Thirty-eight of the fifty-one tears of the articular surface were of the so-called critical area of the supraspinatus insertion, ten were of the supraspinatus and infraspinatus, two were of the infraspinatus alone, and one was of the supraspinatus and the subscapularis. The tear on the bursal surface was of the supraspinatus insertion. Sixteen of the twenty-seven tears that involved both surfaces were of the supraspinatus insertion alone, and eleven were of the supraspinatus and the infraspinatus. No significant association was detected, with the numbers available, between either the side of the partial-thickness tear ($p = 0.64$) or the tendon or tendons involved ($p = 0.75$) and the success or failure of the procedure.

In forty-six (58 per cent) of the seventy-nine shoulders, no osseous procedure was performed in the subacromial space. Acromial osteophytes were debrided in twenty shoulders (25 per cent), both acromial and clavicular osteophytes were debrided in twelve (15 per cent), and clavicular osteophytes were debrided in one. No significant association was detected between the performance of an exostectomy or its location and the success or failure of the procedure ($p = 0.40$).

All sixty-five patients who were involved in athletic activities had pain with these activities preoperatively, and twenty of these patients (31 per cent) continued to have such pain postoperatively. Preoperatively, sixty-five shoulders (82 per cent) overall had pain with activities of daily living, forty-five (57 per cent) had pain at rest, and fifty-two (66 per cent) had pain at night. Postoperatively, seven shoulders (9 per cent) had pain with activities of daily living, three (4 per cent) had pain at rest, and fifteen (19 per cent) had pain at night. The severity of the pain was almost always markedly diminished postoperatively.

The average time until the patients returned to usual activities of daily living was twenty-five days (range, one day to five months), the average time until they returned to full activities including sports was four months (range, two weeks to one year), and the average time to maximum improvement was eight months (range, two weeks to three years). Of the sixty-five patients who were involved in athletic activities preoperatively, fifty-two (80 per cent) were able to return to the same level of competition postoperatively. Most of these patients were recreational athletes, although some were engaged in competitive tennis.

Two shoulders had a decreased range of active and passive motion postoperatively. One was manipulated with the patient under anesthesia at seven months postoperatively, and the other was manipulated with the patient under anesthesia and was treated with an arthroscopic débridement of adhesive capsulitis at seven months postoperatively. At the most recent follow-up examination, both shoulders had excellent motion without sequelae. The result, according to the rating scale of the University of California at Los Angeles[16], was excellent for one shoulder and good for the other.

At the most recent follow-up evaluation, the result for sixty-nine (87 per cent) of the seventy-nine shoulders was considered satisfactory by the patient. With use of the rating scale of the University of California at Los Angeles[16], there were forty-three (54 per cent) excellent, twenty-five (32 per cent) good, six (8 per cent) fair, and five (6 per cent) poor results. According to the functional score of Constant and Murley[13], twenty-seven shoulders (34 per cent) had the maximum score of 100 points, thirty-one (39 per cent) had a score of 90 to 99 points, ten (13 per cent) had a score of 80 to 89 points, six (8 per cent) had a score of 70 to 79 points, three (4 per cent) had a score of 69 points or less, and two (3 per cent) did not have sufficient data to be rated with this system.

Forty-two shoulders were evaluated with the new rotator-cuff score developed by two of us (maximum score, 100 points), and the score was 90 to 100 points (excellent) for thirty-one, 80 to 89 points (good) for three, 70 to 79 points (fair) for four, and 69 points or less (poor) for four.

The success or failure of the arthroscopic débridement of the rotator cuff was found to be independent of the age of the patient (p = 0.85) and the duration of follow-up (p = 0.49), with the numbers available.

Eight patients had made a Workers' Compensation claim. According to the rating scale of the University of California at Los Angeles[16], the result of the procedure was excellent for three of them, good for two, fair for one, and poor for two. With these eight patients excluded from the analysis, sixty-four (90 per cent) of the remaining seventy-one shoulders had a result that was considered satisfactory by the patient and sixty-three shoulders (89 per cent) had a good or excellent result according to the rating scale of the University of California at Los Angeles.

One patient in the long-term follow-up group (followed for at least five years) had a second operation. The result after the second operation was good, according to the rating scale of the University of California at Los Angeles[16]. The first operation was considered an objective failure, even though the patient rated the result of both operations as excellent. Another patient had, after the index operation, an open débridement of the rotator cuff with an exostectomy of the greater tuberosity, and the result was considered excellent.

A full-thickness tear developed in two patients (both of whom had made a Workers' Compensation claim), and the procedure was considered a failure. The tear was repaired in one patient and debrided (because the tear was not retracted) in the other. Both of the subsequent operations were performed forty-two months after the initial procedure, thereby emphasizing the need for long-term follow-up. Of the other patients in whom the procedure was considered a failure, one had avascular necrosis of the humeral head without collapse, and arthroscopic débridement of the rotator cuff was performed because it was believed that the symptoms originated from the rotator cuff. This may have been a failure in diagnosis. One patient who had bilateral involvement may have had rheumatic disease. In addition to bilateral pain related to the rotator cuff, she had bilateral tennis elbow, bilateral generalized pain involving multiple joints in the hand, and an elevated erythrocyte sedimentation rate. Tests for rheumatoid factor and antinuclear antibodies were negative. The patient refused to see a rheumatologist. As no definitive diagnosis could be made, the result for both shoulders was considered a failure.

Discussion

The short-term (two to less than five-year) results of arthroscopic débridement of the rotator cuff in our series were as good as those reported after open or arthroscopic subacromial decompression; the overall rate of good and excellent results was 89 per cent, and the rate when the patients who had made a Workers' Compensation claim were excluded was 93 per cent. It should be noted that our short-term follow-up is still longer than the follow-up in most reported studies of arthroscopic subacromial decompression, except for those by Payne et al.[44] and Roye et al.[48], and is longer than the follow-up in most reported studies of open subacromial decompression, except for those by Hawkins et al.[29], Neviaser et al.[37], and Stuart et al.[54].

Our long-term follow-up (minimum, five years) is the longest of which we are aware in a study of the arthroscopic treatment of abnormalities of the rotator cuff. The long-term results of arthroscopic débridement of the rotator cuff in the present study (an 81 per cent rate of good and excellent results overall and an 83 per cent rate when the patients who had made a Workers' Compensation claim were excluded) are similar to the short-term results reported for open subacromial decompression; no comparable follow-up data on open débridement are available.

It is possible that the short-term results in our study were better than the long-term results for two reasons: first, our operative technique became more refined as we gained experience with the procedure and, second, the results may deteriorate with time.

Arthroscopic débridement of the rotator cuff is probably not as technically demanding as arthroscopic subacromial decompression. It is, however, more intellectually demanding in that the surgeon must be able to identify the abnormal areas of the rotator cuff accurately. Mere visualization of the undersurface of the cuff is not enough; the surgeon must routinely test the suspicious areas with a motorized shaver. We do this in all arthroscopic procedures on the shoulder. A motorized shaver with a five-millimeter meniscal blade will not damage healthy tissue on either the articular or the bursal side; however, tissue that appears superficially normal or areas where the abnormal tissue is covered by synovial tissue will be débrided away. Once healthy tissue is exposed, the shaver is no longer effective and the débridement is complete. The shaver will not create a full-thickness tear through healthy, functional tissue.

It is our belief that impingement syndrome in the absence of a full-thickness tear of the rotator cuff is most often secondary to a partial-thickness tear. That tear usually becomes apparent after the initial débridement but may be missed if the surgeon does not perform a meticulous dissection. We have found a sweeping motion of the shaver to be most effective for débridement of the rotator cuff. An angled shaver makes it easier to reach the more posterior infraspinatus insertion in the humeral head; internal rotation also makes this area accessible. If the more posterior structures need to be debrided, it may be necessary to reverse the portals (by placing the arthroscope anteriorly and the instrumentation posteriorly). We performed all arthroscopic débridements of the rotator cuff with the patient in the lateral decubitus position with ten to fifteen pounds (4.5 to 6.8 kilograms) of traction on the arm. Of technical note, we have found it extremely difficult to fully inspect and debride the posterior insertion of the cuff with the patient in the beach-chair position.

Glenohumeral Instability Associated with Abnormality of the Rotator Cuff

Glenohumeral instability, especially anterior instability, subjects the rotator cuff to increased eccentric tension loads, predisposing to overuse, injury, and dysfunction[38]. This overuse leads to weakness, which allows secondary impingement and subsequent development of symptoms. The difficulty with diagnosing instability when it is associated with disease of the rotator cuff is that the more dramatic signs and symptoms related to the cuff often obscure the subtle signs of instability[5]. Therefore, a high index of suspicion of glenohumeral instability must be maintained during examinations of patients who have symptoms related to the rotator cuff, especially young patients who are involved in activities such as swimming, throwing, racquet sports, and other athletic activities that require overhead use of the upper limb. The underlying instability may be subtle, and often careful physical and diagnostic arthroscopic examinations are required to make the diagnosis. These patients often need a glenohumeral stabilization procedure in order for treatment to be effective. Our results with arthroscopic débridement of the rotator cuff without glenohumeral stabilization for patients who have had symptoms related to the rotator cuff and underlying glenohumeral instability have been uniformly poor.

Many authors have commented on the high prevalence of posterosuperior labral fraying in combination with lesions on the articular side of the rotator cuff. Altchek and Carson[2] noted a 40 per cent prevalence in fifty throwing athletes who had pain in the anterior aspect of the shoulder that was refractory to non-operative treatment. These lesions are often attributed to internal impingement. As described by Davidson et al.[14], internal impingement occurs with the arm cocked in 90 degrees of abduction and full external rotation. In this position, the posterior portion of the supraspinatus can be pinched between the humeral head and the posterosuperior part of the glenoid rim[14]. It has been noted that the increased anterior humeral translation associated with anterior glenohumeral instability intensified internal impingement with the arm in a position of abduction and external rotation[14,31]. However, we have found superior labral fraying during most operations for partial-thickness tears on the articular side of the rotator cuff, regardless of whether or not the patient engaged in a sport that involved throwing. Most patients who have this combination of lesions do not participate in athletic activities that require overhead movement and do not often assume the position of abduction and external rotation; therefore, they are unlikely to be subjected to substantial internal impingement forces. A more plausible hypothesis is that, in most patients, the superior labral degeneration is due to the superior shear forces imparted by the relatively unopposed deltoid on the humeral head, not by impingement or impaction forces. Because of this force-couple imbalance, the humeral head is repetitively sheared across the superior portion of the labrum during active elevation of the arm. The superior labral degeneration caused by the subtle superior instability associated with a lesion of the rotator cuff is analogous to the anteroinferior fraying of the labrum seen in patients who have chronic anteroinferior glenohumeral instability.

Halbrecht[28] found that contact between the posterosuperior aspect of the glenoid and the rotator cuff may be physiological with the arm in maximum abduction and external rotation. Anterior glenohumeral instability would then appear to decrease internal impingement. In addition, most shoulders with both a tear on the articular side of the rotator cuff and posterior labral fraying are not lax or unstable. Davidson et al.[14] as well as Halbrecht reported that patients who had this combined abnormality without glenohumeral instability were managed successfully with arthroscopic débridement of the rotator cuff combined with débridement of the areas of labral degeneration and postoperative rehabilitation.

Interestingly, it has been our experience that, in the presence of dysfunction of the rotator cuff, the anterosuperior portion of the labrum degenerates more often than the posterosuperior portion does. The reason may be that the resultant instability caused by the dysfunction tends to be anterosuperior in direction[11,43]. In the present series, sixty-one (77 per cent) of seventy-nine shoulders had an abnormality of the labrum; fifty-four

(68 per cent) had anterosuperior labral degeneration, whereas only twenty-five (32 per cent) had posterosuperior labral degeneration. We refer to these lesions as supraspinatus labral instability patterns, or SLIP lesions[26]. Some shoulders had no labral lesions.

Before the present study, we observed SLIP lesions in 90 per cent of patients who had a partial-thickness tear of the rotator cuff; 66 per cent of the lesions occurred anterosuperiorly, and only 11 per cent occurred posterosuperiorly[26].

Evaluation of Patients

It is unfortunate that our geographical location is characterized by a transient population, as this made it difficult for us to personally examine some of our patients for the follow-up data. However, while a personal examination is obviously more desirable, we do not believe that our inability to perform one for some of our patients affected our results. Patients convey their sense of satisfaction, or lack thereof, as well over the telephone as they do in person.

The rating scale of the University of California at Los Angeles[16], which was used as a more objective indicator of success in our study as well as in several others[16,18,48,49,52,53,57], contains five items (Table I). The information on patient satisfaction is purely subjective, and the data on pain and function are gathered from the patient's history. Active flexion is rated on a scale of 5 points, but the maximum score is given as long as the patient can actively flex more than 150 degrees. (This is also the case with the functional score of Constant and Murley[13].) In other words, a lack of less than 30 degrees of flexion is allowed before the score is affected. We believe that a lack of 30 degrees produces a substantial functional deficit. Strength of flexion is also rated on a scale of 5 points. When the grade was determined on the basis of a telephone interview, any suspected weakness was given a grade of 4 points and major weakness was given a grade of 3 points. No patient who was interviewed or examined was unable to raise the arm against gravity (which would indicate a grade of 0, 1, or 2 points).

The cutoff for a successful result, according to the rating scale of the University of California at Los Angeles[16], is 28 points; a score of 27 points or less is considered a failure. No patient who had a score of 28 points had a score of 5 points for strength; thus, it was not possible that, because of a subtle undiagnosed weakness, a patient who was thought to have a successful result on the basis of a telephone interview actually had a failure. All patients who had a borderline successful score denied that they had extreme or substantial weakness. It is unlikely that a patient would not notice or admit to a strength deficit that would warrant a score of 3 points (indicating the ability to raise the arm against gravity but not against resistance). Therefore, we are confident that the nature of the result (satisfactory or unsatisfactory) was determined accurately for the pa-

tients who were interviewed by telephone with use of the scale of the University of California at Los Angeles.

Despite our confidence in the rating scale of the University of California at Los Angeles[16] for the present study, we have noted certain deficiencies. As such, we developed an assessment scale that is specific to the rotator cuff (Table III). We plan to use this scale for future outcome studies of patients who have rotator cuff disease.

Return to Activities of Daily Living

The average time until patients have returned to activity after arthroscopic subacromial decompression has varied. Roye et al.[48] reported a return to activities of daily living within two weeks, whereas Speer et al.[53] noted that the average was three months (range, three weeks to seven months). Altchek et al.[3] reported an average of four months until full recovery. Snyder et al.[52], in a study involving thirteen shoulders treated with arthroscopic débridement of the rotator cuff and eighteen treated with arthroscopic débridement and with arthroscopic subacromial decompression, reported an average time to maximum improvement of six months; the time did not differ between the patients who had a decompression and those who did not.

The patients in the present study returned to activities of daily living in an average of twenty-five days. This seems long to us, as patients who have been managed more recently have appeared to progress more rapidly because of improved operative technique. An example of an activity of daily living examined in the present study was shampooing of the hair. This task requires moderate power of the arm in full abduction and external rotation, and the ability to perform it probably takes longer to return than the ability to perform other activities. The time to return to full activity (four months) after the arthroscopic débridement of the rotator cuff may sometimes have been due to overly intensive postoperative physical therapy; the weakened cuff may have been subjected to too much activity too soon. When asked about their postoperative course, many patients stated that they felt better immediately but then had a great deal of pain and aching during and after physical therapy. Many stated that they finally became symptom-free when they abandoned our intensive postoperative exercise program. This may be an appropriate subject for future research. The average time to maximum improvement was eight months. Patients should be warned about the duration of the recovery period; this applies especially to athletes, who will most likely be unable to play for a season.

It should also be noted that there is currently no evidence that débridement for tendinosis of the rotator cuff actually stimulates a healing response. We have had the opportunity to perform second-look arthroscopy on three of the shoulders in which the procedure had failed. We did not find any signs of healing of the rotator cuff.

We have not had the opportunity to perform a repeat arthroscopy on any of the shoulders for which the procedure was a success. It is possible that débridement of the abnormal tissue may merely remove the primary abnormality, a situation that is analogous to débridement of pathological or ischemic tissue in other areas of the body, thereby allowing functional recovery when there is appropriate rest and rehabilitation.

Overview

Débridement of the rotator cuff without subacromial decompression is an effective long-term treatment for partial-thickness tendinosis or tears of the rotator cuff. The success of this treatment as well as the present review of the pertinent literature supports the concept that primary failure of the rotator cuff most likely occurs by eccentric tension overload rather than by compression overload by impingement from aberrant acromial morphology. The procedure of débridement of the cuff without acromioplasty has the clear advantage of addressing identifiable pathoanatomy of the cuff while avoiding iatrogenic harm to the coracoacromial arch, including the likely destabilization of the glenohumeral joint secondary to disruption of the important stabilizing effect of the acromion and the coracoacromial ligament.

NOTE: The authors thank Stephen J. Brannen, Ph.D., for help with the statistical analysis.

References

1. **Adolfsson, L.,** and **Lysholm, J.:** Results of arthroscopic acromioplasty related to rotator cuff lesions. *Internat. Orthop.,* 17: 228-231, 1993.
2. **Altchek, D. W.,** and **Carson, E. W.:** Arthroscopic acromioplasty. Current status. *Orthop. Clin. North America,* 28: 157-168, 1997.
3. **Altchek, D. W.; Warren, R. F.; Wickiewicz, T. L.; Skyhar, M. J.; Ortiz, G.;** and **Schwartz, E.:** Arthroscopic acromioplasty. Technique and results. *J. Bone and Joint Surg.,* 72-A: 1198-1207, Sept. 1990.
4. **Andrews, J. R.; Broussard, T. S.;** and **Carson, W. G.:** Arthroscopy of the shoulder in the management of partial tears of the rotator cuff: a preliminary report. *Arthroscopy,* 1: 117-122, 1985.
5. **Beach, W. R.,** and **Caspari, R. B.:** Arthroscopic management of rotator cuff disease. *Orthopedics,* 16: 1007-1015, 1993.
6. **Bigliani, L. U.; Morrison, D. S.;** and **April, E. W.:** The morphology of the acromion and its relationship to rotator cuff tears. *Orthop. Trans.,* 10: 216, 1986.
7. **Bigliani, L. U.; D'Alessandro, D. F.; Duralde, X. A.;** and **McIlveen, S. J.:** Anterior acromioplasty for subacromial impingement in patients younger than 40 years of age. *Clin. Orthop.,* 246: 111-116, 1989.
8. **Burkhart, S. S.:** Arthroscopic debridement and decompression for selected rotator cuff tears. Clinical results, pathomechanics, and patient selection based on biomechanical parameters. *Orthop. Clin. North America,* 24: 111-123, 1993.
9. **Burkhart, S. S.:** Congenital subacromial stenosis. *Arthroscopy,* 11: 63-68, 1995.
10. **Burkhead, W. Z., Jr.; Burkhart, S. S.; Gerber, C.; Harryman, D. T., II; Morrison, D. S.; Uhthoff, H. K.;** and **Williams, G. R., Jr.:** Symposium: the rotator cuff: debridement versus repair — part I. *Contemp. Orthop.,* 31: 262-271, 1995.
11. **Burkhead, W. Z., Jr.; Burkhart, S. S.; Gerber, C.; Harryman, D. T., II; Morrison, D. S.; Uhthoff, H. K.;** and **Williams, G. R., Jr.:** Symposium: the rotator cuff: debridement versus repair — part II. *Contemp. Orthop.,* 31: 313-326, 1995.
12. **Codman, E. A.:** *The Shoulder. Rupture of the Supraspinatus Tendon and Other Lesions in or about the Subacromial Bursa,* pp. 65-177. Boston, privately printed, 1934.
13. **Constant, C. R.,** and **Murley, A. H.:** A clinical method of functional assessment of the shoulder. *Clin. Orthop.,* 214: 160-164, 1987.
14. **Davidson, P. A.; Elattrache, N. S.; Jobe, C. M.;** and **Jobe, F. W.:** Rotator cuff and posterior-superior glenoid labrum injury associated with increased glenohumeral motion: a new site of impingement. *J. Shoulder and Elbow Surg.,* 4: 384-390, 1995.
15. **Deutsch, A.; Altchek, D. W.; Schwartz, E.; Otis, J. C.;** and **Warren, R. F.:** Radiologic measurement of superior displacement of the humeral head in the impingement syndrome. *J. Shoulder and Elbow Surg.,* 5: 186-193, 1996.
16. **Ellman, H.:** Arthroscopic subacromial decompression: analysis of one- to three-year results. *Arthroscopy,* 3: 173-181, 1987.
17. **Ellman, H.:** Diagnosis and treatment of incomplete rotator cuff tears. *Clin. Orthop.,* 254: 64-74, 1990.
18. **Esch, J. C.; Ozerkis, L. R.; Helgager, J. A.; Kane, N.;** and **Lilliott, N.:** Arthroscopic subacromial decompression: results according to the degree of rotator cuff tear. *Arthroscopy,* 4: 241-249, 1988.
19. **Fu, F. H.; Harner, C. D.;** and **Klein, A. H.:** Shoulder impingement syndrome. A critical review. *Clin. Orthop.,* 269: 162-173, 1991.
20. **Fukuda, H.; Craig, E. V.;** and **Yamanaka, K.:** Surgical treatment of incomplete thickness tears of rotator cuff: long-term follow-up. *Orthop. Trans.,* 11: 237-238, 1987.
21. **Gartsman, G. M.:** Arthroscopic subacromial decompression for stage II impingement: the first 100 consecutive cases. *Orthop. Trans.,* 12: 673, 1988.
22. **Gartsman, G. M.:** Arthroscopic acromioplasty for lesions of the rotator cuff. *J. Bone and Joint Surg.,* 72-A: 169-180, Feb. 1990.
23. **Gartsman, G. M.:** Arthroscopic treatment of rotator cuff disease. *J. Shoulder and Elbow Surg.,* 4: 228-241, 1995.
24. **Gartsman, G. M.,** and **Milne, J. C.:** Articular surface partial-thickness rotator cuff tears. *J. Shoulder and Elbow Surg.,* 4: 409-415, 1995.
25. **Goldie, I.:** Epicondylitis lateralis humeri (epicondylalgia or tennis elbow). A pathogenetical study. *Acta Chir. Scandinavica,* Supplementum 339, pp. 77-113, 1964.
26. **Guidi, E. J.; Olivierre, C. O.; Nirschl, R. P.;** and **Pettrone, F. A.:** Supraspinatus labrum instability pattern (SLIP) lesions of the shoulder. *Orthop. Trans.,* 18: 750, 1994.
27. **Ha'eri, G. B.,** and **Wiley, A. M.:** Shoulder impingement syndrome. Results of operative release. *Clin. Orthop.,* 168: 128-132, 1982.
28. **Halbrecht, J. L.:** Internal impingement of the shoulder. Read at the Annual Meeting of the Arthroscopy Association of North America, San Francisco, California, Feb. 16, 1997.
29. **Hawkins, R. J.; Brock, R. M.; Abrams, J. S.;** and **Hobeika, P.:** Acromioplasty for impingement with an intact rotator cuff. *J. Bone and Joint Surg.,* 70-B(5): 795-797, 1988.
30. **Hawkins, R. J.; Saddemi, S. R.; Moor, J. T.;** and **Hawkins, A.:** Arthroscopic subacromial decompression: a 2-year follow-up study [abstract]. *Arthroscopy,* 8: 409, 1992.
31. **Jobe, C. M.:** Superior glenoid impingement. Current concepts. *Clin. Orthop.,* 330: 98-107, 1996.

32. **Johansson, J. E.,** and **Barrington, T. W.:** Coracoacromial ligament division. *Am. J. Sports Med.,* 12: 138-141, 1984.
33. **Lazarus, M. D.; Chansky, H. A.; Misra, S.; Williams, G. R.;** and **Iannotti, J. P.:** Comparison of open and arthroscopic subacromial decompression. *J. Shoulder and Elbow Surg.,* 3: 1-11, 1994.
34. **Loehr, J. F.,** and **Uhthoff, H. K.:** The pathogenesis of degenerative rotator cuff tears. *Orthop. Trans.,* 11: 237, 1987.
35. **Lohr, J. F.,** and **Uhthoff, H. K.:** The microvascular pattern of the supraspinatus tendon. *Clin. Orthop.,* 254: 35-38, 1990.
36. **Neer, C. S., II:** Anterior acromioplasty for the chronic impingement syndrome in the shoulder. A preliminary report. *J. Bone and Joint Surg.,* 54-A: 41-50, Jan. 1972.
37. **Neviaser, T. J.; Neviaser, R. J.; Neviaser, J. S.;** and **Neviaser, J. S.:** The four-in-one arthroplasty for the painful arc syndrome. *Clin. Orthop.,* 163: 107-112, 1982.
38. **Nirschl, R. P.:** Shoulder tendonitis. In *American Academy of Orthopaedic Surgeons. Symposium on Upper Extremity Injuries in Athletes,* pp. 322-337. Edited by F. A. Pettrone. St. Louis, C. V. Mosby, 1986.
39. **Nirschl, R. P.:** Rotator cuff tendinitis: basic concepts of pathoetiology. In *Instructional Course Lectures, American Academy of Orthopaedic Surgeons.* Vol. 38, pp. 439-445. Rosemont, Illinois, American Academy of Orthopaedic Surgeons, 1989.
40. **Nirschl, R. P.:** Rotator cuff surgery. In *Instructional Course Lectures, American Academy of Orthopaedic Surgeons.* Vol. 38, pp. 447-462. Rosemont, Illinois, American Academy of Orthopaedic Surgeons, 1989.
41. **Ogilvie-Harris, D. J.,** and **Wiley, A. M.:** Arthroscopic surgery of the shoulder. A general appraisal. *J. Bone and Joint Surg.,* 68-B(2): 201-207, 1986.
42. **Ozaki, J.; Fujimoto, S.; Nakagawa, Y.; Masuhara, K.;** and **Tamai, S.:** Tears of the rotator cuff of the shoulder associated with pathological changes in the acromion. A study in cadavera. *J. Bone and Joint Surg.,* 70-A: 1224-1230, Sept. 1988.
43. **Paulos, L. E.,** and **Franklin, J. L.:** Arthroscopic shoulder decompression. Development and application. A five year experience. *Am. J. Sports Med.,* 18: 235-244, 1990.
44. **Payne, L. Z.; Altchek, D. W.; Craig, E. V.;** and **Warren, R. F.:** Arthroscopic treatment of partial rotator cuff tears in young athletes. A preliminary report. *Am. J. Sports Med.,* 25: 299-305, 1997.
45. **Penny, J. N.,** and **Welsh, R. P.:** Shoulder impingement syndromes in athletes and their surgical management. *Am. J. Sports Med.,* 9: 11-15, 1981.
46. **Post, M.,** and **Cohen, J.:** Impingement syndrome. A review of late stage II and early stage III lesions. *Clin. Orthop.,* 207: 126-132, 1986.
47. **Rothman, R. H.,** and **Parke, W. W.:** The vascular anatomy of the rotator cuff. *Clin. Orthop.,* 41: 176-186, 1965.
48. **Roye, R. P.; Grana, W. A.;** and **Yates, C. K.:** Arthroscopic subacromial decompression: two- to seven-year follow-up. *Arthroscopy,* 11: 301-306, 1995.
49. **Ryu, R. K.:** Arthroscopic subacromial decompression: a clinical review. *Arthroscopy,* 8: 141-147, 1992.
50. **Sampson, T. G.; Nisbet, J. K.;** and **Glick, J. M.:** Precision acromioplasty in arthroscopic subacromial decompression of the shoulder. *Arthroscopy,* 7: 301-307, 1991.
51. **Siekanowicz, A. J.,** and **Nirschl, R. P.:** Open repair of full thickness rotator cuff tears with preservation of the acromion and coracoacromial ligament. *Orthop. Trans.,* 20: 401, 1996.
52. **Snyder, S. J.; Pachelli, A. F.; Del Pizzo, W.; Friedman, M. J.; Ferkel, R. D.;** and **Pattee, G.:** Partial thickness rotator cuff tears: results of arthroscopic treatment. *Arthroscopy,* 7: 1-7, 1991.
53. **Speer, K. P.; Lohnes, J.;** and **Garrett, W. E., Jr.:** Arthroscopic subacromial decompression: results in advanced impingement syndrome. *Arthroscopy,* 7: 291-296, 1991.
54. **Stuart, M. J.; Azevedo, A. J.;** and **Cofield, R. H.:** Anterior acromioplasty for treatment of the shoulder impingement syndrome. *Clin. Orthop.,* 260: 195-200, 1990.
55. **Thorling, J.; Bjerneld, H.; Hallin, G.; Hovelius, L.;** and **Hagg, O.:** Acromioplasty for impingement syndrome. *Acta Orthop. Scandinavica,* 56: 147-148, 1985.
56. **Uhthoff, H. K.; Hammond, D. I.; Sarkar, K.; Hooper, G. J.;** and **Papoff, W. J.:** The role of the coracoacromial ligament in the impingement syndrome — a clinical, radiological and histological study. *Internat. Orthop.,* 12: 97-104, 1988.
57. **Van Holsbeeck, E.; DeRycke, J.; Declercq, G.; Martens, M.; Verstreken, J.;** and **Fabry, G.:** Subacromial impingement: open versus arthroscopic decompression. *Arthroscopy,* 8: 173-178, 1992.
58. **Warner, J. J.; Kann, S.;** and **Maddox, L. M.:** The "arthroscopic impingement test." *Arthroscopy,* 10: 224-230, 1994.

Arthroscopic Management of Rotator Cuff Disease

Gary M. Gartsman, MD

Abstract

Rotator cuff disease (stage 2 impingement, partial-thickness tears, complete cuff tears, and irreparable tears) is as yet only partially understood, and the role of arthroscopy in its management is still under debate. Stage 2 impingement can be managed satisfactorily with arthroscopic techniques. Arthroscopy allows a complete inspection of the glenohumeral joint, enabling the surgeon to diagnose and treat coexisting intra-articular lesions. A thorough bursectomy, coraco-acromial ligament resection, and acromioplasty can be performed without the need for deltoid detachment. Arthroscopic technique appears to offer advantages over open technique in the management of partial-thickness tears by allowing accurate inspection of the articular surface of the rotator cuff. The depth and size of the tear can be determined precisely, allowing an appropriate selection of debridement, decompression, and/or tendon repair. The management of complete tears is currently under investigation, with some advocating complete arthroscopic repair and some preferring arthroscopic acromioplasty and "mini-open" repair; there are merits to both approaches. The arthroscopic management of irreparable tears appears to offer the advantages of an open decompression with decreased morbidity. However, the surgeon's ability to accurately determine reparability may be less precise with arthroscopy.

J Am Acad Orthop Surg 1998;6:259-266

This article summarizes the present state of knowledge on arthroscopic surgical management of rotator cuff disease. Four distinct stages of rotator cuff disease are reviewed: stage 2 disease (subacromial impingement syndrome), partial rotator cuff tears, complete tears, and irreparable tears.

Literature Review

A number of reports in the orthopaedic surgery literature have described the arthroscopic management of stage 2 rotator cuff disease. Several authors have reported 70% to 90% success rates with arthroscopic acromioplasty.[1-4] All stress that arthroscopic surgery is suc-cessful when impingement is due to extrinsic compression on the tendon by the structures of the coraco-acromial arch but is not successful when the "impingement" is due to glenohumeral subluxation.

Other studies have compared the open and arthroscopic techniques. Lazarus et al[5] found that while the open technique produced a slightly higher success rate, the return to function was superior with arthroscopic treatment. Norlin[6] found that the arthroscopic technique produced better results and a more rapid return of function. Van Holsbeeck et al[7] reported marginally better results with the open technique but advised arthroscopic decompression for patient convenience and satisfaction.

Three options are available for the treatment of partial-cuff tears: (1) debridement of the partial-thickness tear alone, (2) debridement of the tear with arthroscopic decompression, and (3) open or arthroscopic repair of the partial-thickness tear combined with subacromial decompression. Andrews et al[8] reported 85% good or excellent results in a group of throwing athletes (average age, 22) treated with arthroscopic debridement alone without decompression. Snyder et al[9] found 47 partial tears in a group of 600 patients and advocated debridement without decompression if the tear was confined to the articular surface. Arthroscopic subacromial decompression was added if the tear was present on both the articular and the bursal surfaces. Esch et al[10] reported 85% good or excellent

Dr. Gartsman is Clinical Associate Professor, Department of Orthopaedics, University of Texas Medical School, Houston, and is in private practice with Fondren Orthopedic Group, Texas Orthopedic Hospital, Houston.

Reprint requests: Dr. Gartsman, Fondren Orthopedic Group, Texas Orthopedic Hospital, 7401 South Main Street, Houston, TX 77030.

The author or the departments with which he is affiliated have received something of value from a commercial or other party related directly or indirectly to the subject of this article.

results in 34 patients treated with arthroscopic subacromial decompression. Gartsman[3] reported good results in 80% of 40 patients with an average age of 40; decompression was performed in all cases.

There are also three options for the treatment of complete rotator cuff tears: (1) arthroscopic decompression without cuff repair, (2) arthroscopic decompression with "mini-open" repair, and (3) arthroscopic repair. A number of studies have reported on the use of arthroscopic decompression without cuff repair. Esch et al[10] reported satisfactory results in 20 of 26 (77%) patients treated with arthroscopic subacromial decompression without cuff repair. The results were excellent in all 4 patients in whom the tear was smaller than 1 cm. Levy et al[11] reported 84% excellent or good results in 25 patients. Ellman[2] reported good results in 9 of 10 patients with tears measuring 2 cm or less, but only 3 of 6 patients had good results if the tear was 2 to 4 cm. Gartsman[3] reported satisfactory results in 10 of 20 patients. In a comparison study of open repair versus arthroscopic treatment, Montgomery et al[12] found 78% good results in 50 patients treated with open repair but only 39% satisfactory results in 38 patients treated with arthroscopic decompression without repair. Burkhart et al[13] reported 90% good or excellent results in 72 patients, with follow-up ranging from 6 to 72 months. In that study, patients with good external rotation strength and good subscapularis strength had been carefully selected for arthroscopic treatment alone.

Levy et al[14] described 80% excellent or good results with arthroscopic decompression followed by a mini-open repair. Liu and Baker[15] reported 84% good or excellent results in 44 patients with an average 4.2-year follow-up. Paulos and Kody[16] reported 89% good or excellent results in 18 patients treated with a similar technique.

Another possible approach for the patient with a complete tear is arthroscopic repair. This technique is the most recent and necessarily the one with the least documentation in the literature. Snyder and Bachner[17] recently reported on a preliminary series of 47 patients. Forty-one patients (83%) had excellent or good results. Gartsman et al[18] reported that 66 of their 73 patients (90%) had excellent or good results with a minimum 2-year follow-up.

Little has been written about the treatment of patients with irreparable tears. Ellman and Gartsman[19] have achieved good pain relief with arthroscopic treatment in a limited number of patients, with reasonable pain relief documented in most patients followed up for as long as 5 years. They emphasize that thorough debridement and synovectomy accompanied by removal of any downward-protruding acromial or acromioclavicular joint spurs is necessary. Burkhart et al[13] reported that 25 patients with massive irreparable tears had 88% good or excellent results after arthroscopic repair; those results have not deteriorated with the passage of time.

Indications

The indications for arthroscopic treatment and open surgery are identical. These include pain or weakness that interferes with work, sports, or activities of daily living and that is unresponsive to an appropriate nonoperative treatment. The usual nonoperative regimen consists of a number of elements, including oral anti-inflammatory medication, cortisone injections into the subacromial space (two or three spaced 2 months apart), activity modification, selective rest, and a rehabilitation program. That program is designed to restore or maintain movement and to improve strength in the deltoid, the scapular stabilizers, and the rotator cuff. The recommended duration for this nonoperative approach varies in different publications, but it seems reasonable to consider surgery if the patient's pain continues for a period of 12 months or is increasing in severity after 6 months.

Diagnosis

The classic history of stage 2 impingement is one of shoulder pain with activities that place the shoulder in the painful arc of 70 to 100 degrees of elevation or abduction. The pain is localized to the subacromial region and radiates to the area of the deltoid insertion and often anteriorly into the biceps. Night pain is regularly noted. The role of trauma is variable; some patients present with symptoms after a major injury, but in the majority the pain occurs after repetitive activities without trauma or antecedent injury.

Physical examination demonstrates a full or nearly normal range of passive motion. Localized tenderness in the area of the supraspinatus insertion is infrequent. Acromioclavicular joint tenderness should alert the examiner that this joint may be the primary source of pathology. Acromioclavicular joint arthritis may mimic stage 2 impingement or may exist in addition to the primary impingement process.

The physician should carefully examine younger patients (less than 40 years old) for the presence of glenohumeral instability. In these patients, subacromial pain may be the result of traction tendinitis rather than true stage 2 impingement.

Three impingement signs consistent with stage 2 impingement have been described. The primary sign involves the examiner placing the shoulder in maximum elevation.[20] With the secondary sign, the shoulder is elevated 80 degrees and then maximally internally rotated.[21] The tertiary sign is subacromial pain with the shoulder in 90 degrees of abduction. The signs are recorded as positive when subacromial pain is produced. The location of the pain during these maneuvers should be carefully noted. A patient with soft-tissue pain from rhomboid-trapezius spasm may have increased pain when each of these maneuvers is performed, but the pain will not be localized to the subacromial region.

After the physical examination, an impingement test may be performed. The test consists of the subacromial injection of a local anesthetic into the subacromial space and repetition of the maneuvers that produced the impingement signs. If the pain is eliminated or substantially reduced, the test is recorded as positive. The physician must remain aware that a positive test only confirms that the structures producing pain lie within the subacromial space and is not, in and of itself, diagnostic of impingement syndrome.

Glenohumeral instability may result in secondary traction tendinitis and a positive impingement test. Successful surgical management does not involve shoulder decompression, but rather the treatment of the underlying glenohumeral instability. The diagnosis of impingement syndrome is clinical, and arthroscopy does not routinely play a role.

A number of conditions that mimic the clinical presentation of impingement are best diagnosed with arthroscopic techniques.

Glenohumeral instability, articular-surface partial rotator cuff tears, labrum tears, small areas of degenerative arthritis, posterior glenoid-cuff impingement, and lesions of the rotator interval are examples. Other conditions that may mimic stage 2 impingement syndrome but that cannot be diagnosed with arthroscopic technique include acromioclavicular joint arthritis, cervical spine disease, and suprascapular neuropathy.

Arthroscopy is particularly valuable in the diagnosis and management of partial-thickness tears of the rotator cuff (Fig. 1). The vast majority of partial-thickness tears are on the articular surface[22] and are not visible during inspection of the bursal surface of the cuff, such as occurs during an open procedure. It would seem, therefore, that the incidence of partial tears has been underestimated in the literature dealing with open surgery.

Techniques proposed to deal with this issue during open procedures include saline injection, methylene blue injection, and division of the tendon and visual inspection. The techniques that involve injection of fluid into the glenohumeral joint depend on the surgeon's ability to appreciate fluid egress from the cuff (saline injection) or staining of the cuff tissues with blue dye (methylene blue injection). These events signal a partial tear and should prompt the surgeon to split the cuff longitudinally to find the defect. Some surgeons will incise the rotator cuff longitudinally if no defect is found but a tear is suspected on the basis of the clinical or radiologic evaluation. However, exposure is limited, and the articular surface of the cuff is not well visualized. Inspection of the articular surface is better performed with arthroscopic technique, as the entire cuff can be easily inspected and the location, size, and depth of the tear can be appreciated. The tear can be marked with a suture, so that the precise area can be found on subacromial inspection and repair.

For patients with complete tears, the findings from the clinical examination are most commonly compared with those from radiologic studies (arthrography or magnetic resonance [MR] imaging [Fig. 2]) to make the diagnosis. The arthroscope can be used as well to diagnose the presence and size of a complete rotator cuff tear[23] (Fig. 3), although no authors have suggested that this be used routinely. The arthroscope is most useful in diag-

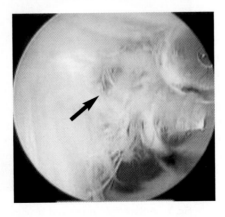 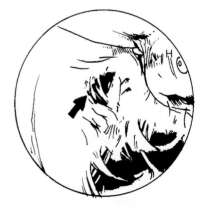

Fig. 1 Arthroscopic image and accompanying line drawing of a partial-thickness rotator cuff tear (arrow) viewed from the articular surface (glenohumeral joint). H = humeral head.

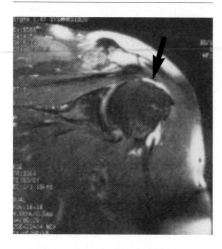

Fig. 2 Coronal T2-weighted spin-echo MR image demonstrating a full-thickness rotator cuff tear (arrow).

before an arthroscopic subacromial decompression to examine for any unsuspected lesion or to determine the status of the intra-articular structures. This clearly is an advantage to the arthroscopic approach. The knowledge gained may alter the postoperative management and may serve to explain why some patients do better than others. "Impingement syndrome" is a clinical diagnosis and is therefore somewhat imprecise. The increased knowledge gained by arthroscopic joint examination will likely serve to further subdivide and clarify this syndrome and allow more effective treatment.

The subacromial findings in stage 2 impingement are variable. The space may be clear, or a dense fibrous reaction may exist. The dense fibrous tissue is reactive bursitis. Impingement syndrome may exist even in the presence of a clear, well-defined subacromial space. In some individuals, the contact between the rotator cuff and the acromion produces pain but does not incite an inflammatory bursitis reaction. Tendon erosion, fraying, or partial-thickness tears may be found on the superior or bursal surface of the cuff.

Erosions on the acromial undersurface near the anterior edge are frequently noted, as are small areas of inflammation. Interestingly, the literature does not document consistent abnormalities of the coracoacromial ligament. While these findings are suggestive of subacromial impingement, they are not necessarily diagnostic.

nosing complete tears in patients who have false-negative imaging studies. False-negative results occur most frequently with arthrography, particularly if the synovial lining remains intact, or with MR imaging if the tear is smaller than 1 cm.

It is difficult for surgeons to determine whether a large, retracted rotator cuff tear is reparable. This is as true for arthroscopic technique as it is for conventional open technique. If the tendon is mobile and can be advanced to its anatomic location, the tear is reparable. However, if the tendon does not meet these criteria, it is not necessarily irreparable. Subacromial, subdeltoid, and intra-articular adhesions may limit cuff excursion. The ability to release these adhesions and determine definitively whether the tear can be repaired is, for most surgeons, better in an open procedure than in an arthroscopic setting.

Findings

Most authors include an examination of the glenohumeral joint

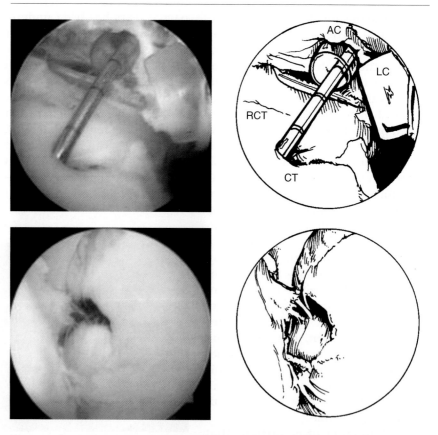

Fig. 3 Arthroscopic images and accompanying line drawings of full-thickness rotator cuff tears viewed from the subacromial space **(top)** and from the glenohumeral joint **(bottom)**. AC = anterior capsule; CT = cuff tear; LC = lateral cannula; RCT = rotator cuff tendon.

The diagnosis of subacromial impingement is made clinically on the basis of the history and the findings from the physical examination, impingement testing, and imaging studies.

The clinical findings in patients with partial tears are related both to delineation of the tear and to the characteristics of other areas of the joint. Most tears are located on the articular surface; approximately 75% are in the supraspinatus, 20% in the infraspinatus, and 5% in the teres minor.[19] The depth or severity is grade 1 (less than one fourth of the tendon thickness) in 45% of cases, grade 2 (less than one half of tendon thickness) in 40%, and grade 3 (more than one half of tendon thickness) in 15%.[19] The finding of chondral defects in the humeral head or glenoid, labrum tears, or separations is suggestive of glenohumeral instability and should prompt the surgeon to consider whether the partial rotator cuff tear is coexistent with other clinical diagnoses.

The intra-articular lesions in patients with complete tears found during open rotator cuff repair are poorly documented, precluding adequate comparison with the arthroscopic findings. Most arthroscopic studies report abnormalities that may include areas of synovitis, partial biceps-tendon tears, arthritic changes in the humeral head or glenoid, labrum tears, and loose bodies.[24] More complete documentation of glenohumeral findings may promote better understanding of the postoperative performance of patients and further delineate the category "rotator cuff tear." It is uncertain whether these changes are brought about by the cuff tear or merely accompany the cuff tear and occur as a natural consequence of aging.

As irreparable tears generally occur in older patients, the arthroscopic findings include arthritic changes, synovitis, and biceps tendon tears. Not surprisingly, these findings occur with a higher frequency than is noted in patients with partial or complete rotator cuff tears.

Treatment

Arthroscopic treatment of stage 2 impingement involves examination under anesthesia to document range of motion and instability, followed by an inspection of the glenohumeral joint and treatment, if indicated, of any coexisting intra-articular lesions. Subacromial treatment includes excision of the pathologic bursa to (1) inspect the surface of the tendons, (2) remove the space-occupying lesion, and (3) remove an inflamed, pain-producing structure. In most cases, treatment of the coracoacromial ligament involves resection from the lateral border to the medial acromial border. Some surgeons prefer to divide, rather than resect, the ligament.

An inferior acromioplasty is performed, with the goal being to convert the acromion to a flat (type 1) structure (Fig. 4). This may be accomplished with a power burr placed in either the lateral or the posterior portal, depending on the surgeon's preference. Anterior acromial recession is more controversial. This step involves removing the anterior acromial osteophyte or protuberance (i.e., all of the anterior acromion that projects anterior to the anterior border of the acromioclavicular joint). This part of the procedure is performed by some but not by others.

The acromioclavicular joint contributes to the impingement syndrome by two mechanisms: formation of inferior acromioclavicular joint osteophytes and acromioclavicular joint arthritis. Inferior osteophytes may project downward into the rotator cuff tendons and cause or exacerbate impingement.

Determination of the presence of these osteophytes is made radiologically on plain films or an MR imaging study. The osteophytes can be removed arthroscopically.

Acromioclavicular joint arthritis may also coexist with subacromial impingement. If the patient is symptomatic from acromioclavicular joint arthritis as determined on the preoperative clinical examination, acromioclavicular joint resection is performed. Acromioclavicular resection may be performed through the subacromial approach, although some surgeons prefer a direct approach into the acromioclavicular joint itself.

Three factors must be considered in the arthroscopic management of partial-thickness rotator cuff tears: (1) size and depth of the tear, (2) patient activity level, and (3) bone structure. No one factor

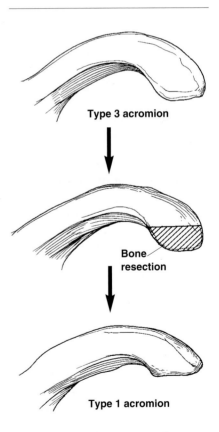

Fig. 4 Steps in inferior acromioplasty.

solely determines treatment; it is the clinician's ability to analyze the effects of all the factors involved that leads to appropriate management.

The most critical determination that must be made is whether the tear can be treated by arthroscopic decompression alone or whether the decompression must be accompanied by tendon repair. There is no general agreement on how the area of the tear should influence the surgeon. There is some agreement on the role of tendon depth, with most authors recommending repair if 50% or more of the tendon substance is involved. Sedentary patients with partial tears are more likely to do well with decompression alone; active patients are more likely to benefit from tendon repair. Patients with structural bone abnormalities (e.g., hooked acromion, inferior acromioclavicular joint osteophytes, anterior acromial spurs) are more likely to benefit from decompression. However, patients with partial tears and no extrinsic structural bone abnormalities are more likely to benefit from repair if the lesion is more than 50% of the tendon thickness and from debridement alone if the lesion is less than 50% of the tendon thickness.

These factors are then considered in light of patient preference. Some patients will prefer an open approach if it can more reliably effect a cure; others may chose arthroscopic surgery because that approach offers fewer lifestyle inconveniences. At each end of the decision-making spectrum, treatment is less controversial. Active individuals with normal bone shape and tears involving more than 50% of the tendon thickness are best treated with surgical repair. Sedentary patients with a hooked acromion and tears involving less than 50% of the tendon thickness can be treated successfully with arthroscopic decompression alone. It is in the middle area that treatment is less well defined; surgeon experience and patient preference, rather than scientific data, appear to dictate treatment.

There are three options for arthroscopic management of complete rotator cuff tears: (1) arthroscopic decompression without repair, (2) arthroscopic decompression and mini-open repair, and (3) arthroscopic decompression and repair of the torn tendon with the use of arthroscopic techniques alone. The surgeon may elect to perform an arthroscopic subacromial decompression without any attempt to repair the torn tendon. Debridement of tendon flap tears, synovectomy, and leveling of a prominent greater tuberosity may accompany this procedure. A second option is to perform the arthroscopic decompression and then make a small lateral incision and repair the tendon tear with conventional open technique; the advantage is that the incision is smaller and deltoid detachment is not needed, as the acromioplasty is performed arthroscopically. The third option is to perform the decompression and tendon repair entirely with the use of arthroscopic techniques.

Arthroscopic technique allows intra-articular inspection and loose-body removal, synovectomy, labrum debridement, and repair of partial biceps lesions if necessary. The advantages of decreased pain from smaller incisions and improved cosmesis are important to patients.

The greatest difficulty with arthroscopic treatment of the seemingly irreparable cuff tear is the possibility of misdiagnosis. Often a massive cuff tear is retracted and appears irreparable, but after release of adhesions on both its bursal and articular surfaces, the defect is reparable. In many instances, arthroscopic inspection will lead to an inaccurate assessment of irreparability. Magnetic resonance imaging, which some surgeons do not use routinely in the older patient, is often of great value in this clinical setting. The amount of tendon retraction is more clearly defined than on arthrography and, perhaps more important, the degree of atrophy in the rotator cuff muscles can be appreciated. If a patient has grade 3 rotator cuff strength or less and the MR study demonstrates retraction of the tendon to the glenoid rim with severe muscular atrophy, the cuff defect is almost certainly irreparable. The arthroscopic approach is then the technique of choice, as it combines the thorough decompression afforded by open debridement with the advantages of arthroscopic surgery.

The technique of subacromial decompression is altered if the tendons are irreparable. As Nirschl[25] and Flatow et al[26] have reported, removal of the coracoacromial arch in patients without any functioning rotator cuff can result in the devastating complication of superomedial humeral head dislocation. The coracoacromial ligament is not resected, and a minimal acromioplasty is performed. The goal is to shape or sculpt the acromion, rather than flattening its inferior surface. Interposed soft-tissue fragments of tendon are removed. If the greater tuberosity is prominent, it can be contoured and smoothed.

Comparison of Open and Arthroscopic Approaches

Arthroscopy appears to have certain theoretical advantages over conventional open surgery. The skin incisions are smaller, and the cosmetic result is better. The procedure can be performed on an outpatient basis, which is more convenient for the patient and less expensive for the third-party payer. Most patients can perform activities of daily living and return to a sedentary job within days. Since the deltoid is not detached from the acromion, active range-of-motion exercises can be started as soon as tolerated.

Perhaps more important is the fact that the glenohumeral joint can be inspected. Although clinically important intra-articular lesions are not common, glenohumeral instability, labrum tears, partial-thickness articular-surface rotator cuff tears, biceps lesions, and arthritic changes in the glenoid and/or humeral head can be identified. These might well be overlooked with a conventional open approach; their accurate diagnosis and eventual treatment can clearly be of benefit in achieving the most optimal functional result for the patient.

Arthroscopic subacromial decompression can be a difficult skill for many individuals to master, and it is certainly harder to teach than open acromioplasty. Better hand-eye coordination is required. The ability to triangulate and manipulate power instruments within millimeters of each other can be challenging.

The cost difference between outpatient arthroscopic surgery and inpatient open procedures may not be as great as perceived by patients, surgeons, and insurance carriers. Certainly the cost of a hospital stay is avoided with arthroscopic surgery, but this is at least partially offset by the increased cost of the arthroscopic setup. The price of disposable instruments, tubing, and saline is an important consideration. The operating room, recovery room, surgeon's, and anesthesiologist's fees constitute the largest portion of the hospital cost. These charges are similar for both arthroscopic and open acromioplasty.

It would seem logical that the arthroscopic approach allows patients to more rapidly return to a job that does not require heavy labor. This should have a substantial impact in cost analyses that take into account days lost from work; however, studies that systematically address that issue have not been performed. Furthermore, it appears that even in this area, the differences are slight. Many patients do not have manual-labor jobs and can return to work when pain is adequately controlled. The ability to return to work seems to be less heavily influenced by the lesions found at the time of surgery; more important are social, emotional, and economic concerns, which are not influenced by the surgical technique.

Deltoid management differs between the open and arthroscopic approaches. The open approach requires a small amount of deltoid detachment and reattachment, and the deltoid must be protected and allowed to heal in order to avoid the debilitating complication of deltoid dehiscence. In contrast, the arthroscopic technique allows immediate active motion. Advocates of open techniques state that very little deltoid removal from the acromion is required and that reliable techniques exist for the secure reattachment of the deltoid. Advocates of the arthroscopic approach argue that deltoid detachment is avoided with the arthroscopic approach; however, the arthroscopic technique also has the potential for deltoid injury. The deltoid fascial origin can be disrupted if an overly aggressive anterior or anterolateral acromioplasty is performed.

The rehabilitation programs after arthroscopic and open repair of the rotator cuff are identical, with most authors recommending 6 weeks of passive motion while the tendon-bone junction is uniting, followed by a similar period of time for active motion. Strengthening of the repaired tendon may begin about 3 months after sur-

gery. Arthroscopic treatment cannot overcome the principles of tendon biology. Postoperative management after decompression for stage 2 impingement and irreparable tears progresses more rapidly after arthroscopic surgery because active motion can be started immediately without fear of deltoid detachment.

Current Status

In cases of stage 2 impingement, arthroscopic and open techniques produce equivalent results. Therefore, the selection of the appropriate technique depends on surgeon and patient preference.

In patients with partial tears, arthroscopy appears to offer the advantages of open technique in allowing the surgeon to evaluate the size, location, and depth of the tear. The decision to perform debridement, debridement and decompression, or debridement, decompression, and repair should be based on tear depth, patient activity level, and the existence of correctable structural bone abnormalities. There is no evidence to document the superiority of the open, arthroscopic, or combined technique.

The current data support tendon repair over arthroscopic debridement alone as the treatment of choice for complete tears. The results of mini-open repair after arthroscopic debridement are promising. Total arthroscopic management of the complete rotator cuff tear is currently in a state of rapid development, and it is difficult to draw firm conclusions. It has not yet been established whether arthroscopic decompression and tendon repair is a successful procedure with long-lasting results, and whether the technical complexity of the procedure limits its usefulness. Further clinical investigation should be directed at critically analyzing the efficacy of the various treatment options. Currently, surgeons treat a patient with a full-thickness tear on the basis of their personal experience with open and arthroscopic techniques.

For irreparable tears, arthroscopic debridement appears to combine the completeness of open debridement with the advantages of arthroscopic treatment. However, further documentation is needed.

Summary

The best treatment for rotator cuff disease continues to be controversial. Rotator cuff disease and its management are only partially understood, and decisions are currently made on the basis of the individual surgeon's clinical experience rather than firm scientific data and experiential analysis.

Central to this debate on the best treatment for rotator cuff disease is the lack of prospective, controlled clinical studies that clearly define the patient population, surgical technique, and evaluation method. Patient outcome studies are vital. Until these are performed, the orthopaedic surgeon must base treatment decisions on personal experience and suggestions from the literature.

References

1. Altchek DW, Warren RF, Wickiewicz TL, Skyhar MJ, Ortiz G, Schwartz E: Arthroscopic acromioplasty: Technique and results. *J Bone Joint Surg Am* 1990;72:1198-1207.

2. Ellman H: Arthroscopic subacromial decompression: Analysis of one- to three-year results. *Arthroscopy* 1987;3: 173-181.

3. Gartsman GM: Arthroscopic acromioplasty for lesions of the rotator cuff. *J Bone Joint Surg Am* 1990;72:169-180.

4. Ryu RK: Arthroscopic subacromial decompression: A clinical review. *Arthroscopy* 1992;8:141-147.

5. Lazarus MD, Chansky HA, Misra S, Williams GR, Iannotti JP: Comparison of open and arthroscopic subacromial decompression. *J Shoulder Elbow Surg* 1994;3:1-11.

6. Norlin R: Arthroscopic subacromial decompression versus open acromioplasty. *Arthroscopy* 1989;5:321-323.

7. Van Holsbeeck E, DeRycke J, Declercq G, Martens M, Verstreken J, Fabry G: Subacromial impingement: Open versus arthroscopic decompression. *Arthroscopy* 1992;8:173-178.

8. Andrews JR, Broussard TS, Carson WG: Arthroscopy of the shoulder in the management of partial tears of the rotator cuff: A preliminary report. *Arthroscopy* 1985;1:117-122.

9. Snyder SJ, Pachelli AF, Del Pizzo W, Friedman MJ, Ferkel RD, Pattee G: Partial thickness rotator cuff tears: Results of arthroscopic treatment. *Arthroscopy* 1991;7:1-7.

10. Esch JC, Ozerkis LR, Helgager JA, Kane N, Lilliott N: Arthroscopic subacromial decompression: Results according to the degree of rotator cuff tear. *Arthroscopy* 1988;4:241-249.

11. Levy HJ, Gardner RD, Lemak LJ: Arthroscopic subacromial decompression in the treatment of full-thickness rotator cuff tears. *Arthroscopy* 1991;7:8-13.

12. Montgomery TJ, Yerger B, Savoie FH III: Management of rotator cuff tears: A comparison of arthroscopic debridement and surgical repair. *J Shoulder Elbow Surg* 1994;3:70-78.

13. Burkhart SS, Nottage WM, Ogilvie-Harris DJ, Kohn HS, Pachelli A: Partial repair of irreparable rotator cuff tears. *Arthroscopy* 1994;10:363-370.

14. Levy HJ, Uribe JW, Delaney LG: Arthroscopic assisted rotator cuff repair: Preliminary results. *Arthroscopy* 1990; 6:55-60.

15. Liu SH, Baker CL: Arthroscopically assisted rotator cuff repair: Correlation of functional results with integrity of the cuff. *Arthroscopy* 1994;10:54-60.

16. Paulos LE, Kody MH: Arthroscopically enhanced "miniapproach" to rotator cuff repair. *Am J Sports Med* 1994;22:19-25.

17. Snyder SJ, Bachner EJ: Arthroscopic fixation of rotator cuff tears with miniature screw anchors and permanent mattress sutures: A preliminary report. Presented at the American Shoulder and Elbow Surgeons Annual Meeting, Williamsburg, Va, October 30, 1993.

18. Gartsman GM, Brinker MR, Khan M: Early effectiveness of arthroscopic repair for full-thickness tears of the rotator cuff: An outcome analsis. *J Bone Joint Surg Am* 1998;80:33-40.

19. Ellman H, Gartsman GM: *Arthroscopic Shoulder Surgery and Related Procedures.* Philadelphia: Lea & Febiger, 1993, pp 203-218.

20. Neer CS II: Impingement lesions. *Clin Orthop* 1983;173:70-77.

21. Hawkins RJ, Abrams JS: Impingement syndrome in the absence of rotator cuff tear (stages 1 and 2). *Orthop Clin North Am* 1987;18:373-382.

22. Gartsman GM, Milne JC: Articular surface partial-thickness rotator cuff tears. *J Shoulder Elbow Surg* 1995;4: 409-415.

23. Gartsman GM: Arthroscopic assessment of rotator cuff tear reparability. *Arthroscopy* 1996;12:546-549.

24. Gartsman GM, Taverna E: The incidence of glenohumeral joint abnormalities associated with full-thickness, reparable rotator cuff tears. *Arthroscopy* 1997;13:450-455.

25. Nirschl R: Rotator cuff surgery. *Instr Course Lect* 1989;38:447-462.

26. Flatow EL, Connor PM, Levine WN, Arroyo JS, Pollock RG, Bigliani LU: Coracoacromial arch reconstruction for anterosuperior subluxation after failed rotator cuff surgery: A preliminary report. Presented at the 13th Annual Meeting of the American Shoulder and Elbow Surgeons, Amelia Island, Fla, October 20, 1996.

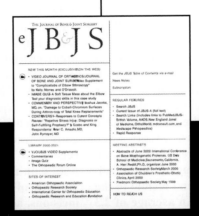

Arthroscopic Repair of Full-Thickness Tears of the Rotator Cuff*

BY GARY M. GARTSMAN, M.D.†, MYRNA KHAN, M.S.‡, AND STEVEN M. HAMMERMAN, M.D.†, HOUSTON, TEXAS

Investigation performed at Texas Orthopedic Hospital, Houston

ABSTRACT: We present the results of arthroscopic repair of full-thickness tears of the rotator cuff in seventy-three patients (thirty-nine men and thirty-four women). The average age of the patients at the time of the operation was 60.7 years (range, thirty-one to eighty-two years). All of the patients were followed for at least two years (average, thirty months; range, twenty-four to forty months). The shoulders were evaluated with the rating scale of the University of California at Los Angeles, the shoulder index of the American Shoulder and Elbow Surgeons, and the functional rating scale of Constant and Murley. In addition, the patients completed the Short-Form 36 Health Survey (SF-36) preoperatively and at the yearly follow-up evaluations.

Eleven tears were small (less than one centimeter in length), forty-five were medium (one to three centimeters), eleven were large (more than three to five centimeters), and six were massive (more than five centimeters). The average length of the tear was twelve millimeters, and the average width was twenty-seven millimeters. Sixty-nine tendons were repaired anatomically, and four were repaired an average of three millimeters (range, two to eight millimeters) medial to the anatomical insertion of the tendon. An average of 2.3 (range, one to four) suture anchors were used in the repair. Sixty-three glenohumeral joints were normal, and ten had an intra-articular lesion. Seven patients had a concomitant resection of the acromioclavicular joint. The average duration of the operation was fifty-six minutes (range, thirty-five to ninety minutes).

The active and passive ranges of motion improved significantly after the procedure (p = 0.0001). The strength of resisted elevation improved from 7.5 to 14.0 pounds (3.4 to 6.3 kilograms) (p = 0.0001). The average total score according to the rating scale of the University of California at Los Angeles improved from 12.4 to 31.1 points; the average total score according to the shoulder index of the American Shoulder and Elbow Surgeons, from 30.7 to 87.6 points; and the average absolute score according to the rating system of Constant and Murley, from 41.7 to 83.6 points (p = 0.0001 for all comparisons). The average score for the pain component of the rating scale of the University of California at Los Angeles improved from 2.4 to 8.6 points; fifty-seven (78 per cent) of the seventy-three patients rated the relief of pain as good or excellent on the visual-analog scale. The average score for satisfaction improved from 0.4 to 4.6 points; sixty-six patients (90 per cent) rated their satisfaction as good or excellent at the time of the most recent examination. None of the shoulders were rated as good or excellent before the operation, whereas sixty-one (84 per cent) were so rated at the most recent follow-up evaluation after the index procedure. In addition, significant improvements (p = 0.0015) were noted in the scales and summary measures of the SF-36.

Arthroscopic repair of full-thickness tears of the rotator cuff produced satisfactory results with regard to traditional orthopaedic criteria as well as with regard to patient-assessed criteria such as satisfaction, pain relief, and general health. The arthroscopic method offers several advantages, including smaller incisions, access to the glenohumeral joint for the inspection and treatment of intra-articular lesions, no need for detachment of the deltoid, and less soft-tissue dissection. However, these advantages must be considered against the technical difficulty of the method, which limits its application to surgeons who are skilled in both open and arthroscopic procedures on the shoulder.

Operative skills have advanced sufficiently so that full-thickness tears of the rotator cuff can be repaired with arthroscopic techniques. The proposed advantages of the arthroscopic method are that it involves smaller skin incisions, provides access to the glenohumeral joint for the inspection and treatment of intra-articular lesions, does not require detachment of the deltoid, and necessitates less soft-tissue dissection. The purpose of this study was to evaluate the results of arthroscopic repair performed by one surgeon at one institution.

Materials and Methods

Seventy-eight consecutive patients had arthroscopic repair of a full-thickness tear of the rotator cuff between

*No benefits in any form have been received or will be received from a commercial party related directly or indirectly to the subject of this article. No funds were received in support of this study.

†Texas Orthopedic Hospital, Fondren Orthopedic Group, 7401 South Main Street, Houston, Texas 77030. E-mail address for Dr. Gartsman: gary@fondren.com.

‡Computing Resource Center, Academic Information Services, One Baylor Plaza, Suite M216, Houston, Texas 77030.

January and December 1994. The criterion for inclusion in this study was a full-thickness, reparable tear of at least one rotator-cuff tendon. A tear was considered to be reparable if the tendon could be restored to, or within ten millimeters of, its anatomical insertion when traction was applied to the tendon. If the tendon could not be positioned appropriately, sites at which its mobility was limited were inspected and released as necessary. Mobility of the tendon was limited by the contracture of a number of anatomical structures, including the superior aspect of the glenohumeral joint capsule and the coracohumeral ligament. Adhesions to the inferior surface of the acromion and to the inferior aspect of the deltoid fascia also limited the ability to free the retracted tendon. If the torn tendon could not be mobilized adequately or if the tendon was absent, the lesion was considered to be irreparable. A more detailed description of the determination of the repairability of tears of the rotator cuff has been published[13].

The uniformity of the study group was maintained as much as possible so that the effects of this new procedure could be investigated. Thus, individuals who had had a previous procedure on the shoulder, those who had a partial-thickness tear of the rotator cuff, and those who had an irreparable tear were excluded. Patients who had filed a Workers' Compensation claim were also excluded because various issues may have affected their outcome; Misamore et al.[21] recently documented inferior results among patients who had filed such a claim. Patients who had an acute tear were also excluded because they had often sustained substantial trauma with additional osseous or soft-tissue damage.

A minimum of two years of follow-up was required for inclusion in the study. Five patients who had been followed for less than two years were excluded. However, a review of the demographic data and operative findings demonstrated that these patients were representative of the entire patient population. Two of the five patients could not be located, one had died of an unrelated cause, and two were evaluated one year postoperatively but were lost to follow-up before the two-year minimum. Therefore, seventy-three patients (thirty-nine men and thirty-four women) who had had a unilateral procedure on the shoulder were evaluated. The average duration of follow-up was thirty months (range, twenty-four to forty months). The patients were evaluated at six weeks; at three, six, nine, and twelve months; and yearly thereafter.

The average age at the time of the operation was 60.7 years (range, thirty-one to eighty-two years). Fifty-two patients had involvement of the dominant shoulder, and twenty-one had involvement of the non-dominant shoulder. The average duration of the symptoms before the operation was eighteen months (range, six to 144 months). Fifty-two patients had had an average of 1.7 (range, one to eight) preoperative subacromial injections of cortisone, administered by either the referring physician or one of us (G. M. G.).

Preoperative Assessment

In order to allow the results of the present study to be compared with those of others in the literature, data were collected with use of the rating scale of the University of California at Los Angeles[8], the rating system of Constant and Murley[5], and the shoulder index of the American Shoulder and Elbow Surgeons[27]. The rating scale of the University of California at Los Angeles is a 35-point scale with 10 points for pain, 10 points for function, and 5 points each for motion, strength, and patient satisfaction. The rating system of Constant and Murley is a 100-point scale with 15 points for pain, 20 points for function, 40 points for active range of motion, and 25 points for strength. The shoulder index of the American Shoulder and Elbow Surgeons consists of a pain score and a section including ten self-assessed activities of daily living. Pain is assessed by the patient on a 10-point visual-analog scale (with 0 points indicating no pain and 10 points, unbearable pain). This score is subtracted from 10, and the resulting number is multiplied by 5 for a maximum total of 50 points. The ten activities of daily living are each scored from 0 to 3 points (with 0 points indicating an inability to perform the task and 3 points, normal function); the total of these ten scores is multiplied by 5/3 for a maximum total of 50 points. Thus, the total possible score for the entire index is 100 points. In addition, the patients completed the Short-Form 36 Health Survey (SF-36)[33,34] preoperatively and at the yearly examinations.

The active ranges of motion were measured with the system of Constant and Murley and included forward elevation, abduction, external rotation with the arm in abduction, and internal rotation behind the back. Passive elevation and external rotation (with the arm in adduction) were measured to the nearest 5 degrees by the examiner with a handheld goniometer. Internal rotation behind the back was recorded as the most cephalad vertebral level reached by the extended thumb. The operating surgeon recorded all measurements during the initial physical examination and subsequent follow-up visits. No attempt was made to increase the precision of the measurements by requiring the evaluation to be performed by a blinded examiner, evaluating test-retest validity, measuring interobserver and intraobserver reliability, instructing the patient before the measurements, or asking the patient to perform warm-up exercises before the evaluation.

The strength of resisted elevation was measured with a dynamometer with the arm elevated 90 degrees in the scapular plane and internally rotated; the result was recorded in pounds. Lidocaine was not injected into the subacromial space before the shoulder was examined, so it was not possible to quantify how much of the loss of strength was due to pain.

Anteroposterior glenoid, axillary, and supraspinatus outlet radiographs were made routinely. Imaging studies (magnetic resonance imaging or arthrography) were performed if necessary. Sixty patients had preoperative imaging studies: sixteen had arthrography and forty-four had magnetic resonance imaging. There were no false-negative arthrograms or magnetic resonance images.

The primary indication for the operation was persistent pain in the shoulder that had not responded to a minimum of six months of non-operative treatment consisting of avoidance of painful activities, use of non-steroidal anti-inflammatory medication, and participation in a home physical-therapy program designed to maintain or improve the range of motion of the shoulder and to increase the strength of the uninvolved muscles[11]. Cortisone was injected into the subacromial space if pain had not decreased after two to three months of oral administration of non-steroidal anti-inflammatory medication or if the use of such medication was contraindicated.

Rights of the Patients

In order to maintain patient confidentiality throughout the investigation, each patient was assigned a unique identification number. The identification number was kept separate from the name so that the statistician did not know the patient's identity. Before the start of the investigation, statistical analysis was performed to quantify the number of patients that would be required in order for statistically valid conclusions to be drawn. All patients provided written, informed consent stating that they understood the purpose of the study as well as the potential risks and benefits of the operation. Patients were informed that they had the right to operative or non-operative care other than that proposed in the study. They were also informed that they had the right not to participate in the study even if they chose the type of care described in the study. The patient's understanding of these rights was documented in writing.

Operative Technique

Before the administration of the general anesthetic, an interscalene block was given in order to diminish postoperative pain. The patient was placed in the sitting position. The glenohumeral joint was inspected, and intra-articular lesions were treated as necessary.

The arthroscope was then removed from the joint and was redirected into the subacromial space. Any bursal tissue that impeded a clear view of the torn tendon was removed. The length of the tear as well as any medial retraction was recorded. The tendon was grasped with a surgical instrument, and the repairability of the tendon (the ability of the tissue to hold sutures and thus to be used in the repair) was determined[13]. The tendon must be sufficiently mobile to allow it to be attached to the humerus. Occasionally, there were adhesions between the tendon and the superior aspect of the gleno-humeral joint capsule, the coracohumeral ligament, the acromion, the deltoid fascia, or a combination of these, that limited excursion. Adhesions were removed with a motorized shaver or electrocautery until full excursion was possible, and then the arthroscopic subacromial decompression was completed[11].

The purpose of the acromioplasty was to create adequate space for the rotator-cuff tendons. As the thickness and shape of the acromions varied, the amount of bone removed during the acromioplasty also varied. The goal was to achieve a flat acromial undersurface. As all of the patients in the present study had a chronic tear of the rotator cuff, impingement was considered to be part of the pathological process regardless of whether or not it was the cause of the tear. Osteophytes in the inferior part of the acromioclavicular joint were removed if necessary, as determined on the basis of preoperative radiographs or by inspection at the time of the operation. The acromioclavicular joint was removed only if the patient had had preoperative localized pain or tenderness of the joint on physical examination[12].

A cancellous bed was prepared at the site of the repair by removal of a thin layer of cortical bone with a power burr. No trough was utilized. A suture anchor was inserted lateral to the cancellous bone surface in the denser metaphyseal bone. A number-2 braided, non-absorbable suture was placed approximately five millimeters from the margin of the tendon. The number of suture anchors varied with the length of the tear. After all repair sutures were inserted, an additional suture was placed in the margin of the tendon and traction was applied to reduce the tendon to its repair site and to allow the suture to be tied without tension. The tendon was repaired with the arm at the side. If this could not be accomplished, the tendon was repaired medially[20]. Abduction of the arm was not necessary for any of the repairs. The number-2 sutures were tied so that the knot was on the bursal surface of the tendon. Absorbable sutures were not used. The traction suture was removed after all of the repair sutures were tied. Longitudinal tears were repaired with simple monofilament sutures, as dictated by the geometry of the tear.

It is recommended that two surgeons be present during the procedure, as this technique requires many complicated maneuvers. A detailed description of the operative technique has been published previously[15].

Postoperative Management

The arm was maintained in a sling in 15 degrees of abduction, and an ice-pack wrap was used to decrease swelling and pain in the shoulder. Passive elevation and external rotation were started on the afternoon of the operation and were continued at home for six weeks. The patient was discharged to home on the morning after the operation. Active range-of-motion exercises were begun at six weeks and were continued until the twelfth week, at which point strengthening exercises

TABLE I
SCORES FOR THE SHOULDER-RATING SYSTEMS*

	Preoperative (points)	Most Recent (points)
Rating scale of University of California at Los Angeles[8]		
Total score	12.4 ± 4.2	31.1 ± 3.2
Pain	2.4 ± 1.7	8.6 ± 1.6
Function	3.7 ± 2.2	8.9 ± 1.2
Flexion	3.6 ± 2.2	4.9 ± 0.3
Strength	2.3 ± 1.0	4.1 ± 0.9
Satisfaction	0.4 ± 0.5	4.6 ± 0.9
Shoulder index of American Shoulder and Elbow Surgeons[27]		
Total score	30.7 ± 15.7	87.6 ± 12.8
Pain	7.7 ± 1.7	1.4 ± 1.6
Function	11.4 ± 5.7	26.8 ± 8.0
Rating scale of Constant and Murley[5]		
Absolute score	41.7 ± 12.8	83.6 ± 9.0
Age-adjusted score†	43.3 ± 11.6	84.0 ± 7.5
Pain	3.6 ± 2.6	12.9 ± 2.3
Function	3.4 ± 1.9	18.8 ± 1.5
Elevation	7.6 ± 2.5	9.8 ± 0.6
Abduction	6.2 ± 2.6	9.6 ± 1.1
External rotation	6.8 ± 2.2	9.5 ± 1.2
Internal rotation	6.7 ± 2.1	9.1 ± 1.2
Strength	7.5 ± 4.7	14.0 ± 5.4

*The values are given as the average and the standard deviation. The differences between the preoperative and the most recent scores were significant (p = 0.0001), according to the Wilcoxon signed-rank test.

†The age-adjusted score is an average of the age-stratified data.

with rubber tubing were begun. The strengthening exercises were designed to strengthen the deltoid, the infraspinatus, the supraspinatus, the scapular rotators, and the biceps. The range-of-motion and strengthening exercises were continued for one year.

At each follow-up examination, the patient assessed the pain in and function of the shoulder as well as his or her level of satisfaction with the three shoulder-rating systems. The examiner documented the active and passive ranges of motion as well as the strength of resisted elevation. At the yearly follow-up examinations, after arrival in the clinic but before the examination, the patient completed the SF-36. No postoperative imaging studies (ultrasound, magnetic resonance imaging, or arthrography) were performed.

Statistical Analysis

The Wilcoxon signed-rank test was used to evaluate the preoperative and most recent scores for significant differences. The Wilcoxon rank-sum test was used to test for preoperative and postoperative differences between the patients who had a normal glenohumeral joint and those who had an abnormal glenohumeral joint. The Spearman rank correlation was used to determine the relationships between several independent variables, including the preoperative and postoperative overall scores on the rating scale of the University of California at Los Angeles; the preoperative and postoperative strength of resisted elevation; the age of the patient; and the length, width, and total area of the tear. Standard statistical software (SAS, Cary, North Carolina) was used to analyze the data.

Results

Operative Findings

Sixty-three glenohumeral joints were normal, and ten had an intra-articular lesion. Serious intra-articular abnormalities were defined as those that needed operative treatment or that were expected to alter the postoperative rehabilitation or the outcome[17]. Three patients had osteoarthrosis of the humeral head; three had osteoarthrosis of the humeral head and the glenoid; two had a partial tear of the biceps tendon; one had osteoarthrosis of the humeral head, a tear of the anterior aspect of the glenoid labrum, and a partial tear of the biceps; and one had a proliferative synovitis.

As the tendons of the supraspinatus, infraspinatus, and teres minor blend together to form the rotator cuff, identification of the involved tendons is somewhat arbitrary. Nonetheless, we used our best clinical judgment to determine the pattern of the tear. Forty patients had a tear of the supraspinatus; twenty-five, a tear of the supraspinatus and the infraspinatus; five, a tear of the supraspinatus, infraspinatus, and teres minor; and three, a tear of the supraspinatus, infraspinatus, and superior portion of the subscapularis.

The size of the tear was measured with a calibrated arthroscopic probe. All shoulders were positioned in 15 degrees of abduction, 10 degrees of elevation, and 5 degrees of external rotation for the measurement. The length of the tear was measured as the distance from the anterior border of the greater tuberosity at the bicipital

TABLE II
SCORES FOR ACTIVITIES OF DAILY LIVING ACCORDING TO THE SHOULDER INDEX OF THE AMERICAN SHOULDER AND ELBOW SURGEONS[27]*

	Preoperative (points)	Most Recent (points)
Putting on coat	1.55 ± 0.76	2.93 ± 0.30
Sleeping	0.96 ± 0.95	2.62 ± 0.70
Reaching behind back	1.01 ± 0.79	2.70 ± 0.46
Toileting	2.39 ± 0.84	2.97 ± 0.16
Combing hair	1.59 ± 0.96	2.89 ± 0.36
Reaching high shelf	0.96 ± 0.95	2.67 ± 0.58
Lifting 10 lbs. (4.5 kg) above shoulder	0.53 ± 0.78	2.22 ± 0.99
Throwing overhead	0.55 ± 0.80	2.34 ± 0.90
Working	1.33 ± 1.05	2.81 ± 0.99
Sports activities	0.52 ± 0.82	2.67 ± 0.73

*The values are given as the average and the standard deviation. The differences between the preoperative and the most recent scores were significant (p = 0.0001), according to the Wilcoxon signed-rank test.

TABLE III
PASSIVE RANGE OF MOTION*

	Preoperative	Most Recent
Elevation (degrees)	135 ± 22	149 ± 4
External rotation (degrees)	66 ± 12	78 ± 10
Internal rotation	L1 ± 4 levels	T9 ± 3 levels

*The values are given as the average and the standard deviation. The differences between the preoperative and the most recent values were significant (p = 0.0001), according to the Wilcoxon signed-rank test.

groove to the intact portion of the tendon posteriorly on the greater tuberosity. Eleven tears were small (less than one centimeter long), forty-five were medium (one to three centimeters long), eleven were large (more than three to five centimeters long), and six were massive (more than five centimeters long). The average length was twelve millimeters (range, five to sixty millimeters). The width of the tear was measured as the distance from the margin of the lateral border of the greater tuberosity to the edge of the tendon. The average width was twenty-seven millimeters (range, zero to thirty millimeters). The average area of the tear was 324 square millimeters (range, fifty to 1255 square millimeters). In terms of the area, seventeen tears were small (twenty-five to 100 square millimeters), twenty-five were medium (101 to 350 square millimeters), eighteen were large (351 to 600 square millimeters), and thirteen were massive (more than 600 square millimeters).

Sixty-nine tendons were repaired anatomically, and four were repaired an average of three millimeters (range, two to eight millimeters) medial to the anatomical insertion of the tendon. Side-to-side repair was performed as dictated by the geometry of the tear. An average of 2.3 (range, one to four) suture anchors were used. During the period of this study, a wide variety of suture anchors (including metallic screw-in anchors, metallic expandable anchors, and polyethylene expandable anchors) were used. We currently use metallic screw-in anchors exclusively. The average duration of the operation was fifty-six minutes (range, thirty-five to ninety minutes). Seven patients had resection of the acromioclavicular joint.

Complications

There were no intraoperative or perioperative complications. No patient had a neural injury, wound infection, or drainage from the wound. The suture anchors did not cause any complications. No patient needed manipulation for postoperative stiffness.

Shoulder-Rating Systems

All three rating systems reflected significant improvement in the status of the shoulder when the preoperative scores were compared with the scores at the time of the most recent follow-up (p = 0.0001) (Table I). The average total score increased from 12.4 to 31.1

points with use of the rating scale of the University of California at Los Angeles and from 30.7 to 87.6 points with use of the shoulder index of the American Shoulder and Elbow Surgeons. The average absolute score with use of the system of Constant and Murley improved from 41.7 to 83.6 points, and the average age-adjusted score (an average of the age-stratified data[4]) improved from 43.3 to 84.0 points.

Satisfaction: The rating scale of the University of California at Los Angeles was used to rate the level of satisfaction. The average score for satisfaction was 0.4 point preoperatively and 4.6 points postoperatively. Preoperatively, none of the patients rated their satisfaction as good or excellent (a score of 4 or 5 points). Postoperatively, sixty-six (90 per cent) of the seventy-three patients rated their satisfaction as good or excellent and seven (10 per cent) rated it as fair or poor (a score of 0 to 3 points).

Pain: The procedure resulted in a significant reduction in pain (p = 0.0001). Preoperatively, no patient had no or minimum pain (a score of 0, 1, or 2 points on the visual-analog scale). Postoperatively, fifty-seven patients (78 per cent) had no or minimum pain, eleven (15 per cent) had moderate pain (3 or 4 points), and five (7 per cent) had severe pain (5 to 10 points).

Function: Function of the shoulder was assessed with the function component of the rating scale of the University of California at Los Angeles (Table I) and the scores for the ten activities of daily living included in the shoulder index of the American Shoulder and Elbow Surgeons (Table II). Preoperatively, three patients (4 per cent) rated the function as good or excellent (8, 9, or 10 points) and seventy patients (96 per cent) rated it as fair or poor (0 to 7 points) according to the rating scale of the University of California at Los

TABLE IV
SCORES FOR THE SHORT-FORM 36 (SF-36) HEALTH SURVEY[33,34]*

	Preoperative (points)	Most Recent (points)
Physical function	57.2 ± 25.7	76.6 ± 27.1
Physical role function	24.6 ± 37.4	75.7 ± 40.4
Bodily pain	27.7 ± 19.7	68.2 ± 24.1
General health	70.8 ± 28.7	72.4 ± 21.8
Vitality	50.6 ± 24.2	62.8 ± 18.4
Social function	57.5 ± 31.2	84.0 ± 25.5
Emotional role function	62.1 ± 43.8	82.4 ± 34.3
Mental health	70.3 ± 22.2	78.2 ± 19.3
Physical component summary	34.1 ± 9.1	46.6 ± 10.8
Mental component summary	48.7 ± 13.1	52.6 ± 9.4

*All values are given as the average and the standard deviation. The differences between the preoperative and the most recent scores were significant (p = 0.0015), according to the Wilcoxon signed-rank test, except for the general health score and the mental component summary score.

TABLE V

SPEARMAN RANK CORRELATIONS FOR COMPARISON OF VARIOUS PARAMETERS*

	University of California at Los Angeles[8]		Strength of Resisted Elevation		Length of Tear	Width of Tear	Area of Tear	Age of Patient
	Preoperative Score	Most Recent Score	Preoperative	Most Recent				
University of California at Los Angeles								
Preoperative score	1.00	0.081	0.417 (0.0002)	0.067	0.067	−0.049	0.015	−0.157
Most recent score		1.00	0.309 (0.008)	0.515 (0.0001)	−0.161	−0.092	−0.122	−0.043
Strength of resisted elevation								
Preoperative			1.00	0.456 (0.0001)	−0.244 (0.037)	−0.131	−0.199	−0.448 (0.0001)
Most recent				1.00	−0.407 (0.0003)	−0.310 (0.008)	−0.373 (0.001)	−0.368 (0.001)
Length of tear					1.00	0.676 (0.0001)	0.906 (0.0001)	0.336 (0.004)
Width of tear						1.00	0.912 (0.0001)	0.292 (0.012)
Area of tear							1.00	0.346 (0.003)
Age of patient								1.00

*The values are given as the r values, with the p values in parentheses.

Angeles; postoperatively, sixty-seven patients (92 per cent) rated the function as good or excellent and six (8 per cent) rated it as fair or poor. There was significant improvement in all ten activities of daily living that were assessed with the shoulder index of the American Shoulder and Elbow Surgeons (p = 0.0001).

Range of motion: The active and passive ranges of motion were significantly improved at the most recent follow-up evaluation (p = 0.0001) (Tables I and III).

Strength: The strength of resisted elevation improved 87 per cent, from an average of 7.5 pounds (3.4 kilograms) preoperatively to an average of 14.0 pounds (6.3 kilograms) at the most recent follow-up evaluation. This improvement was significant (p = 0.0001).

General health: All of the scores according to the SF-36, with the exception of the score for general health and the mental component summary score, improved significantly (p = 0.0015) (Table IV).

Correlation of Variables

Age was not significantly correlated with either the preoperative (r = −0.157) or the postoperative (r = −0.043) overall score according to the rating scale of the University of California at Los Angeles, but it was correlated with the preoperative (r = −0.448, p = 0.0001) and postoperative (r = −0.368, p = 0.001) strength of resisted elevation as well as with the area of the tear (r = 0.346, p = 0.003) (Table V).

Effect of Glenohumeral Abnormalities

The average preoperative score according to the rating scale of the University of California at Los Angeles was 23.7 points for the sixty-three patients who had a normal glenohumeral joint and 10.9 points for the ten who had a serious glenohumeral lesion (p = 0.22). The average postoperative scores were 31.2 and 29.9 points, respectively (p = 0.23). These differences were not found to be significant, with the numbers available. This comparison indicates that the identification and treatment of intra-articular lesions leads to results that are similar to those for patients who do not have an intra-articular lesion.

Analysis of Unsatisfactory Results

Twelve patients had a fair or poor result (a total score of less than 29 points according to the rating scale of the University of California at Los Angeles) at the most recent examination after the index procedure and before any subsequent procedures. Symptomatic arthrosis of the acromioclavicular joint developed in two patients within one year postoperatively. One patient had subsequent arthroscopic resection of the acromioclavicular joint, and the result was excellent at the most recent evaluation. The other patient refused an additional operation. The remaining ten patients did not demonstrate any consistent pattern to account for the fair or poor results.

Discussion

During the last decade, the operative repair of full-thickness tears of the rotator cuff has gradually shifted through three phases: open repair, combined open and arthroscopic repair (so-called mini-open repair), and, most recently, arthroscopic repair alone. Successful results have been documented after arthroscopic repair of stage-2 impingement and partial-thickness tears[6,7,10,11,16,31]. Orthopaedic surgeons now use arthroscopic techniques for many of the elements that make up the operative repair of a full-thickness tear — namely, acromioplasty, release of the coracoacromial ligament, bursal resection, and removal of adhesions.

However, several authors have reported poor results when patients who had a full-thickness tear were managed with arthroscopic subacromial decompression without repair of the defect in the cuff[9,11,25,28]. Most investigations have supported the concept that subacromial decompression must be combined with repair of the tendon in patients who have a chronic full-thickness tear[22,37].

The mini-open method involves arthroscopic evaluation of the glenohumeral joint and arthroscopic acromioplasty combined with open repair of the full-thickness tear[14]. In initial studies, Blevins et al.[2] found that fifty-seven (89 per cent) of sixty-four patients were satisfied and Paulos and Kody[26] reported that sixteen of eighteen patients had a good or excellent result. Both sets of authors were careful to point out that the limited incision used in the repair restricts the use of this technique to the treatment of smaller, less retracted tears located in the anterior portion of the rotator cuff (the anterior one-half of the infraspinatus and the supraspinatus).

As orthopaedists have performed the mini-open repair, they have gained familiarity with the arthroscopic appearance of full-thickness tears of the rotator cuff. There have also been improvements in arthroscopic instruments, suturing techniques, suture anchors, and knot-tying. The ability to arthroscopically measure the tear and assess the quality of the tendon and its repairability has improved[13]. By performing arthroscopic operations for glenohumeral instability, orthopaedic surgeons have also developed expertise in other applicable techniques, such as preparing bone for soft-tissue attachment[29,35]. These developments have allowed the open portion of the mini-open technique to be eliminated and the repair to be performed exclusively with the arthroscopic technique.

Snyder et al.[30] and Gazielly et al.[18] documented their results with arthroscopic methods similar to those described in the present study. Snyder et al. reported an excellent or good result for forty-one (87 per cent) of forty-seven patients. Gazielly et al., in a study of fifteen patients, reported that the average score according to the system of Constant and Murley improved from 58.1 to 87.6 points. The present study documents our experience with the arthroscopic repair of full-thickness tears of the rotator cuff.

We noted substantial improvement in the scores of all three shoulder-rating systems when the preoperative scores were compared with the scores at the most recent evaluation. Although neither the system of Constant

and Murley nor the shoulder index of the American Shoulder and Elbow Surgeons specifically defines an excellent or poor score, Ellman et al.[8] defined a score of 34 or 35 points according to the rating scale of the University of California at Los Angeles as excellent, a score of 29 to 33 points as good, and a score of less than 29 points as fair or poor. Ellman et al. also stated that good and excellent results correspond with Neer's[23,24] definition of a satisfactory result and that fair and poor results correspond with Neer's definition of an unsatisfactory result. Accordingly, in the present study, sixty-one patients (84 per cent) had a good or excellent result and twelve (16 per cent) had a fair or poor result.

There was also marked improvement in each of the components of the shoulder-rating systems. At the most recent evaluation, sixty-six patients (90 per cent) rated their satisfaction with the shoulder as good or excellent compared with no patients preoperatively. The average pain score on the visual-analog scale of the shoulder index of the American Shoulder and Elbow Surgeons improved from 7.7 to 1.4 points. Fifty-seven patients (78 per cent) rated the postoperative relief of pain as good or excellent. The function of the shoulder improved according to the scores for all ten activities of daily living included in the shoulder index of the American Shoulder and Elbow Surgeons, and sixty-seven patients (92 per cent) rated the function of the shoulder as good or excellent at the most recent follow-up. Patients were particularly pleased with the improved ability to sleep comfortably. The active range of motion improved in all measured planes; the average preoperative score for the motion component of the system of Constant and Murley was 27.2 (of a possible 40) points, whereas the average postoperative score was 37.9 points. The increases in the passive range of motion were smaller but also were significant. The strength of resisted elevation improved significantly from 7.5 pounds (3.4 kilograms) preoperatively to 14.0 pounds (6.3 kilograms) postoperatively. There was improvement in all scales and summary measures of the SF-36, with the exception of the general health score and the mental component summary score.

Direct comparison of the results of the present study with those of previous studies on the open repair of full-thickness tears of the rotator cuff is difficult because of the various rating systems used. Bigliani et al.[1] summarized the results of a number of articles on open repair and reported good or excellent results in terms of both pain relief (85 to 100 per cent of patients) and function (70 to 95 per cent of patients). Good or excellent results were reported for forty-two (84 per cent) of fifty patients in the study by Ellman et al.[8], for sixty-four (51 per cent) of 126 patients in the study by Vastamaki[32], and for forty-five (69 per cent) of sixty-five patients in the study by Wolfgang[36]. Hawkins et al.[19] reported that eighty-six (86 per cent) of their 100 patients had relief of pain. The level of improvement of the various parameters described in the present study suggests that arthroscopic repair of full-thickness tears produces equivalent results.

Currently, we treat full-thickness tears of the rotator cuff arthroscopically; no open operations are performed. The use of the arthroscopic technique allows us to inspect the glenohumeral joint and to avoid detaching the origin of the deltoid. The size of the tear is not a factor; we have more difficulty repairing chronic retracted tears, regardless of size, than we do repairing large or massive mobile tears. Although we cannot document our impressions statistically, we believe that arthroscopic repair results in an improved cosmetic appearance, decreased pain postoperatively, and more rapid gains in motion compared with open operative treatment of similar lesions.

The present study has a number of weaknesses. Although the investigation was prospective, the patients were not randomized and the investigator was not blinded. In addition, the follow-up period was relatively short; we are continuing to follow these patients so that we can evaluate the results after longer periods of time. There is evidence, however, that the maximum improvement occurs in the first year after repair of the rotator cuff and that additional improvement is unlikely. We found, as did Misamore et al.[21] and Bokor et al.[3], that improvement occurred only during the first year after the operation. We excluded patients for whom the repair was a revision operation and those who had filed a Workers' Compensation claim; this selection bias may have improved our overall results. We also excluded patients who had an irreparable tear. The determination of repairability remains a challenge not only during arthroscopic operations but also during traditional open repair.

Caution is advised for orthopaedic surgeons who are considering the transition from open to arthroscopic techniques. The orthopaedic surgeon not only must master each of the individual elements described here but also must perform them in a precise and timely fashion. Experience is required in order to recognize the pattern of the tear as viewed through the arthroscope. Mobilization of the tendon can be difficult in a patient who has a retracted tear. Suture anchors must be placed accurately so that the repaired tendon rests in the desired location. The orthopaedist must manage multiple strands of suture material within the tight confines of the subacromial space and tie secure knots with use of arthroscopic tools.

Orthopaedic surgeons who attempt this technique will find it useful to have a skilled assistant surgeon present. In an era of declining reimbursement, this is a disadvantage compared with the traditional open technique.

The present report is based on our experience; therefore, it must be assumed that a learning curve affected the results. Because this study took place at a time when the techniques and equipment of arthroscopic repair of the rotator cuff were evolving, additional refinements will invariably occur as the procedure is used more widely.

At present, these techniques can be recommended only for use by experienced orthopaedic surgeons who are familiar with the normal and abnormal anatomy seen during both open and arthroscopic operations on the shoulder. A thorough understanding of the various conditions that produce pain in the shoulder is also necessary. An orthopaedic surgeon who performs open repairs infrequently should not attempt the arthroscopic procedure. The open operation is relatively simple and has a documented history of success[8,19-21,36]. In contrast, the arthroscopic technique is technically demanding and is still in the developmental stage.

References

1. **Bigliani, L. U.; Cordasco, F. A.; McIlveen, S. J.;** and **Musso, E. S.:** Operative repairs of massive rotator cuff tears: long-term results. *J. Shoulder and Elbow Surg.,* 1: 120-130, 1992.
2. **Blevins, F. T.; Warren, R. F.; Cavo, C.; Altchek, D. W.; Dines, D.; Palletta, G.;** and **Wickiewicz, T. L.:** Arthroscopic assisted rotator cuff repair: results using a mini-open deltoid splitting approach. *Arthroscopy,* 12: 50-59, 1996.
3. **Bokor, D. J.; Hawkins, R. J.; Huckell, G. H.; Angelo, R. L.;** and **Schickendantz, M. S.:** Results of nonoperative management of full-thickness tears of the rotator cuff. *Clin. Orthop.,* 294: 103-110, 1993.
4. **Constant, C. R.:** Age related recovery of shoulder function after injury. Thesis, University College, Cork, Ireland, 1986.
5. **Constant, C. R.,** and **Murley, A. H.:** A clinical method of functional assessment of the shoulder. *Clin. Orthop.,* 214: 160-164, 1987.
6. **Ellman, H.:** Arthroscopic subacromial decompression: analysis of one- to three-year results. *Arthroscopy,* 3: 173-181, 1987.
7. **Ellman, H.:** Diagnosis and treatment of incomplete rotator cuff tears. *Clin. Orthop.,* 254: 64-74, 1990.
8. **Ellman, H.; Hanker, G.;** and **Bayer, M.:** Repair of the rotator cuff. End-result study of factors influencing reconstruction. *J. Bone and Joint Surg.,* 68-A: 1136-1144, Oct. 1986.
9. **Ellman, H.; Kay, S. P.;** and **Wirth, M.:** Arthroscopic treatment of full-thickness rotator cuff tears: 2- to 7-year follow-up study. *Arthroscopy,* 9: 195-200, 1993.
10. **Esch, J. C.; Ozerkis, L. R.; Helgager, J. A.; Kane, N.;** and **Lilliott, N.:** Arthroscopic subacromial decompression: results according to the degree of rotator cuff tear. *Arthroscopy,* 4: 241-249, 1988.
11. **Gartsman, G. M.:** Arthroscopic acromioplasty for lesions of the rotator cuff. *J. Bone and Joint Surg.,* 72-A: 169-180, Feb. 1990.
12. **Gartsman, G. M.:** Arthroscopic resection of the acromioclavicular joint. *Am. J. Sports Med.,* 21: 71-77, 1993.
13. **Gartsman, G. M.:** Arthroscopic assessment of rotator cuff tear reparability. *Arthroscopy,* 12: 546-549, 1996.
14. **Gartsman, G. M.:** Combined arthroscopic and open treatment of tears of the rotator cuff. *J. Bone and Joint Surg.,* 79-A: 776-783, May 1997.
15. **Gartsman, G. M.,** and **Hammerman, S. M.:** Full-thickness tears: arthroscopic repair. *Orthop. Clin. North America,* 28: 83-98, 1997.

16. **Gartsman, G. M.,** and **Milne, J. C.:** Articular surface partial-thickness rotator cuff tears. *J. Shoulder and Elbow Surg.,* 4: 409-415, 1995.

17. **Gartsman, G. M.,** and **Taverna, E.:** The incidence of glenohumeral joint abnormalities associated with full-thickness, reparable rotator cuff tears. *Arthroscopy,* 13: 450-455, 1997.

18. **Gazielly, D. F.; Gleyze, P.; Montagnon, C.;** and **Thomas, T.:** Arthroscopic repair of distal supraspinatus tears with Revo screw and permanent mattress sutures — a preliminary report. Read at the Annual Meeting of the American Shoulder and Elbow Surgeons, Amelia Island, Florida, Oct. 20, 1996.

19. **Hawkins, R. J.; Misamore, G. W.;** and **Hobeika, P. E.:** Surgery for full-thickness rotator-cuff tears. *J. Bone and Joint Surg.,* 67-A: 1349-1355, Dec. 1985.

20. **McLaughlin, H. L.:** Repair of major cuff ruptures. *Surg. Clin. North America,* 43: 1535-1540, 1963.

21. **Misamore, G. W.; Ziegler, D. W.;** and **Rushton, J. L., II:** Repair of the rotator cuff. A comparison of results in two populations of patients. *J. Bone and Joint Surg.,* 77-A: 1335-1339, Sept. 1995.

22. **Montgomery, T. J.; Yerger, B.;** and **Savoie, F. H.:** Management of rotator cuff tears: a comparison of arthroscopic debridement and surgical repair. *J. Shoulder and Elbow Surg.,* 3: 70-78, 1994.

23. **Neer, C. S., II:** Anterior acromioplasty for the chronic impingement syndrome in the shoulder. A preliminary report. *J. Bone and Joint Surg.,* 54-A: 41-50, Jan. 1972.

24. **Neer, C. S., II:** Impingement lesions. *Clin. Orthop.,* 173: 70-77, 1983.

25. **Ogilvie-Harris, D. J.,** and **Demazière, A.:** Arthroscopic debridement versus open repair for rotator cuff tears. A prospective cohort study. *J. Bone and Joint Surg.,* 75-B(3): 416-420, 1993.

26. **Paulos, L. E.,** and **Kody, M. H.:** Arthroscopically enhanced "miniapproach" to rotator cuff repair. *Am. J. Sports Med.,* 22: 19-25, 1994.

27. **Richards, R. R.; An, K. N.; Bigliani, L. U.; Friedman, R. J.; Gartsman, G. M.; Gristina, A. G.; Iannotti, J. P.; Mow, V. C.; Sidles, J. A.;** and **Zuckerman, J. D.:** A standardized method for the assessment of shoulder function. *J. Shoulder and Elbow Surg.,* 3: 347-352, 1994.

28. **Seitz, W. H., Jr.,** and **Froimson, A. I.:** Comparison of subacromial arthroscopic decompression in partial and full thickness rotator cuff tears. *J. Bone and Joint Surg.,* 74-B (Supplement III): 294, 1992.

29. **Snyder, S. J.:** Shoulder instability. In *Shoulder Arthroscopy,* pp. 179-214. New York, McGraw-Hill, 1994.

30. **Snyder, S. J.; Mileski, R. A.;** and **Karzel, R. P.:** Results of arthroscopic rotator cuff repair. Read at the Annual Meeting of the American Shoulder and Elbow Surgeons, Amelia Island, Florida, Oct. 20, 1996.

31. **Snyder, S. J.; Pachelli, A. F.; Del Pizzo, W.; Friedman, M. J.; Ferkel, R. D.;** and **Pattee, G.:** Partial thickness rotator cuff tears: results of arthroscopic treatment. *Arthroscopy,* 7: 1-7, 1991.

32. **Vastamaki, M.:** Factors influencing the operative results of rotator cuff rupture. *Internat. Orthop.,* 10: 177-181, 1986.

33. **Ware, J. E., Jr.:** Standards for validating health measures: definition and content. *J. Chronic Dis.,* 40: 473-480, 1987.

34. **Ware, J. E., Jr.,** and **Sherbourne, C. D.:** The MOS 36-item short-form health survey (SF-36). I. Conceptual framework and item selection. *Med. Care,* 30: 473-483, 1992.

35. **Wolf, E. M.; Cheng, J. C.;** and **Dickson, K.:** Humeral avulsion of glenohumeral ligaments as a cause of anterior shoulder instability. *Arthroscopy,* 11: 600-607, 1995.

36. **Wolfgang, G. L.:** Surgical repair of tears of the rotator cuff of the shoulder. Factors influencing the result. *J. Bone and Joint Surg.,* 56-A: 14-26, Jan. 1974.

37. **Zvijac, J. E.; Levy, H. J.;** and **Lemak, L. J.:** Arthroscopic subacromial decompression in the treatment of full thickness rotator cuff tears: a 3- to 6-year follow-up. *Arthroscopy,* 10: 518-523, 1994.

Full-Thickness Rotator Cuff Tears: Factors Affecting Surgical Outcome

Joseph P. Iannotti, MD, PhD

Abstract

Eighty-five percent to 95% of patients who undergo primary surgical repair of full-thickness rotator cuff tears have a significant decrease in shoulder pain and improvement in shoulder function. The results of surgery are dependent on the surgical technique, the extent of pathologic changes in the rotator cuff, and the postoperative rehabilitation protocol. Preoperative factors associated with a less favorable result are the size of the tear, the quality of the tissues, the presence of a chronic rupture of the long head of the biceps tendon, and the degree of preoperative shoulder weakness. Surgical factors associated with a less favorable result include inadequate acromioplasty, residual symptomatic acromioclavicular arthritis, inadequate rotator cuff tissue mobilization, deltoid detachment or denervation, and failure of rotator cuff healing. Clinical evaluation and preoperative imaging of the shoulder will improve patient selection and counseling. Meticulous surgical technique and postoperative rehabilitation will optimize the final result.

J Am Acad Orthop Surg 1994;2:87-95

Disorders of the rotator cuff constitute the most common source of shoulder pain. The wide spectrum of pathologic conditions includes rotator cuff tendinitis, partial- and full-thickness tears, and calcific tendinopathy. Many etiologic factors underlie these conditions, but the pathogenesis remains controversial. Important factors include age-related degeneration of the tendons, mechanical impingement on the rotator cuff by subacromial and acromioclavicular joint spurs, and changes in the vascularity of the rotator cuff tendon. However, the natural history and progression of rotator cuff disease from simple tendinitis to partial- and full-thickness rotator cuff tears remain poorly understood and are an area of considerable debate.

In this article I will review the preoperative evaluation of full-thickness rotator cuff tears, the surgical management of primary rotator cuff repair, and the factors that influence the postoperative functional outcome.

Preoperative Evaluation

History

The presence of preinjury rotator cuff symptoms correlates with the degree of tendon degeneration and can be an important factor in predicting the outcome of surgical management. The combination of long-standing rotator cuff symptoms and a large full-thickness cuff tear following low-velocity trauma is generally indicative of an acute extension of a chronic degenerative rotator cuff defect. The acute extension is usually associated with pain and weakness. Tears often are associated with fair- or poor-quality degenerative tissue, a significant degree of tendon retraction, peritendinous adhesions, and soft-tissue capsular contracture.

Full-thickness rotator cuff tears associated with high-velocity trauma, particularly in younger individuals, are rarer. When younger patients are treated with early surgery, degenerative changes in the tendons usually do not occur. The prognosis is also better, as measured by greater active postoperative elevation of the arm compared with that after late repair.[1]

Physical Examination

The physical examination should assess the range of motion and the degree of weakness of the rotator cuff musculature. The disparities in active and passive arcs of shoulder elevation are measured. Rotator cuff weakness is then defined by evaluation of muscle strength in both external rotation and internal rotation. The degree of muscular atrophy of the supraspinous and infraspinous fossae is also noted. External rotation strength can be tested in various positions of arm elevation but is least affected by pain when tested

Dr. Iannotti is Associate Professor of Orthopaedic Surgery and Chief, Shoulder Service, Department of Orthopaedic Surgery, University of Pennsylvania School of Medicine, Philadelphia.

Reprint requests: Dr. Iannotti, 3400 Spruce Street, Philadelphia, PA 19104.

with the arm placed at the side. Internal rotation is evaluated by the lift-off test.

Significant weakness (grade 3 or less) of external rotation and significant muscular atrophy are associated with larger chronic full-thickness tears, which extend well into the infraspinatus tendon and are, on average, more difficult to repair. Not surprisingly, these tears are associated with a higher occurrence of persistent postoperative full-thickness defects of the rotator cuff and postoperative weakness.[2,3]

A less favorable prognosis for functional recovery following surgery also should be anticipated in patients with the constellation of large chronic rotator cuff defects, chronic rupture of the long head of the biceps tendon, marked weakness of forward flexion, chronic atrophy of the deltoid, and cephalic migration of the humeral head when active elevation of the arm is attempted. These clinical findings often are associated with massive chronic ruptures of the rotator cuff that are not reparable by primary suturing techniques. These cases may require reconstructive procedures using local or distant tendon transfer to achieve coverage of the humeral head.

Local Anesthetic Injections

The response to local anesthetic injections into the subacromial space or acromioclavicular joint has diagnostic and prognostic value. A marked temporary decrease in shoulder pain associated with the impingement signs helps to confirm the diagnosis of an intrinsic shoulder disorder localized to the rotator cuff and is usually a reflection of the level of pain improvement that can be expected following rotator cuff surgery.[4] In some cases, improvement of active arcs of shoulder motion is also observed.

A significant decrease in shoulder pain with local anesthetic injection is also helpful in distinguishing between true weakness of external rotation or elevation and weakness due to pain. Pain in the acromioclavicular joint that persists following subacromial injection of a local anesthetic suggests significant concomitant acromioclavicular arthropathy and is an indication to assess pain relief by means of a subsequent anesthetic injection into the acromioclavicular joint. If a further significant decrease in shoulder pain is observed and the imaging studies demonstrate significant degenerative changes in the acromioclavicular joint, primary distal clavicular resection is indicated. Lack of improvement with either injection test suggests that an alternative cause for the shoulder pain should be considered.

Imaging Studies

The plain radiographic examination should include an anteroposterior (AP) view in the plane of the scapula and an axillary view of the shoulder. Specialized views are taken to evaluate the degree of acromioclavicular arthritis and supraspinatus outlet narrowing. These include the AP coronal 30-degree caudal-tilt view (Fig. 1, A), the supraspinatus outlet view (10- to 15-degree caudal-tilt lateral scapular view) (Fig. 1, B), and the AP coronal 10- to 30-degree cephalic-tilt view to evaluate the acromioclavicular joint (Fig. 1, C). When properly obtained, these views can be used to define the degree of anterior extension of the acromion beyond the anterior border of the clavicle (Fig. 1, A), the morphology and size of the spur associated with the undersurface of the acromion (Fig. 1, B), and the presence of cystic and degenerative changes in the acromioclavicular joint (Fig. 1, C).

Additional imaging studies useful in the diagnosis of a full-thickness tear of the rotator cuff include arthrography, ultrasonography, and magnetic resonance (MR) imaging. Arthrography has been considered the standard study, with a reported accuracy greater than 95% in the diagnosis of full-thickness cuff tears[5] (Fig. 2), but it has not been universally reported to have a high degree of accuracy in determining the size of a full-thickness tear or the presence of a partial-thickness tear. Arthrography of the shoulder is easily performed and interpreted but is an invasive procedure associated with transient synovitis and a very small potential for infection.

Ultrasonography of the shoulder has been reported to be an accurate and cost-effective noninvasive screening tool for the diagnosis of full-thickness rotator cuff tears[6,7] (Fig. 3). The accuracy of ultrasonography is highly dependent on the experience of the ultrasonographer and the type of equipment used. Its accuracy is significantly improved by obtaining dynamic images through the range of shoulder motion. Using only static images results in decreased accuracy in the diagnosis of full-thickness rotator cuff tears. Ultrasonography has been used to measure the size of the tear and the degree of tendon retraction. Ultrasonography has not yet achieved widespread use in North America as a routine imaging study of the rotator cuff and is most likely to be used in the centers with the most experience in its performance and interpretation.

Magnetic resonance imaging of the shoulder has also been shown to be highly accurate for the diagnosis of full-thickness rotator cuff tears[8] (Fig. 4). The advantages of MR imaging, in addition to its noninvasiveness, include the capacity to accurately measure the size of the cuff defect, the magnitude of tendon retraction, and the degree of supraspinatus and infraspinatus muscular atrophy. The presence of acromioclavicular joint arthritis and acromial spur formation can be determined. Magnetic resonance imaging is also helpful in defining

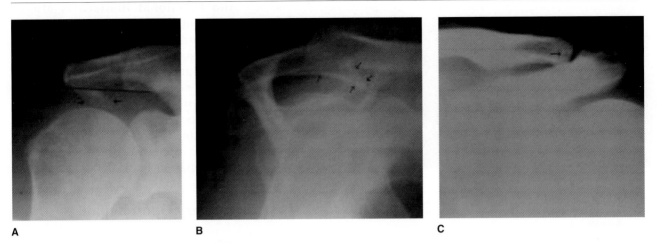

A   **B**   **C**

Fig. 1   Specialized radiographic views of the shoulder. **A,** An AP coronal 30-degree caudal-tilt (Rockwood tilt) view demonstrating anterior extension of the acromion (arrows) beyond the anterior border of the clavicle (line). **B,** Supraspinatus outlet view demonstrating a large anteroinferior acromial osteophyte (arrows). (Reproduced with permission from Iannotti JP [ed]: *Rotator Cuff Disorders: Evaluation and Treatment.* American Academy of Orthopaedic Surgeons Monograph Series. Rosemont, Ill: American Academy of Orthopaedic Surgeons, 1991, p 15.) **C,** An AP coronal 15-degree cephalic-tilt view (Zanca view) demonstrating cystic changes at the distal end of the clavicle (arrow).

other associated pathologic conditions, including glenohumeral arthritis, capsular and labral pathologic changes, rupture of the long head of the biceps tendon, and ganglion cysts. Ganglion cysts can simulate the clinical findings of a chronic full-thickness rotator cuff tear by extrinsic compression of the suprascapular nerve. The accuracy of MR imaging is dependent on the experi-

ence of the reader, the technique of MR sequencing, and the equipment utilized.

Certain anatomic findings that can be depicted on MR imaging studies correlate with less favorable functional outcomes following rotator cuff repair, among them large tears involving the subscapularis and the infraspinatus and teres minor, chronic rupture of the long head of the biceps

tendon, cephalic migration of the humeral head, early degenerative changes of the glenohumeral articulation, and moderate to severe atrophy of the supraspinatus and infraspinatus musculature. These pathologic findings are easily identified by experienced MR imagers and often correlate well with the clinical findings.[8]

Goals and Indications for Surgical Intervention

The primary goal of surgical intervention for the vast majority of patients with rotator cuff tears is to decrease pain, including rest pain, night pain, and pain with activities of daily living. Additional goals of surgery are to improve shoulder function and to limit the progression of rotator cuff tendinopathy.

The indications for surgical intervention must be individualized and are dependent on the patient's age and physical demands, the size of the rotator cuff tear, the mechanism of injury, and the progression of pain. It is my preference to advise initial nonoperative treatment for patients who

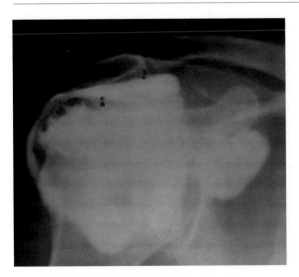

Fig. 2   An AP single-contrast arthrogram demonstrating a full-thickness rotator cuff tear with contrast material within the subacromial space (arrows). (Reproduced with permission from Iannotti JP [ed]: *Rotator Cuff Disorders: Evaluation and Treatment.* American Academy of Orthopaedic Surgeons Monograph Series. Rosemont, Ill: American Academy of Orthopaedic Surgeons, 1991, p 19.)

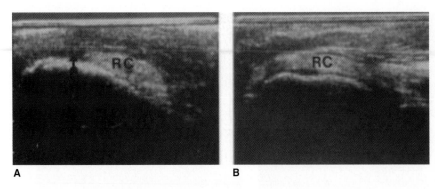

Fig. 3 Longitudinal sonograms of both shoulders. **A,** Image of the right shoulder depicts a full-thickness tear (arrow) of the rotator cuff (RC). **B,** Image of the left shoulder shows an intact rotator cuff.

have good active arcs of shoulder motion and strength at the time of their initial presentation and who have either a chronic rotator cuff tear or an acute extension of a small tear superposed on chronic symptoms. Such patients generally have minimal involvement of the posterior aspect of the rotator cuff (infraspinatus and teres minor). For patients with less severe symptoms, nonoperative treatment may simply be modification of activity and a home exercise program. For patients with more severe symptoms, nonoperative treatment includes oral anti-inflammatory medication, occasional subacromial injection of corticosteroids, and supervised physical therapy.

The length of nonoperative treatment must be individualized on the basis of the pathologic changes, the patient's response to treatment, and his or her functional demands and expectations. If pain persists despite compliance with a well-supervised nonoperative treatment program, surgical intervention can be recommended, provided the pain level

and functional limitations are sufficiently serious. Early surgical intervention is indicated in patients who sustain acute trauma associated with significant weakness of the shoulder and posterior cuff involvement, particularly in younger patients with higher functional demands. Patients with acute tears or large extensions of chronic cuff tears can be included in this group.

Primary Open Repair

With a few exceptions, all operative procedures described in the recent literature for primary repair of chronic rotator cuff tears include the use of an anteroinferior acromioplasty to provide adequate decompression of the subacromial space.[9-17] Almost all patients with chronic full-thickness rotator cuff tears have significant subacromial outlet narrowing, and an adequate acromioplasty has been shown to be an important element in the subsequent relief of shoulder pain.[14-16]

The presence of clinically significant acromioclavicular joint arthritis, as defined by clinical examination, injection testing, and imaging studies, serves as the indication for concomitant formal distal clavicle resection. Informal surveys of shoulder surgeons indicate that 5% to 20% of patients meet this criterion. Without this primary indication for distal clavicle resection, an adequate decompression of only the undersurface of the acromioclavicular joint is generally performed when there is significant impingement in this area. Anterior acromioplasty may not be necessary in the rare case of a young patient with an acute traumatic rotator cuff tear, but it is sometimes performed to aid in surgical exposure. In patients with massive tears and a proximally migrated humerus, preservation and repair of the coracoacromial ligament is con-

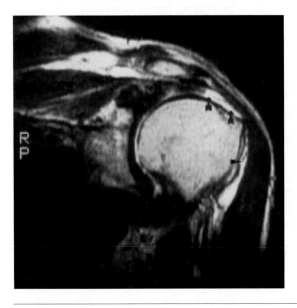

Fig. 4 Coronal oblique T2-weighted (repetition time = 2,000 msec; echo time = 80 msec) MR image (16-cm field of view, 4-mm section thickness) depicts synovial fluid within a full-thickness defect of the supraspinatus tendon (arrows). Synovial fluid extends into the subdeltoid space (arrowhead). There is minimal atrophy of the supraspinatus muscle belly.

sidered, and distal clavicle resection and aggressive acromioplasty are avoided.

Technique

Most surgeons prefer an anterosuperior approach to the shoulder performed within Langer's lines (Fig. 5). The approach is usually performed in association with detachment of a small portion of the anterior deltoid from the acromioclavicular joint to the anterolateral corner of the acromion, with splitting of the fibers of the middle deltoid for a distance of 3 to 4 cm. An anteroinferior acromioplasty is performed as described by Neer.[4]

Mobilization of the cuff tendons requires release of all adhesions in the subacromial space, the coracohumeral ligament at the base of the coracoid, and occasionally the intraarticular portion of the capsule when it is contracted (Fig. 6). To avoid injury of the suprascapular nerve, dissection of the supraspinatus and infraspinatus musculature medial to the glenoid margin should not exceed 1.5 to 2.0 cm. Debridement of the edges of the rotator cuff tendon should remove only tissue that is mechanically unsound. Relaxing incisions at the rotator interval may also improve lateral mobilization of the tendon for repair to a bone trough with the arm held at the patient's side (Fig. 7).

Most tears require direct suturing of the tendon edge to a bone trough in the greater tuberosity. A shallow bone trough is made to expose the bleeding cancellous bone of the tuberosity, and care is taken to preserve the cortical bone of the lateral portion of the greater tuberosity (Fig. 8, A). The primary repair of the rotator cuff tear is performed utilizing heavy nonabsorbable suture (No. 2 or larger). The technique for repair is dictated by the configuration of the tendon tear.

Horizontal mattress sutures are placed through drill holes in the tuberosity and passed through the lateral edge of the cuff tendon (Fig. 8, B and C). In most cases, tendon-to-tendon repair is also performed along

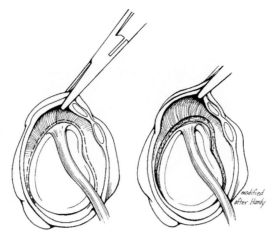

Fig. 6 Technique of capsular advancement in patients with fixed, retracted rotator cuff tears.

with suturing of the lateral tendon edge to a bone trough. The deltoid is sutured back to the acromion through drill holes and to the deltotrapezius aponeuroses. Routine skin closure includes subcuticular suturing.

Postoperative management after primary repair of full-thickness cuff tears must be individualized to

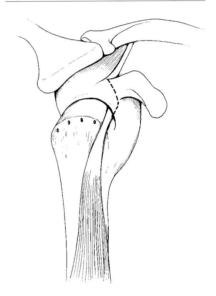

Fig. 7 Incision in the rotator cuff interval from the edge of the tear to the base of the coracoid releases the coracohumeral ligament and supraspinatus tendon as a unit, allowing lateral mobilization of tissue toward the greater tuberosity.

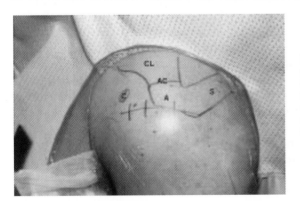

Fig. 5 Anterosuperior incision for open acromioplasty and rotator cuff repair. A = acromion; AC = acromioclavicular joint; C = coracoid; CL = distal clavicle; S = spine of the scapula.

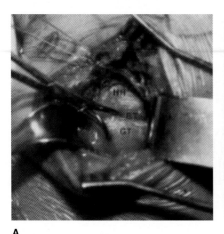 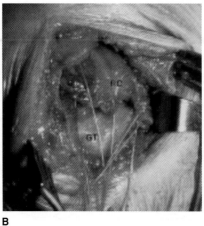 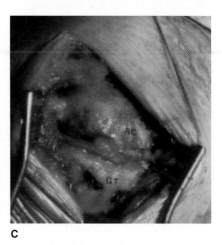

A   B   C

Fig. 8 Suturing procedure. **A,** Bone trough (BT) between the humeral head (HH) and the greater tuberosity (GT). The hole made by passing a towel clip from the bone trough through the lateral wall of the greater tuberosity is used to pass suture for tendon-to-bone repair. **B,** Traction sutures placed within the rotator cuff (RC) are used to mobilize the tendon edges and then pulled laterally to the bone trough within the greater tuberosity. **C,** Horizontal mattress sutures are passed from the greater tuberosity through the rotator cuff and tied over a bone bridge in the greater tuberosity.

account for the size of the tear, the quality of the tissues, the difficulty of repair, and the patient's goals. In general, supine active assisted motion is started on the first postoperative day. Waist-level use of the hand can in most cases be started immediately after surgery. Active range-of-motion exercises and isotonic strengthening are usually started 6 to 8 weeks after surgery. Progression of the strengthening program must be individualized; the period required for full rehabilitation ranges from 6 to 12 months after surgery.

Results

The overall clinical results with respect to shoulder pain have been reported to be satisfactory in 85% to 95% of patients who have undergone open repair of full-thickness tears.[2-4,9-13] If an early satisfactory result is obtained, the pain relief and functional improvement appear to be lasting. Analysis of the 7- to 15-year follow-up of patients who underwent primary rotator cuff repair demonstrates maintenance of satisfactory clinical results without

significant deterioration of function or recurrence of shoulder pain.[9,18,19] Improvement in pain level is highly correlated with patient satisfaction.

Several recent retrospective studies of rotator cuff repair also report that 85% to 95% of patients have significant improvement in shoulder function following primary rotator cuff repair.[2,3,9-13] The degree of functional improvement reported is difficult to compare among these studies due to the wide variation in techniques utilized to define function and to measure shoulder strength and functional outcome. Most reports indicate that improvement in pain level correlates with the adequacy of acromioplasty and subacromial decompression.[14-17] Improvement of function is correlated with improvement in pain level as well as adequacy of the rotator cuff repair and healing of the rotator cuff defect.[2,16] Postoperative strength and function correlate with the preoperative size of the tear, the quality of the tendon tissue, and the ease of tissue mobilization.[3]

Significant postoperative weakness on forward flexion and difficulty

with use of the arm at or above shoulder level are usually seen in the following circumstances: (1) failure of repair of a full-thickness cuff tear or a postoperative tear, particularly when the tear involves the posterior aspect of the rotator cuff (infraspinatus and teres minor); (2) deltoid detachment or denervation; and (3) rupture of the long head of the biceps tendon.[20-22]

It may still be possible to achieve active elevation of the arm above shoulder level in the presence of a postoperative full-thickness cuff tear as long as there is significant improvement in the postoperative pain level, full rehabilitation of the deltoid, and sufficient anterior and posterior rotator cuff musculature to maintain containment of the humeral head within the glenoid fossa during elevation of the arm.[2] In such cases, however, patients often have decreased strength of external rotation and abduction. Despite the persistence of weakness in patients with postoperative rotator cuff defects, improvement of the pain level and concomitant improvement of shoulder function often result in a high level of patient satisfaction.[2,23]

Arthroscopic Repair

The preliminary results and short-term follow-up after arthroscopic subacromial decompression in conjunction with arthroscopic rotator cuff repair or arthroscopically assisted rotator cuff repair have recently been reported.[23,24] The principles of arthroscopically assisted rotator cuff repair and subacromial decompression are the same as those of open procedures. An adequate decompression must be carried out beneath the acromion and the acromioclavicular joint. When indicated, arthroscopic resection of the distal clavicle may be necessary. Mobilization of rotator cuff tissue, release of adhesions and scar tissue, and repair of the tendon to a well-prepared bleeding bone trough are required.

Arthroscopic techniques appear to provide acceptable clinical results, particularly in patients with small rotator cuff tears involving a single tendon with good- to excellent-quality tissue and minimal tissue retraction and scarring. The challenge of arthroscopic surgery for rotator cuff repair lies in proper patient selection and improvement of the techniques for tendon-to-bone repair.

Technique

After adequate arthroscopic subacromial decompression, the anterolateral portal is utilized for preparing a bone trough for tendon repair. The techniques for arthroscopic rotator cuff repair to a bone trough include percutaneous insertion of absorbable tacks and metallic staples. Use of single- or double-point fixation, tacks, or staples carries the potential for loss of fixation, particularly in patients with soft cancellous bone. Loss of fixation can result in failure of tendon repair as well as mechanical irritation caused by these devices in the subacromial space. An alternative technique is arthroscopically assisted rotator cuff repair using standard suture techniques through a lateral deltoid-splitting incision.[24,25] This technique requires an open procedure to split the deltoid, but generally does not require detachment of the deltoid from the acromion, particularly in patients with small cuff tears of the supraspinatus tendon.

Results

The recently reported results of arthroscopically assisted techniques have been favorable.[24,25] However, the results are not directly comparable with the results of traditional open surgery because studies involving open techniques include larger numbers of patients, many of whom have large chronic tears requiring extensive soft-tissue mobilization. Arthroscopically assisted techniques for cuff repair have not been thoroughly evaluated for these more difficult cases. Further refinement of arthroscopic techniques for rotator cuff repair and analysis of long-term follow-up data will facilitate definition of the appropriate indications for arthroscopic rotator cuff repair. At the present time, arthroscopic techniques for rotator cuff repair remain an area for further development and careful consideration.

Repair of Massive Tears Not Amenable to Primary Repair

Surgical options for treatment of patients with massive full-thickness rotator cuff tears that are not amenable to primary repair include subacromial decompression and debridement of nonviable rotator cuff tissue without attempts at rotator cuff reconstruction, the use of autogenous or allograft tendon grafts, and the use of active tendon transfers.

Rockwood et al[23] analyzed the data on a large group of patients treated by subacromial decompression and debridement of mechanically nonviable rotator cuff tissue. The results were satisfactory in 85% of their patients, as measured by excellent improvement in pain level and active elevation of the arm above shoulder level. The patients with the best results had a well-compensated and well-rehabilitated deltoid, an intact long head of the biceps tendon, and significant improvement in pain level. Quantitative measurements of shoulder strength were not reported in this series; therefore, these results cannot be compared with those in patients who underwent rotator cuff repair.

The use of prosthetic materials or allograft tissue for rotator cuff repair has been reported to have variable results.[26,27] Improvement in pain level and function has been reported with the use of freeze-dried allograft in selected cases.[27] Use of these materials will require further experimental and clinical evaluation and cannot be strongly advocated at this time.

Tendon transfers may involve the subscapularis, latissimus dorsi, deltoid, or trapezius. Transfer of the upper two thirds of the subscapularis tendon is a commonly performed tendon transfer and is particularly useful for irreparable defects of the supraspinatus tendon.[28] It is best performed in patients with an intact or reparable posterior rotator cuff and an intact long head of the biceps tendon. Transfer of the subscapularis requires maintenance of the inferior glenohumeral capsular ligaments and the inferior third of the subscapularis muscle. This procedure can be performed for isolated reconstruction of the rotator cuff and is also used in prosthetic shoulder replacement associated with rotator cuff tears and deficient superior coverage of the humeral head.

Latissimus dorsi transfer is a difficult and extensive operative procedure, which is primarily indicated for patients with loss of external rotational power and irreparable defects of the posterior portion of the rotator cuff involving the infraspinatus and teres minor tendons.[29,30] The best results occur in patients with an intact subscapularis and long head of the biceps tendon and well-compensated deltoid function. Latissimus dorsi transfer is a demanding operative procedure, and at the present time there is limited experience in the United States.

Use of a portion of the middle deltoid as a tissue transfer in patients with irreparable rotator cuff tears also has been reported.[31] This technique has had limited use in Europe and has not yet been widely accepted in the United States, nor has it been adequately evaluated.

Trapezius transfers for repair of massive rotator cuff tears are now of purely historic interest and are no longer performed.

Summary

Clinical evaluation of patients with full-thickness rotator cuff tears can define many of the prognostic factors that influence the long-term functional outcome of rotator cuff repair. Plain radiographs remain the most important diagnostic tool for evaluating the degree of subacromial outlet narrowing and acromioclavicular joint disease. Although arthrography, ultrasonography, and MR imaging are all accurate for the diagnosis of full-thickness rotator cuff tears in specific clinical settings, MR imaging appears to be the most useful in evaluating the prognostic factors that influence the functional outcome following surgical repair.

A carefully conducted trial of nonoperative treatment should generally precede surgery. Surgical treatment of full-thickness rotator cuff tears yields patient satisfaction in a large percentage of patients and significant improvement in pain and function levels, which appear to be maintained over a 7- to 15-year follow-up period. Subacromial decompression and appropriate management of clinically significant acromioclavicular disease will, in most cases, decrease pain associated with impingement. Successful repair and healing of full-thickness cuff tears are highly correlated with improvement in shoulder strength.

Clinical, radiographic, and operative factors that are associated with a higher incidence of less favorable results include the presence of large and massive rotator cuff tears involving the infraspinatus and teres minor, significant preoperative weakness of external rotation and abduction, chronic rupture of the long head of the biceps tendon, anterior deltoid denervation or detachment, poor-quality tendon tissue, and difficulty with intraoperative tissue mobilization. These factors are interrelated and can be helpful both in the diagnosis and in preoperative patient counseling.

References

1. Bassett RW, Cofield RH: Acute tears of the rotator cuff: The timing of surgical repair. *Clin Orthop* 1983;175:18-24.
2. Harryman DT II, Mack LA, Wang KY, et al: Repairs of the rotator cuff: Correlation of functional results with integrity of the cuff. *J Bone Joint Surg Am* 1991;73:982-989.
3. Iannotti JP, Bernot M, Kuhlman J, et al: Prospective evaluation of rotator cuff repair. *J Shoulder Elbow Surg* 1993;2:S9.
4. Neer CS II: Anterior acromioplasty for the chronic impingement syndrome in the shoulder: A preliminary report. *J Bone Joint Surg Am* 1972;54:41-50.
5. Mink JH, Harris E, Rappaport M: Rotator cuff tears: Evaluation using double-contrast shoulder arthrography. *Radiology* 1985;157:621-623.
6. Crass JR, Craig EV, Thompson RC, et al: Ultrasonography of the rotator cuff: Surgical correlation. *J Clin Ultrasound* 1984;12:487-491.
7. Mack LA, Nyberg DA, Matsen FR III, et al: Sonography of the postoperative shoulder. *AJR* 1988;150:1089-1093.
8. Iannotti JP, Zlatkin MB, Esterhai JL, et al: Magnetic resonance imaging of the shoulder: Sensitivity, specificity and predictive value. *J Bone Joint Surg Am* 1991;73:17-29.
9. Bigliani LU, Cordasco FA, McIlveen SJ, et al: Operative repair of massive rotator cuff tears: Long term results. *J Shoulder Elbow Surg* 1992;1:120-130.
10. Gore DR, Murray MP, Sepic SB, et al: Shoulder-muscle strength and range of motion following surgical repair of full-thickness rotator cuff tears. *J Bone Joint Surg Am* 1986;68:266-272.
11. Ellman H, Hanker G, Bayer M: Repair of the rotator cuff: End result study of factors influencing reconstruction. *J Bone Joint Surg Am* 1986;68:1136-1144.
12. Björkenheim JM, Paavolainen P, Ahovuo J, et al: Surgical repair of the rotator cuff and surrounding tissues: Factors influencing the results. *Clin Orthop* 1988;236:148-153.
13. Hawkins RJ, Misamore GW, Hobeika PE: Surgery for full-thickness rotator cuff tears. *J Bone Joint Surg Am* 1985;67:1349-1355.
14. Ogilvie-Harris DJ, Demaziere A: Arthroscopic debridement versus open repair for rotator cuff tears. *J Bone Joint Surg Br* 1993;75:416-420.
15. Packer NP, Calvert PT, Bayley JI, et al: Operative treatment of chronic ruptures of the rotator cuff of the shoulder. *J Bone Joint Surg Br* 1983;65:171-175.
16. Rockwood CA Jr, Williams GR: The shoulder impingement syndrome: Management of surgical treatment failures. *Orthop Trans* 1992;16:739-740.
17. Flugstad D, Matsen FA, Larry I, et al: Failed acromioplasty: Etiology and prevention. *Orthop Trans* 1986;10:229.
18. Neer CS II, Flatow EL, Lech O: Tears of

the rotator cuff: Long term results of anterior acromioplasty and repair. *Orthop Trans* 1988;12:673-674.

19. Adamson GJ, Tibone JE: Ten year assessment of primary rotator cuff repairs. *J Shoulder Elbow Surg* 1993;2: 57-63.

20. Bigliani LU, McIlveen SJ, Cordasco FA, et al: Operative management of failed rotator cuff repairs. *Orthop Trans* 1988;12:674.

21. DeOrio JK, Cofield RH: Results of a second attempt at surgical repair of a failed initial rotator cuff repair. *J Bone Joint Surg Am* 1984;66:563-567.

22. Neviaser RJ, Neviaser TJ: Re-operation for failed rotator cuff repair: Analysis of 50 cases. *J Shoulder Elbow Surg* 1992;1:283-286.

23. Rockwood CA Jr, Williams GR, Burkhead WZ Jr: Debridement of irreparable degenerative lesions of the rotator cuff. *Orthop Trans* 1992;16:740.

24. Paletta GA Jr, Warner JJP, Altchek DW, et al: Arthroscopic rotator cuff repair: Evaluation of results and a comparison of techniques. Presented at the 60th Annual Meeting of the American Academy of Orthopaedic Surgeons, San Francisco, Feb 18-23, 1993.

25. Weber SC, Schaefer RK: Mini open versus traditional open technique in the management of tears of the rotator cuff. Presented at the 60th Annual Meeting of the American Academy of Orthopaedic Surgeons, San Francisco, Feb 18-23, 1993.

26. Nasca RJ: The use of freeze-dried allografts in the management of global rotator cuff tears. *Clin Orthop* 1988; 228:218-226.

27. Neviaser JS, Neviaser RJ, Neviaser TJ: The repair of chronic massive ruptures of the rotator cuff of the shoulder by use of a freeze-dried rotator cuff. *J Bone Joint Surg Am* 1978;60:681-684.

28. Cofield RH: Subscapular muscle transposition for repair of chronic rotator cuff tears. *Surg Gynecol Obstet* 1982;154: 667-672.

29. Gerber C, Vinh TS, Hertel R, et al: Latissimus dorsi transfer for the treatment of massive tears of the rotator cuff: A preliminary report. *Clin Orthop* 1988; 232:51-61.

30. Gerber C: Latissimus dorsi transfer for the treatment of irreparable tears of the rotator cuff. *Clin Orthop* 1993;275: 152-160.

31. Augereau B: Rekonstruktion massiver Rotatorenmanschettenrupturen mit einem Deltoidlappen. *Orthopade* 1991; 20:315-319.

Transfer of the Pectoralis Major Muscle for the Treatment of Irreparable Rupture of the Subscapularis Tendon[*]

BY H. RESCH, M.D.†, P. POVACZ, M.D.†, E. RITTER, M.D.†, AND W. MATSCHI, PH.D.†, SALZBURG, AUSTRIA

Investigation performed at General Hospital Salzburg, Salzburg

Abstract

Background: The clinical diagnosis of a tear of the subscapularis tendon is difficult, and the resulting delays frequently cause a major time-lapse before repair is attempted. Diagnostic delay often means that surgical repair is no longer possible. In twelve patients who had an irreparable tear of the subscapularis tendon, the superior one-half to two-thirds of the tendon of the pectoralis major muscle was used as a substitute for the subscapularis tendon. In order to adapt the orientation of the transferred muscle to that of the subscapularis, it was routed behind the conjoined tendon of the coracobrachialis muscle and the short head of the biceps to the lesser tuberosity.

Methods: The operations were performed between May 1993 and June 1997. The average age of the twelve patients was sixty-five years old (range, forty-nine to eighty-one years old). Eight patients had an isolated rupture of the subscapularis tendon, and four had a concomitant lesion in the form of either a partial or a complete rupture of the supraspinatus tendon. The dominant symptoms were anterior shoulder pain and weakness that had responded poorly to nonoperative therapy. Four patients also had signs of recurrent anterior instability.

Results: After an average follow-up interval of twenty-eight months (range, twenty-four to fifty-four months), nine of the twelve patients assessed the final result as excellent or good; three, as fair; and none, as poor. Pain was reduced, with the score improving from an average of 1.7 points (of a maximum of 15 points) preoperatively to an average of 9.6 points postoperatively. The patients' subjective functional evaluation improved from an average score of 20 points preoperatively to an average of 63 points postoperatively. The average functional rating with use of the Constant and Murley score increased from 26.9 to 67.1 percent of normal. All four preoperatively unstable shoulders were stable at the time of the latest follow-up.

Conclusions: This repair technique can be recommended as a reconstructive procedure for elderly patients who have an irreparable tear of the subscapularis tendon.

The symptoms of a tear of the subscapularis tendon as described in the literature are anterior shoulder pain with dysfunction and weakness and a poor response to nonoperative therapy[6,9,10,15,19]. Both the pain and the dysfunction may be caused by a loss of balance between the anterior and posterior elements of the rotator cuff, which changes the kinematic pattern of the shoulder[1,2]. There is also agreement in the literature that the clinical diagnosis of a subscapularis tendon tear is difficult, often leading to a delay of months or even years before surgical repair is attempted[6,9].

Unlike an isolated rupture of the supraspinatus tendon, a rupture of the tendon of the subscapularis muscle can be followed by retraction of the tendon, which is unhindered by intact tendon tissue alongside of the rupture site. After a delay of several months or years, this retraction makes repair very difficult. Gerber et al. reported significantly better results in patients who had had only a short delay between the traumatic event and the repair compared with those who had had a considerable delay before the operation[10]. The average time between the injury and the operation in their series was fifteen months (range, one to fifty-six months)[10].

Compared with tears of the supraspinatus and infraspinatus tendons, rupture of the subscapularis tendon is rare. Codman reported involvement of the subscapularis tendon in only 3.5 percent of 200 rotator cuff tears[3]. Deutsch et al. found major involvement of the subscapularis tendon in fourteen (4 percent) of 350 rotator cuff tears[6], and Frankle and Cofield reported involvement of the subscapularis tendon in twenty-five (8 percent) of 301 full-thickness rotator cuff tears[7]. Hauser[12], Neviaser et al.[15], and Wirth and Rockwood[19] described subscapularis tendon tears following anterior traumatic dislocation of the shoulder. In the series of Neviaser et al., of thirty-one patients with a rotator cuff tear following dislocation of the shoulder, eight had a subscapularis tendon tear with consequent recurrent shoulder instability[15]. In the series of Wirth and Rockwood, of 221 patients who were operated on because of anterior instability, eighteen had a subscapularis tendon tear[19]. In 1991, Gerber and Krushell described sixteen patients with an isolated tear of the subscapularis tendon, which was clearly

*No benefits in any form have been received or will be received from a commercial party related directly or indirectly to the subject of this article. No funds were received in support of this study.

†General Hospital Salzburg, Unfallchirurgie, Müllner-Hauptstraße 48, A-5020 Salzburg, Austria. Please address requests for reprints to H. Resch.

the result of trauma involving hyperextension of the arm or extreme external rotation of the adducted arm[9]. In 1997, Deutsch et al. reported on fourteen patients who had an isolated rupture of the subscapularis tendon[6]; eleven patients had the same mechanism of injury as described by Gerber and Krushell[9].

The delay caused by difficulties in diagnosis leads to a situation in which mobilization of the retracted tendon is no longer possible or repair is not indicated because of the degree of atrophy in the muscle. On the other hand, persistent pain with shoulder dysfunction and, in some cases, pronounced anterior instability call for some form of surgical intervention. The irreparable subscapularis tendon can be replaced with the superior portion of the pectoralis major tendon. Wirth and Rockwood detached the superior half of the tendon of the pectoralis major from the humerus and transferred it superiorly to the humeral head[19]. However, with use of this procedure, the course of the subscapularis muscle is not followed and soft tissue is not interposed between the humeral head and the coracoid process.

The aim of the current study was to find a muscle-tendon unit to replace an irreparably torn subscapularis tendon and to evaluate the results following surgery.

Materials and Methods

Between May 1993 and June 1997, twelve patients who had a chronic, irreparable rupture of the tendon of the subscapularis muscle were operated on with use of a portion of the tendon of the pectoralis major muscle as a substitute. At the time of the intervention, the patients (ten men and two women) had an average age of sixty-five years (range, forty-nine to eighty-one years). The right shoulder was involved in seven patients and the left shoulder, in five. Eight patients had involvement of the dominant shoulder. Nine patients had sustained a definite injury. Three of them sustained the injury in a downhill-skiing accident, one was injured in a cross-country-skiing accident, two fell on a level surface, one fell from a ladder, one slipped on ice, and one had an accident at work. This last patient was the only one who was able to provide a precise description of the mechanism of injury (the adducted arm was subjected to abrupt external rotation). Three patients had no clear memory of a traumatic event. Four patients had a traumatic injury that caused anterior shoulder dislocation followed by recurrent anterior instability. Two patients had symptoms that were so severe they had very little functional use of the arm.

Eight of the twelve patients had been examined initially at an outside institution, where the correct diagnosis had been made for only one. Two patients had had a previous repair of the rotator cuff, which had failed to reveal the rupture of the subscapularis tendon. The average interval from the traumatic event or the onset of the symptoms to the surgical procedure was twenty-seven

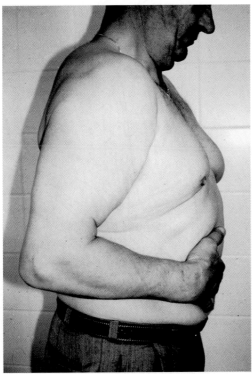

FIG. 1-A   FIG. 1-B

Figs. 1-A and 1-B: Photographs of a patient performing the belly-press test.
Fig. 1-A: Positive result on the injured side. With the hand pressed against the belly, the patient cannot maintain the elbow anterior to the midline of the trunk as seen from the side.
Fig. 1-B: Negative result on the contralateral side. The elbow remains in the frontal plane.

TABLE I
FUNCTIONAL ASSESSMENT SCORE ACCORDING TO
THE SYSTEM OF CONSTANT AND MURLEY[4]

Category	No. of Points
Subjective criteria	
Pain	0-15
Activities of daily life	
Ability to perform professional activities	0-4
Ability to perform leisure activities	0-4
Sleep	0-2
Level at which work can be performed	0-10
Waist	2
Xyphoid	4
Neck	6
Head	8
Above head	10
Objective criteria	
Active flexion without pain	0-10
Active abduction without pain	0-10
>150 degrees	10
121-150 degrees	8
91-120 degrees	6
61-90 degrees	4
31-60 degrees	2
0-30 degrees	0
Functional external rotation	0-10
Hand behind head with elbow forward	2
Hand behind head with elbow backward	2
Hand above head with elbow forward	2
Hand above head with elbow backward	2
Full elevation from last position	2
Functional internal rotation	0-10
With dorsum of hand on back, head of third metacarpal reaches:	
T10 spinous process	10
T8 spinous process	8
L3 spinous process	6
S1 spinous process	4
Ipsilateral buttock	2
Strength of abduction	0-25
(1 lb. [0.45 kg] = 1 point)	

available for only eight patients; in five, it was an average of 10 degrees greater on the injured side than on the contralateral side. Evaluation of internal rotation showed that two patients were able to touch the lumbar spine; three, the sacrum; five, the buttock; and two, the thigh only.

The lift-off test as described by Gerber and Krushell[9] could be used for the five patients who could touch their back. All five had a positive result — that is, they were incapable of maintaining the raised position of the hand behind the back. Eight patients were evaluated with the so-called belly-press test[10], and all eight had a positive result — that is, when they exerted pressure on the stomach they were not able to maintain the elbow anterior to the midline of the trunk as viewed from the side; instead, the elbow dropped back behind the trunk (Figs. 1-A and 1-B). In our study, the test was performed with the examiner's hand inserted between the patient's hand and stomach to assess the pressure exerted on the stomach compared with that exerted by the hand on the uninjured side. All patients demonstrated a difference in the pressure exerted against the stomach compared with that exerted by the hand on the contralateral side. Eight of the twelve patients were able to perform strength tests with the arm in 90 degrees of abduction and 90 degrees

months (range, sixteen to sixty months).

When first seen in our department, all twelve patients reported disabling anterior shoulder pain radiating into the upper arm and down as far as the hand. The pain occurred during the night and during activities of daily living. All patients had pronounced dysfunction and weakness, and two of the four patients with shoulder instability had almost complete loss of arm function.

Active flexion of the involved shoulder was identical to that on the contralateral side in seven patients, and it was reduced by an average of 36 degrees in five. Active flexion in the twelve patients averaged 93 degrees (range, 30 to 170 degrees). In six patients active abduction was the same as that on the uninjured side, and in six it was reduced by an average of 38 degrees. Active abduction in the twelve patients averaged 85 degrees (range, 20 to 170 degrees). Ten patients had the same amount of active external rotation on both sides, and two had less active external rotation on the injured side. Measurements of passive external rotation were

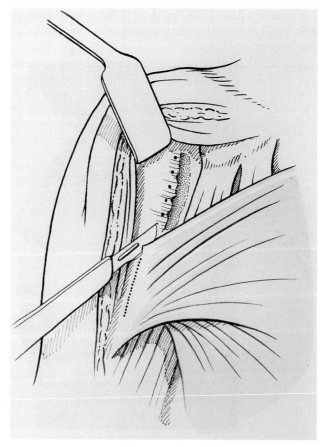

FIG. 2-A

Figs. 2-A, 2-B, and 2-C: Surgical technique.
Fig. 2-A: Schematic view of the detachment of the superior one-half to two-thirds of the pectoralis major tendon from the humerus.

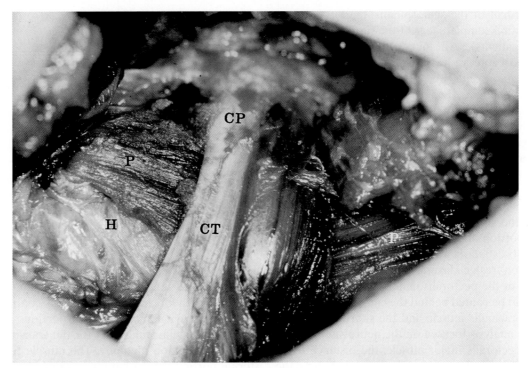

FIG. 2-B

Photograph made after blunt exploration, showing how a portion of the pectoralis major is passed between the pectoralis minor and the conjoined tendon and then behind the conjoined tendon to the lesser tuberosity, where it is attached with bone sutures. CP = coracoid process, CT = conjoined tendon, H = humeral head, and P = pectoralis major muscle (transferred portion).

of flexion; a spring balance was used to measure the force in the wrist in kilograms. The remaining four patients were not able to raise the arm actively to 90 degrees for testing. The spring balance also was used, for all twelve patients, to measure internal rotation strength against manual resistance with the upper arm adducted and the forearm in the neutral position.

Preoperative and postoperative function was assessed with use of the 100-point scoring system of Constant and Murley[4] (Table I). The total score for each patient was recorded and related to age and gender-matched normal values (Table II), as identified by Constant and Murley, which allowed the score to be expressed as a percentage of normal. In addition, the patients were asked to assess the function of the shoulder on a 100-point visual analog scale preoperatively and postoperatively.

Anteroposterior, axillary, and outlet radiographs were made for all patients preoperatively. Ultrasonographic examination of the rotator cuff also was performed for all patients. In each patient, it was possible to determine the full extent of the defect — that is, both the absence of the subscapularis tendon and, where relevant, the partial or complete defect of the supraspinatus tendon. For four patients, ultrasonography was followed by magnetic resonance imaging. This was done not merely to confirm the defect but also to obtain information on the condition of the muscle belly of the subscapularis and, if possible, to measure the distance between the coracoid process and the humeral head[8].

Intraoperative Findings

Eight patients were found to have an isolated rupture of the subscapularis tendon, with avulsion from the lesser tuberosity. In the remaining four patients, the rupture of the subscapularis tendon was combined with a rupture of

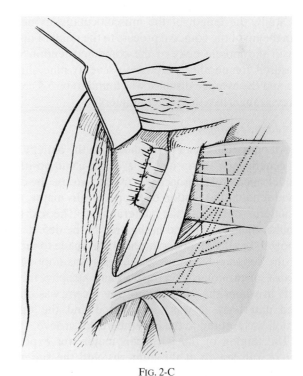

FIG. 2-C

Schematic view of the course of the muscle.

the anterior half of the supraspinatus tendon (two patients) or with a complete tear of the supraspinatus tendon (two patients). All four patients demonstrated clinical signs of anterior instability; two had recurrent anterior dislocation and two, recurrent anterior subluxation. In eight patients, the subscapularis tendon tear was complete, whereas in four, tendinous fibers that were approximately five millimeters wide remained intact at the distal margin. In eight patients, the long head of the biceps had ruptured; in three, it was completely dislocated anteriorly; and in one, it was subluxated anteriorly.

Anatomical Study

Before the surgery was performed, the practicality of using a portion of the pectoralis major muscle to replace the subscapularis was studied in twenty shoulders from fourteen fresh cadavera. The assumption was that the portion of the pectoralis major muscle to be transferred should be routed behind the conjoined tendon of the coracobrachialis muscle and the short head of the biceps. This analysis focused on the neurovascular supply to the pectoralis major muscle, the distance to be bridged by the transferred muscle, the route behind the conjoined tendon, the course of the musculocutaneous nerve, the width of the tendon defect, and the width of the pectoralis major tendon. It has been shown that longitudinal dissection of the clavicular portion of the pectoralis major muscle does not disturb the neurovascular supply in either the dissected or the remaining part of the muscle because of its segmental supply[13]. In all twenty shoulders, a muscle transfer was performed, as will be described. In no shoulder was the muscle transfer impaired by the musculocutaneous nerve. In a previous study, the length of the musculocutaneous nerve from the tip of the coracoid process to the point of insertion in the muscle belly of the conjoined tendon was measured for another purpose in seventy-nine shoulders and the average distance was found to be 5.4 centimeters (range, two to 11.2 centimeters)[16].

Operative Technique

All operations were performed with the patient under general anesthesia and in a beach-chair position. The deltopectoral approach was used to expose the conjoined tendon, the tendon of the pectoralis major, and the anterior surface of the humeral head. The scar-like or bursa-like tissue found in the area of the defect was removed. In all patients, an attempt was made to mobilize the subscapularis muscle, but this was impossible because of pronounced retraction and atrophy. In patients in whom the long head of the biceps was dislocated anteriorly, it was tenotomized and the distal portion was sutured to the intertubercular groove.

The tendon of the pectoralis major was exposed over its full length at the humerus, and the superior one-half to two-thirds of the tendon (depending on the size of the defect) was detached from the humerus (Fig.

TABLE II

AGE AND GENDER-MATCHED NORMAL VALUES
AS IDENTIFIED BY CONSTANT AND MURLEY[4]

Age (yrs.)	No. of Points	
	Male Patients	Female Patients
21-30	98	97
31-40	93	90
41-50	92	80
51-60	90	73
61-70	83	70
71-80	75	69
81-90	66	54
91-99	56	52

2-A). The muscle fibers corresponding to the detached section of the tendon were split by blunt dissection over a length of approximately ten centimeters between the clavicular and sternal portions in order to take only the clavicular part for the transfer, working from the insertion medially. The muscle fibers of the sternal portion that radiate from dorsal into the proximal part of the tendon had to be transected. This left the clavicular portion of the pectoralis major muscle attached to the tendon with the exception of the transected muscle fibers just mentioned. The sternal portion remained intact.

The space between the pectoralis minor and the conjoined tendon was entered, and the area behind the conjoined tendon was exposed with use of the index fingers of both hands. In all patients, it was possible to locate the musculocutaneous nerve in the depths of the wound and also to identify its entrance into the muscle.

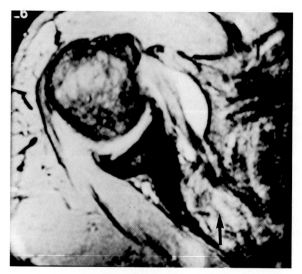

FIG. 3-A

Figs. 3-A, 3-B, and 3-C: Magnetic resonance images of a chronically ruptured subscapularis tendon.
Fig. 3-A: Preoperative image showing osseous impingement between the humeral head and the coracoid process. The subscapularis muscle has a greatly increased signal due to fatty degeneration (arrow).

TABLE III
RESULTS OF PREOPERATIVE AND POSTOPERATIVE CLINICAL EXAMINATION OF THE TWELVE PATIENTS*

	Preoperative	Postoperative
Active flexion *(degrees)*	93 (30-170)	129 (70-170)
Active abduction *(degrees)*	85 (20-170)	113 (70-170)
Active internal rotation *(no. of patients)*		
To lumbar spine	2	8
To sacrum	3	1
To buttock	5	1
To thigh	2	2
Active external rotation *(degrees)*	55 (33-81)	30 (15-65)
Strength *(kg)*		
At 90 degrees of abduction	0.8 (0-4)	2 (1-4)
At 90 degrees of flexion	0.6 (0-2)	2 (0-4)
At 0 degrees of internal rotation	4.5 (2-9)	5.6 (2-12)
Constant and Murley score[4]		
Points	22.6 (2-47)	54.4 (33-81)
Percent†	26.9 (3-51)	67.1 (37-108)
Visual analog scale *(points)*		
Pain (maximum, 15 points)	1.7 (0-5)	9.6 (5-15)
Function (maximum, 100 points)	20 (0-40)	63 (40-100)

*The values are given as the average and the range, except where noted otherwise.
†Adjusted for age and gender-matched normal values.

This is very important for assessment of the space for the transferred muscle when it passes between the nerve and the conjoined tendon. In one patient the interval between the pectoralis minor muscle and the conjoined tendon was opened so that the nerve could be identified visually, whereas in all others the nerve was just palpated. The interval between the nerve and the conjoined tendon was large enough for the muscle to be passed easily between the two structures in all patients. Thus, there was no need to retract the nerve or to protect it with an instrument.

The stay sutures attached to the tendon of the pectoralis major were grasped with curved forceps, the muscle was advanced behind the conjoined tendon but in front of the musculocutaneous nerve, and the tendon was attached to the lesser tuberosity with transosseous, nonabsorbable number-1 sutures. If there was a concomitant partial or complete rupture of the supraspinatus tendon, the tendon was attached not only to the lesser tuberosity but also to the anterior part of the greater tuberosity (Figs. 2-B and 2-C).

In muscular patients and in those in whom the full two-thirds of the tendon was used, it was necessary to reduce the attached muscle belly to avoid putting tension on the nerve. In two patients who had a concomitant partial rupture of the supraspinatus tendon, complete closure of both the anterior and the superior defect was achieved, whereas in two who had an additional, com-

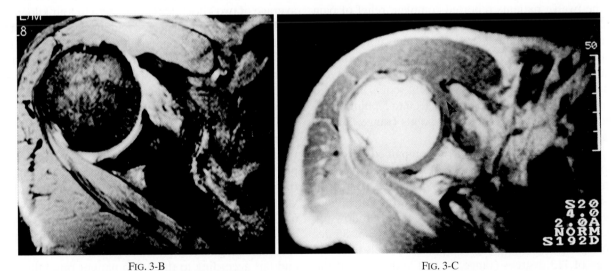

FIG. 3-B   FIG. 3-C

The distance between the humeral head and the coracoid process increased from approximately three millimeters preoperatively (Fig. 3-B) to five millimeters eight months postoperatively (Fig. 3-C); the increase was due to interposed pectoralis major tissue (arrowhead). The interposed tissue has the same signal intensity as the deltoid muscle.

TABLE IV
ELECTROMYOGRAPHIC ACTIVITY OF THE CLAVICULAR PORTION OF THE PECTORALIS MAJOR MUSCLE*

	Amplitudes on Involved Side		Amplitudes on Contralateral Side	
	Per Second	μV	Per Second	μV
Flexion	863 (713-989)	346 (302-450)	815 (536-1075)	378 (314-405)
Internal rotation	962 (920-1117)	432 (348-479)	803 (722-899)	389 (213-465)

*The values are given as the average and the range.

plete rupture of the supraspinatus tendon, complete closure of the superior defect was not possible and the residual defect was left open. In all patients, the tendon was long enough to permit at least 30 degrees of external rotation of the arm after the tendon had been sutured to the lesser tuberosity. Dorsal passage of the substitute muscle caused the conjoined tendon to arch forward slightly.

At the end of the procedure, a final check was performed with the index finger palpating the musculocutaneous nerve and the space between the nerve and the muscle to confirm that there was no tension on the nerve. If such tension is found, the size of the muscle belly must be reduced.

Postoperative Management

The shoulder was immobilized in a sling for six weeks, and passive range-of-motion exercises for abduction, flexion, and internal rotation were begun on the first postoperative day. External rotation was permitted only as far as the neutral position. After six weeks, active range-of-motion exercises were begun in all planes including external rotation. After twelve weeks, full loading was permitted.

Results

Clinical Examination (Table III)

At an average of twenty-eight months (range, twenty-four to fifty-four months) postoperatively, four of the twelve patients reported complete relief of pain and eight, partial relief. The latter group included patients in whom complete coverage of the supraspinatus tendon defect had not been possible. On the 15-point visual analog scale of the scoring system of Constant and Murley[4], the patients' pain-assessment scores improved from an average of 1.7 points (range, 0 to 5 points) preoperatively to an average of 9.6 points (range, 5 to 15 points) at the time of follow-up.

The reduction in pain was accompanied by corresponding increases in the range of motion. Active flexion improved from an average of 93 degrees (range, 30 to 170 degrees) preoperatively to an average of 129 degrees (range, 70 to 170 degrees) at the time of follow-up. Active abduction improved from an average of 85 degrees (range, 20 to 170 degrees) preoperatively to an average of 113 degrees (range, 70 to 170 degrees) at the time of follow-up. Active external rotation was reduced by an average of 25 degrees (range, 0 to 60 degrees), and

no patient had increased passive external rotation at the time of follow-up. Eight patients were able to reach the lumbar spine with the thumb on the involved side and one could touch the sacrum, as compared with two and three patients preoperatively.

Of the five patients who had had a positive lift-off test preoperatively, three had a negative result at the time of follow-up — that is, they could maintain the hand in the raised position behind the back for at least a few seconds. Six patients had a positive result, and three patients could not be assessed. Six of the twelve patients had a positive result on the belly-press test, five had a negative result, and the result was unclear for one patient. None of the four patients who had had anterior instability preoperatively had had a redislocation at the time of follow-up, and three patients had lost the subjective feeling of instability. A seventy-six-year-old patient with pronounced preoperative instability complained of a feeling of uncertainty in flexion and abduction, and she avoided such movements as much as possible.

Strength-testing was performed at 90 degrees of abduction and flexion for all except one patient, for whom it was performed at 70 degrees because the patient was not able to raise the arm higher. Abduction strength improved from an average of 0.8 kilogram (range, zero to four kilograms) preoperatively to an average of two kilograms (range, one to four kilograms) at the time of follow-up, and flexion strength improved from an average of 0.6 kilogram (range, zero to two kilograms) to an average of two kilograms (range, zero to four kilograms). With the upper arm adducted and the elbow flexed to 90 degrees, the strength of internal rotation was tested from the neutral position. The result was an increase from an average of 4.5 kilograms (range, two to nine kilograms) preoperatively to an average of 5.6 kilograms (range, two to twelve kilograms) at the time of follow-up.

The Constant and Murley[4] score improved from an average of 22.6 points (range, 2 to 47 points) preoperatively to an average of 54.4 points (range, 33 to 81 points) at the time of follow-up. The average change in the score adjusted for age and gender-matched normal values was from 26.9 percent (range, 3 to 51 percent) to 67.1 percent (range, 37 to 108 percent).

The postoperative subjective assessment was excellent according to five patients, good according to four, and fair according to three. No patient rated the result as poor. The overall subjective score for the involved shoulder, with use of the 100-point functional visual analog scale, changed from an average of 20 points (range, 0 to 40 points) preoperatively to an average of 63 points (range, 40 to 100 points) at the time of follow-up. This visual analog scale was used as a separate assessment from, and in addition to, the assessment with use of the Constant and Murley[4] score.

Ultrasonography

The follow-up evaluation included dynamic ultrasonography for all patients. The study was performed with the arm in slight external rotation. Satisfactory images of the pectoralis major tendon were obtained for all patients and demonstrated that the transferred muscle was still attached to the lesser tuberosity.

Magnetic Resonance Imaging
(Figs. 3-A, 3-B, and 3-C)

As part of the follow-up, magnetic resonance imaging was performed for seven patients, and good images of the musculotendinous section of the transferred portion of the pectoralis major muscle were obtained for six of them. The course of the transferred muscle to the lesser tuberosity could be identified, demonstrating that the repair was still intact. In six of these seven patients, an abnormal signal was generated by the subscapularis tissue (primarily due to fatty degeneration), whereas the transferred portion of the pectoralis major produced the same signal as the deltoid muscle. Transverse scans of four patients permitted good comparison with the preoperative images with regard to the distance from the coracoid process to the humeral head; in all four, placement of the substitute tissue had caused this distance to increase. The distance was measured at the level of the tip of the coracoid process. After correction of the measured distance with use of the measurement scale of the images, the average distance was 2.5 millimeters preoperatively and 4.5 millimeters postoperatively. The anterior translation of the humeral head that had been noted in two patients preoperatively was no longer present on the follow-up images.

Electromyography

Only six patients consented to have electromyographic analysis with needle electrodes in order to allow comparison between the two sides. The needles were inserted in the clavicular portion of the pectoralis major muscle. The test was performed at 70 degrees of flexion against manual resistance and, for measurement of internal rotation, with the upper arm adducted and the forearm held in the neutral position against manual resistance. Both tests were repeated three times. In all patients, the tests showed almost symmetrical activity between the two sides (Table IV).

Return to Earlier Activities

Because the average age of the twelve patients was sixty-five years, five were no longer working at the time

of the accident or the operation; therefore, at the follow-up evaluation, they were asked whether they had returned to their earlier activities rather than to work. Four patients said that they could perform physical work just as well as they had before the onset of the symptoms, six were able to perform physical tasks but not to the same degree as before, and two said that they were unable to perform any physical work. Five of the seven patients who had been employed at the time of the onset of the symptoms or before the surgery returned to work, at an average of 4.5 months (range, three to eight months) postoperatively.

Complications

No complications were encountered either intraoperatively or postoperatively. Dysfunction of the musculocutaneous nerve was not observed in any patient. No patient had sensory or motor changes or any cosmetic changes caused by the muscle transfer. In very thin patients, a slightly more prominent anterior bulging of the anterior part of the deltoid muscle was seen compared with the other side.

Discussion

Clinical diagnosis of an isolated rupture of the subscapularis tendon is difficult, and until recently there was no reliable clinical test for this lesion[6,9,11,14]. Therefore, correct diagnosis often was delayed for months or even years[6,10]. In the series of Gerber et al., the interval until repair of isolated ruptures of the subscapularis tendon averaged fifteen months (range, one to fifty-six months)[10]. Those authors reported consistently good results in patients who had had early repair and markedly less satisfactory results in those who had had a delayed procedure.

In our experience, a repair of the ruptured tendon after a delay of more than twelve months has been difficult to perform and usually has not led to a favorable result. In the present study, the length of time between the trauma or the onset of pain and the diagnosis averaged twenty-seven months.

Unlike a ruptured supraspinatus tendon that is associated with an intact infraspinatus tendon, a subscapularis tendon that is completely torn can retract unhindered by contact with intact tendon tissue. If the rupture remains untreated for several years, it may no longer be possible to use the subscapularis due to tendon retraction and irreparable changes in the muscle. However, because patients present with disabling pain, a dysfunctional shoulder, and a poor response to nonoperative therapy, sometimes combined with severe shoulder instability, surgical intervention is often indicated in spite of the usually older age of these patients.

The cause of the anterior shoulder pain, and its negligible response to nonoperative treatment, may be subcoracoid impingement[8]. In the current study, magnetic resonance imaging indicated a reduction in the distance between the humeral head and the coracoid process, accompanied by slight translation of the humeral head anteriorly compared with the position on the contralateral side, at least in the patients who had a concomitant lesion of the supraspinatus tendon. This translation appears to be caused by imbalance between the anterior and posterior muscles[1,2]. As pointed out by Burkhart, who performed a fluoroscopic imaging study, a tear that involves most of the anterior or posterior aspect of the cuff causes unstable fulcrum kinematics[1]. Replacement of the subscapularis tendon with a portion of the pectoralis major, following the course of the subscapularis muscle, interposes muscle between the coracoid process and the conjoined tendon on the one side and the humeral head on the other. There is evidence that the transferred portion of muscle acts as an internal rotator, since the electromyographic examinations of the transferred muscle fibers at the point of entry between the pectoralis minor tendon and the conjoined tendon showed almost symmetrical patterns of electrical activity. This assumption is also supported by the finding that, in almost all of our patients in whom magnetic resonance imaging was performed as part of the follow-up, the tissue of the transferred muscle produced the same signal as did other active muscles such as the deltoid, whereas the signal for the ruptured subscapularis muscle was usually different and indicated fatty degeneration.

The only position of the arm in which the subscapularis or the transferred muscle can be tested in isolation is that of maximum passive internal rotation as employed in the lift-off test[9,11]. Unfortunately, this test could not be performed by all of our patients due to a limited range of movement. However, three patients who had not been able to maintain the raised position of the hand behind the back preoperatively were able to do so briefly at the time of follow-up. The belly-press test, which yielded reliable results with regard to subscapularis function in the series of Gerber et al.[10] and in our study, was negative at the time of follow-up for five of our twelve patients; this also suggests involvement of the transferred muscle in internal rotation. Therefore, it can be assumed that the transferred muscle not only acts as a tether but also at least partially balances the infraspinatus-teres minor muscle complex and helps to restore the force couple in the transverse plane[2].

In our anatomical study, we found that transfer of the clavicular portion of the pectoralis major did not compromise the neurovascular supply to the muscle. Segmental ramification of the acromiothoracic artery and the pectoral nerve shortly after they pass beneath the clavicle, forming main branches for the clavicular, sternocostal, and abdominal portions of the pectoralis major, enables the muscle to be split from the periphery to well into the central area without jeopardizing the neurovascular supply. There is also room for the muscle

under the coracoid process, owing to its convex shape. In all patients, there was enough space for passage of the transferred muscle. As the width of the subscapularis tendon is approximately half that of the pectoralis major tendon, it was enough to harvest just the superior half of the tendon in patients who had an isolated rupture of the subscapularis tendon. In those who had a concomitant partial or complete rupture of the supraspinatus tendon, the superior two-thirds of the pectoralis major tendon was harvested to allow at least partial coverage of the supraspinatus defect. However, two-thirds of the substitute tendon is not sufficient to provide full coverage of a combined subscapularis and complete supraspinatus defect; the whole tendon has to be used, which we chose not to do. The goal was to convert a dysfunctional torn cuff to a functional one by restoring the force couple in the transverse plane, with the assumption that a remaining defect would have no influence on the kinematic pattern of the glenohumeral joint[2]. When two-thirds of the tendon was used, it was necessary to reduce the muscle belly to avoid putting tension upon the musculocutaneous nerve. The nerve must always be palpated with the index finger at the end of the procedure and, if there is too much tension on the nerve, the diameter of the muscle belly must be reduced.

The most striking finding of our study was the level of patient satisfaction, which derived primarily from relief of pain. Preoperatively, the patients had had severe pain for an average of twenty-seven months. Because almost all patients reported a reduction in pain just a few days postoperatively, we assume that this pain reduction was due primarily to the interposition of soft tissue between the coracoid process and the humeral head. The improved joint kinematics may also have contributed to the pain relief, though it does not seem likely that it did so in the first few days after the operation. Both of these variables may have helped to prevent subcoracoid impingement. It was not possible, however, to determine the exact degree to which soft-tissue interposition or improved kinematics contributed to this effect.

Reduced pain in turn meant improved function, especially in flexion, abduction, and internal rotation, and fewer problems with premature tiring. The 25-degree average reduction in external rotation resulting from the intervention was not considered a problem by the patients; because their function had been so poor preoperatively, they did not feel impaired by this restriction.

Patient satisfaction also was reflected in the patients' subjective evaluation of arm function with use of the visual analog scale. Their postoperative rating was 43 points higher than the rating before the operation. This change corresponds to the 40 percent increase in the Constant and Murley score[4] at the time of follow-up compared with the preoperative score.

It is difficult to compare the clinical results with

those reported in other studies in the literature[6,8,19], as the average age of the patients was much lower in the other studies (thirty-nine years in the series of Deutsch et al.[6], fifty years in that of Gerber et al.[8], and forty-nine years in that of Wirth and Rockwood[19]) and reconstruction of the subscapularis tendon was possible in most of the patients in those studies. In our patients, reconstruction of the subscapularis tendon was no longer possible, so our results must be interpreted in terms of a salvage operation for elderly patients.

Burkhart et al. emphasized the importance of the transverse-plane force couple for the balance of humeral head motion[1,2]. When the anterior part of the rotator cuff is torn, the posterior part is no longer balanced, which may cause anterior instability. DePalma et al.[5] and Symeonides[17] stressed the buttress effect of the subscapularis muscle against anterior instability. Turkel et al. also mentioned the importance of the subscapularis muscle with regard to anterior stability of the shoulder with the arm in the adducted or slightly abducted position[18]. Neviaser et al. discussed eight patients who presented with anterior instability and concomitant rupture of the subscapularis tendon; stability was restored through repair of the subscapularis tendon[15]. Wirth and Rockwood reported on thirteen patients who were operated on because of anterior instability and an irreparable rupture of the subscapularis[19]. In most procedures, they, like us, used the superior portion of the pectoralis major as a replacement muscle, but, unlike us, they routed the substitute muscle not behind but in front of the conjoined tendon and reinserted it lateral to the bicipital groove. We believe that the route behind the conjoined tendon not only approximates the orientation of the subscapularis muscle but also restores a buttress effect on the humeral head as a result of the tissue interposed between the conjoined tendon and the humeral head. The fact that the interposed muscle belly rests on the conjoined tendon increases anterior stability. As none of our four patients with anterior instability were able to abduct the arm to more than 110 degrees, it cannot be said whether the buttress effect of the transferred muscle as described for the subscapularis[18] would have been lost with increased abduction. However, the fact that all of our patients with instability had marked restriction of external rotation at the time of follow-up can be seen as a contributing stabilizing factor.

All four patients with recurrent anterior instability reported slight or no pain at the time of follow-up; three had subjective stability, and one had a feeling of uncertainty with the arm raised. The introduction of clinical tests (the lift-off test[9] and the belly-press test[10]) as reliable tools for the diagnosis of lesions of the subscapularis tendon[11] should allow detection at an early stage, when direct suturing of the tendon is still possible. Of course, these clinical tests can only raise the suspicion of a torn subscapularis tendon, and the diagnosis must be confirmed by ultrasound or magnetic resonance imaging. Nevertheless, it is to be expected that some patients will continue to present with old, irreparable ruptures. The technique that we have described is a relatively simple and safe way of replacing the traumatized muscle. Even though function is not completely restored in most patients, the technique produces high levels of subjective satisfaction with regard to pain relief, function, and stability.

References

1. **Burkhart, S. S.:** Fluoroscopic comparison of kinematic patterns in massive rotator cuff tears. A suspension bridge model. *Clin. Orthop.,* 284: 144-152, 1992.
2. **Burkhart, S. S.; Nottage, W. M.; Ogilvie-Harris, D. J.; Kohn, H. S.;** and **Pachelli, A.:** Partial repair of irreparable rotator cuff tears. *Arthroscopy,* 10: 363-370, 1994.
3. **Codman, E. A.:** *The Shoulder. Rupture of the Supraspinatus Tendon and Other Lesions In or About the Subacromial Bursa.* Ed. 2, pp. 262-312. Boston, Thomas Todd, 1934.
4. **Constant, C. R.,** and **Murley, A. H.:** A clinical method of functional assessment of the shoulder. *Clin. Orthop.,* 214: 160-164, 1987.
5. **DePalma, A. F.; Cooke, A. J.;** and **Prabhakar, M.:** The role of the subscapularis in recurrent anterior dislocations of the shoulder. *Clin. Orthop.,* 54: 35-49, 1967.
6. **Deutsch, A.; Altchek, D. W.; Veltri, D. M.; Potter, H. G.;** and **Warren, R. F.:** Traumatic tears of the subscapularis tendon. Clinical diagnosis, magnetic resonance imaging findings, and operative treatment. *Am. J. Sports Med.,* 25: 13-22, 1997.
7. **Frankle, M. A.,** and **Cofield, R. H.:** Rotator cuff tears including the subscapularis. In *Proceedings of the Fifth International Conference on Surgery of the Shoulder.* Paris, International Conference of Surgery of the Shoulder, 1992.
8. **Gerber, C.; Terrier, F.;** and **Ganz, R.:** The role of the coracoid process in the chronic impingement syndrome. *J. Bone and Joint Surg.,* 67-B(5): 703-708, 1985.
9. **Gerber, C.,** and **Krushell, R. J.:** Isolated rupture of the tendon of the subscapularis muscle. Clinical features in 16 cases. *J. Bone and Joint Surg.,* 73-B(3): 389-394, 1991.
10. **Gerber, C.; Hersche, O.;** and **Farron, A.:** Isolated rupture of the subscapularis tendon. Results of operative repair. *J. Bone and Joint Surg.,* 78-A: 1015-1023, July 1996.
11. **Greis, P. E.; Kuhn, J. E.; Schultheis, J.; Hintermeister, R.;** and **Hawkins, R.:** Validation of the lift-off test and analysis of subscapularis activity during maximal internal rotation. *Am. J. Sports Med.,* 24: 589-593, 1996.
12. **Hauser, E. D. W.:** Avulsion of the tendon of the subscapularis muscle. *J. Bone and Joint Surg.,* 36-A: 139-141, Jan. 1954.
13. **Hoffman, G. W.,** and **Elliott, L. F.:** The anatomy of the pectoral nerves and its significance to the general and plastic surgeon. *Ann. Surg.,* 205: 504-507, 1987.
14. **Mendoza Lopez, M.; Cardoner Parpal, J. C.; Samso Bardes, F.;** and **Coba Sotes, J.:** Lesions of the subscapular tendon regarding two cases in arthroscopic surgery. *Arthroscopy,* 9: 671-674, 1993.

15. **Neviaser, R. J.; Neviaser, T. J.;** and **Neviaser, J. S.:** Concurrent rupture of the rotator cuff and anterior dislocation of the shoulder in the older patient. *J. Bone and Joint Surg.,* 70-A: 1308-1311, Oct. 1988.

16. **Resch, H.; Wykypiel, H. F.; Maurer, H.;** and **Wambacher, M.:** The antero-inferior (transmuscular) approach for arthroscopic repair of the Bankart lesion: an anatomic and clinical study. *Arthroscopy,* 12: 309-322, 1996.

17. **Symeonides, P. P.:** The significance of the subscapularis muscle in the pathogenesis of recurrent anterior dislocation of the shoulder. *J. Bone and Joint Surg.,* 54-B(3): 476-483, 1972.

18. **Turkel, S. J.; Panio, M. W.; Marshall, J. L.;** and **Girgis, F. G.:** Stabilizing mechanisms preventing anterior dislocation of the glenohumeral joint. *J. Bone and Joint Surg.,* 63-A: 1208-1217, Oct. 1981.

19. **Wirth, M. A.,** and **Rockwood, C. A., Jr.:** Operative treatment of irreparable rupture of the subscapularis. *J. Bone and Joint Surg.,* 79-A: 722-731, May 1997.

Long-Term Functional Outcome of Repair of Large and Massive Chronic Tears of the Rotator Cuff*

BY ANDREW S. ROKITO, M.D.†, FRANCES CUOMO, M.D.†, MAUREEN A. GALLAGHER, PH.D.†,
AND JOSEPH D. ZUCKERMAN, M.D.†, NEW YORK, N.Y.

*Investigation performed at the Shoulder Service, Department of Orthopaedic Surgery,
New York University, Hospital for Joint Diseases, New York City*

Abstract

Background: There have been conflicting reports regarding the effect of the size of a tear of the rotator cuff on the ultimate functional outcome after repair of the rotator cuff. While some authors have reported that the size of the tear does not adversely affect the overall result of repair, others have reported that the outcome is less predictable after repair of a large tear than after repair of a small tear. The purpose of the present study was to examine the long-term functional outcome and the recovery of strength in thirty consecutive patients who had had repair of a large or massive tear of the rotator cuff.

Methods: Thirty consecutive patients who had operative repair of a large or massive chronic tear of the rotator cuff had a comprehensive isokinetic assessment of the strength of the shoulder preoperatively, twelve months postoperatively, and a mean of sixty-five months (range, forty-six to ninety-three months) postoperatively. The functional outcome was assessed with the University of California at Los Angeles shoulder score.

Results: All patients reported that they were satisfied with the result and had increased strength compared with preoperatively. There was a significant decrease in pain ($p < 0.01$) and significant improvements in function ($p < 0.01$) and the range of motion ($p < 0.01$). The mean University of California at Los Angeles shoulder score increased significantly from 12.3 points preoperatively to 31.0 points at the most recent follow-up examination ($p < 0.01$). The mean peak torque in flexion, abduction, and external rotation increased significantly to 80 percent ($p < 0.01$), 73 percent ($p < 0.01$), and 91 percent ($p < 0.01$), respectively, of that of the uninvolved shoulder by the time of the most recent follow-up examination.

Conclusions: Repair of a large or massive tear of the rotator cuff can have a satisfactory long-term outcome. The results of the present study suggest that more than one year is needed for complete restoration of strength. The strength of the affected shoulders still did not equal that of the unaffected, contralateral shoulders by the time of the long-term follow-up.

*No benefits in any form have been received or will be received from a commercial party related directly or indirectly to the subject of this article. No funds were received in support of this study.

†Shoulder Service, Department of Orthopaedic Surgery, New York University, Hospital for Joint Diseases, 301 East 17th Street, New York, N.Y. 10003.

Operative repair of a large or massive chronic tear of the rotator cuff can be technically challenging because of retraction and inelasticity of the tendons, bursal scarring, muscle atrophy, and fatty degeneration. Intra-articular and extra-articular releases are routinely performed to mobilize the tendons so that they can be attached to the greater tuberosity. While some authors have stated that the size of the tear does not appreciably affect the overall result of the repair[1,19,32], others have reported that the outcome after repair of a large tear is less predictable than that after repair of a small tear[7,9,15,17,18,26-28,42,45,46]. Isokinetic strength-testing has been found to be useful for quantifying the recovery of shoulder strength after repair of the rotator cuff[43,45]. In a previous study, we found a trend between the size of the tear and the recovery of strength of the shoulder after repair[45]. We also found that more than one year is needed for the recovery of strength after repair of a large or massive tear of the rotator cuff[45].

The purpose of the present study was to quantify the long-term isokinetic strength of the shoulder and the functional outcome for thirty patients who had had repair of a large or massive chronic tear of the rotator cuff.

Materials and Methods

Thirty consecutive patients who had a reparable chronic tear of the rotator cuff that was either large (three to five centimeters) or massive (more than five centimeters) were managed operatively between June 1989 and July 1993. All of the patients provided written informed consent to verify that they understood the purpose of the investigation. The size of the tear was graded according to the system of DeOrio and Cofield[18] at the time of the operation. The criterion for inclusion in the study was a large or massive tear that could be attached to the greater tuberosity after appropriate mobilization techniques and repaired with the arm at the side. Seventeen patients had a large tear, and thirteen had a massive tear. The subscapularis tendon was intact in all patients. Patients who had a tear that could not be repaired, who had had a previous procedure involving the shoulder, or who had symptoms in the contralateral shoulder were excluded from the study.

The study group consisted of twenty-one men and nine women with a mean age of fifty-seven years (range, thirty-nine to seventy-eight years). The tear was on the dominant side in twenty-three patients. All patients had substantial pain and functional limitation, with regard to work and activities of daily living, that had lasted for more than six months and that were unresponsive to nonoperative treatment. Nonoperative treatment consisted of a period of relative rest, modification of activity, nonsteroidal anti-inflammatory medication, and a home-exercise program that emphasized range-of-motion exercises and strengthening of the shoulder. Cortisone injections were not used for any patient. The clinical diagnosis of a torn rotator cuff was confirmed with arthrography or magnetic resonance imaging.

Preoperative Assessment

The University of California at Los Angeles shoulder score[20] was used to assess the patients both before and after the operation. In order to eliminate bias, this test was administered by one of us (A. S. R.) who had not been involved in the operative procedures and who was blinded to the operative findings. This system assigns a maximum of 10 points each for pain and function and 5 points each for range of motion, strength of forward elevation, and overall patient satisfaction, for a total possible score of 35 points. The strength of the shoulder was graded from 0 to 5, according to standard manual muscle-testing with the arm in maximum elevation. No patient was satisfied with the results of the nonoperative treatment before the operation.

Isokinetic Strength

Isokinetic strength-testing was done within seven days preoperatively, twelve months postoperatively, and at the time of the most recent long-term follow-up examination. Testing was performed with a modified dynamometer (Biodex, Shirley, New York), with use of a standardized protocol, by one of us (M. A. G.) who was blinded to the operative findings. The instrument was interfaced with an NEC-386 computer (Biodex) and a software package that supplies values for parameters related to torque and displacement. The software allows for normalization of the maximum gravity effect caused by the weight of the arm. The shoulders were tested at 60 degrees per second in three axes of motion: flexion-extension and abduction-adduction with the patient sitting and external-internal rotation with the patient standing.

The axis of rotation for flexion-extension was set at the acromion and was positioned to align with the pivot point of the input arm of the dynamometer. The range-of-motion stops were set at 0 and 120 degrees. The elbow was maintained in full extension, with the

forearm in neutral rotation. The axis of rotation for abduction-adduction of the shoulder approximated the axis of the acromioclavicular joint and was aligned perpendicular to the coronal plane. The range-of-motion stops were set at 0 and 120 degrees. External-internal rotation was tested with the shoulder in neutral, the elbow in 90 degrees of flexion, and the forearm in neutral rotation. The limb was supported by an elbow pad. The range-of-motion stops were set at 30 degrees of internal rotation and 45 degrees of external rotation. Stabilization straps were secured and foot-markers were placed during all testing to ensure a standardized and reproducible protocol.

Three trials were performed at submaximum effort in each axis to acquaint the patient with the testing conditions. These trials were followed by a five-minute rest period. Three trials at maximum effort were then performed in each axis. A five-minute rest period was allowed between each testing sequence. Scores for peak torque were recorded for the three repetitions in each axis of motion. The contralateral shoulder was tested in an identical manner. The mean and standard deviation for the three repetitions were then determined for each axis for each shoulder. Values for peak torque as a percentage of that of the uninvolved, contralateral shoulder were calculated.

Operative Technique

The standardized operative procedure was performed by two of us (F. C. and J. D. Z.). First, a superior incision was made in Langer's lines over the top of the acromion and was continued to just lateral to the coracoid process. Subcutaneous flaps were then raised in all directions, followed by detachment of the anterior part of the deltoid from the acromion and resection of the coracoacromial ligament. The deltoid was split in line with its fibers to the level of the greater tuberosity. Care was taken to ensure that this split was not extended more than five centimeters so as to avoid injury of the axillary nerve. By rotating the humerus, it was possible to gain access to all aspects of the tear without the need for a more posterior split of the deltoid. An anterior-inferior acromioplasty was performed, followed by resection of any spurs on the undersurface of the acromioclavicular joint. The lateral end of the clavicle was not resected because the acromioclavicular joint was thought to be asymptomatic in all patients.

After a partial bursectomy, the tear was measured in centimeters from anterior to posterior at its maximum diameter with the arm at the side. The rotator cuff was then repaired with a combination of tendon-to-tendon and tendon-to-bone techniques. After the traction sutures were placed, the mobility of the tendons was assessed. In some patients, the tendon tissue was of good quality and could be repaired readily without the need for extensive mobilization. In other patients, the quality of the tissue was poor with substantial scarring and extensive mobilization was needed to repair the defect. All defects could be closed after appropriate mobilization techniques had been performed.

Mobilization of the cuff began with blunt dissection of extra-articular and intra-articular adhesions. When necessary, the coracohumeral ligament was divided close to its insertion on the base of the coracoid process. If additional length was needed, an intra-articular release of the superior aspect of the capsule and the rotator cuff from the superior aspect of the labrum was performed with a combination of sharp and blunt dissection. If additional mobilization was needed at this point, the rotator interval was released sharply to the base of the coracoid. The rotator cuff tendons in all patients were mobilized sufficiently to permit a transosseous repair to a bleeding cancellous bed prepared in the greater tuberosity with the arm at the side. The arm was then moved through a gentle range of motion to test the repair and to determine a safe range of motion for rehabilitation. The deltoid was then repaired to the acromion through drill-holes.

Postoperative Care

A standardized postoperative rehabilitation protocol was carried out by occupational therapists for all patients. An arm sling was used for the first six weeks postoperatively. An abduction brace was not used. Passive range-of-motion exercises within the predetermined safe range of motion were initiated on the first postoperative day. Active range-of-motion exercises were begun when the healing of the rotator cuff was thought to be secure, usually six to eight weeks postoperatively. Isometric and isotonic cuff-strengthening exercises were added when at least 80 percent of the active range of motion had returned, usually at approximately twelve weeks postoperatively.

Postoperative Assessment

All thirty patients were reevaluated with isokinetic strength-testing and the University of California at Los Angeles shoulder score[20] at twelve months postoperatively and again at a mean of sixty-five months (range, forty-six to ninety-three months) postoperatively.

Statistical Analysis

The significance of the differences, between the preoperative and postoperative evaluations, in strength for each axis of motion and the clinical findings according to the University of California at Los Angeles shoulder score[20] was determined with a Student t test. A p value of less than 0.05 was considered significant.

Results

The mean preoperative University of California at Los Angeles shoulder score[20] was 12.3 points (range, 6 to 20 points). This value increased significantly to a mean of 28.3 points (range, 13 to 35 points) (p < 0.01)

TABLE I

UNIVERSITY OF CALIFORNIA AT
LOS ANGELES SHOULDER SCORES[20]*

	Preop. Score (points)	Most Recent Score† (points)
Pain	3.0 (1-6)	8.5 (6-10)
Function	2.5 (1-6)	8.4 (2-10)
Active forward elevation	3.5 (0-5)	4.6 (2-5)
Strength of forward elevation	3.3 (2-5)	4.5 (1-5)
Satisfaction	0	5‡
Total§	12.3 (6-20)	31.0 (16-35)

*The values are given as the mean, with the range in parentheses.
†All improvements were significant at p < 0.01.
‡All patients were satisfied and had improvement at the most recent evaluation.
§The maximum possible score for a normal shoulder is 35 points.

at one year postoperatively and to a mean of 31.0 points (range, 16 to 35 points) (p < 0.01) at the most recent follow-up examination (Table I). According to the shoulder score, sixteen patients (53 percent) had an excellent result (a score of 34 or 35 points), seven (23 percent) had a good result (a score of 29 to 33 points), and seven (23 percent) had a poor result (a score of less than 29 points) at the time of the most recent follow-up.

Pain: The mean score for pain improved significantly from 3.0 points (range, 1 to 6 points) preoperatively to 8.5 points (range, 6 to 10 points) at the most recent follow-up evaluation (p < 0.01) (Table I). Sixteen (53 percent) of the thirty patients had no pain, and fourteen (47 percent) had either slight, occasional pain or pain only while performing strenuous or particular activities.

Function: The mean score for function increased significantly from 2.5 points (range, 1 to 6 points) preoperatively to 8.4 points (range, 2 to 10 points) at the most recent follow-up evaluation (p < 0.01) (Table I). At the time of the most recent follow-up, seventeen patients (57 percent) were able to perform all of their normal activities without limitation, eleven (37 percent) had only slight or moderate restriction of activity, and two (7 percent) were able to perform only light activities.

Active forward elevation: The mean score for active forward elevation improved significantly from 3.5 points (range, 0 to 5 points) preoperatively to 4.6 points (range, 2 to 5 points) at the most recent follow-up evaluation (p < 0.01) (Table I). Twenty-three patients (77 percent) had 150 degrees or more of active forward elevation (measured with the patient sitting), four (13 percent) had 120 to 150 degrees, one (3 percent) had 90 to 120 degrees, and two (7 percent) had 45 to 90 degrees at the most recent follow-up evaluation.

Strength of forward elevation: Strength of forward elevation, as determined with manual muscle-testing,

TABLE II
PEAK TORQUE VALUES*

	Preop.	1 Year Postop.	Most Recent Follow-up
Flexion			
Peak torque (N-m)	19.5 (5.3-40.6)	26.3 (4.7-44.5)	29.4 (7.3-53.3)
Percent of uninvolved side	52 (17-82)	70 (13-91)	80 (13-100)
Abduction			
Peak torque (N-m)	13.0 (4.1-32.2)	26.2 (4.0-46.3)	23.3 (6.6-51.6)
Percent of uninvolved side	43 (9-66)	86 (15-90)	73 (15-100)
External rotation			
Peak torque (N-m)	12.6 (4.2-19.3)	18.3 (4.7-25.8)	19.1 (4.7-30.4)
Percent of uninvolved side	57 (15-76)	87 (22-96)	91 (22-100)

*The values are given as the mean, with the range in parentheses.

improved significantly from a mean of 3.3 points (range, 2 to 5 points) preoperatively to a mean of 4.5 points (range, 1 to 5 points) at the most recent follow-up evaluation (p < 0.01) (Table I). Twenty-one patients (70 percent) had grade-5 strength, seven (23 percent) had grade-4 strength, one (3 percent) had grade-2 strength, and one had grade-1 strength at the most recent follow-up evaluation.

Satisfaction: At the most recent follow-up evaluation, all thirty patients reported that they were satisfied and that the condition of the shoulder had improved.

Isokinetic strength: The mean peak torque in flexion, abduction, and external rotation increased significantly during the study period (Table II). The mean peak torque in flexion increased from 19.5 newton-meters (range, 5.3 to 40.6 newton-meters) and 52 percent (range, 17 to 82 percent) of that on the contralateral side preoperatively to 26.3 newton-meters (range, 4.7 to 44.5 newton-meters) and 70 percent (range, 13 to 91 percent) of that on the contralateral side at one year postoperatively and to 29.4 newton-meters (range, 7.3 to 53.3 newton-meters) and 80 percent (range, 13 to 100 percent) of that on the contralateral side at the most recent follow-up evaluation (p < 0.01). The mean peak torque in abduction increased from a mean of 13.0 newton-meters (range, 4.1 to 32.2 newton-meters) and 43 percent (range, 9 to 66 percent) of that on the contralateral side to 26.2 newton-meters (range, 4.0 to 46.3 newton-meters) and 86 percent (range, 15 to 90 percent) of that on the contralateral side at one year postoperatively, but then it decreased to 23.3 newton-meters (range, 6.6 to 51.6 newton-meters) and 73 percent (range, 15 to 100 percent) of that on the contralateral side at the most recent follow-up evaluation. This was still an overall significant improvement (p < 0.01). The mean peak torque in external rotation increased progressively from 12.6 newton-meters (range, 4.2 to 19.3 newton-meters) and 57 percent (range, 15 to 76 percent) of that on the contralateral side preoperatively to 18.3 newton-meters (range, 4.7 to 25.8 newton-meters) and 87 percent (range, 22 to 96 percent) of that on the contralateral side at one year postoperatively and to 19.1 newton-meters (range, 4.7 to 30.4 newton-meters) and 91 per-

cent (range, 22 to 100 percent) of that on the contralateral side at the most recent follow-up evaluation (p < 0.01).

Complications

There were no intraoperative or postoperative complications. Although a recurrent tear was suspected clinically in three patients who had a persistent limitation of active forward elevation and poor strength, no imaging studies were done to confirm the diagnosis. No patient chose to have additional operative treatment.

Discussion

Many authors have reported on the efficacy of acromioplasty and repair of the rotator cuff in reducing pain in the shoulder and in restoring function, with overall good or excellent results documented in most studies[2,8,9,13,15,16,20,22,29,35,36,39,41,42,49]. Fewer studies, however, have critically examined the ultimate functional outcome of repair of the rotator cuff[8,27,28,30,47], and this has been the subject of increased attention[20,28,30,45].

In particular, relatively few reports have examined the functional outcome of repair of large and massive tears of the rotator cuff[6,8,10,12,18,21,24,29,34,39,41,44,48]. Several techniques have been proposed to either repair or reconstruct large defects in the tendons. Reconstructive procedures (including local tendon transposition with the superior portion of the subscapularis[14]; incorporation of the biceps tendon[33]; implantation of fascia[3,4], allograft tissue[37], or synthetic material[40]; and extrinsic tendon transfer with use of the latissimus dorsi[25]) have been proposed as potential treatment options and have had varying degrees of success. Other investigators have recommended attaching the shortened rotator cuff more medially onto the articular surface of the humeral head[31].

While tendon débridement and subacromial decompression, either by open or arthroscopic means[10,11,21,24,44], has been shown to decrease pain and to improve function, the results often do not compare favorably with those in studies in which the tears were repaired[34,39]. Recognizing the importance of anterior and posterior stability of the glenohumeral joint in patients who have a massive tear of the rotator cuff, Burkhart et al.[12] recently recommended partial repair. In general, however, when appropriate mobilization techniques are used, most large and massive tears of the rotator cuff can be repaired completely, rather than partially, with better results[8,34,39].

Several investigators have stated that the size of the tear preoperatively has no substantial influence on the overall results of operative treatment[1,19,32]. More recently, however, a strong association between the size of the tear and the functional outcome has been identified. Bassett and Cofield[2] found that strength on abduction and external rotation after repair of small and medium-size tears was consistently better than that after repair of larger tears. Hawkins et al.[29] found a direct relationship (although not a significant one) between the size of the tear and strength as determined with postoperative manual muscle-testing. In a long-term follow-up study of 105 rotator-cuff repairs, Harryman et al.[28], using ultrasound, found a much higher prevalence of recurrent defects in the cuff in the patients who had had a larger tear. Those authors found that the integrity of the repair was the most important factor affecting the functional result. In a previous report on forty-two patients who had repair of the rotator cuff[45], we found a trend between the size of the tear and the recovery of strength. The twenty-four patients with a small or medium tear had almost complete recovery of strength during the first postoperative year, whereas a longer period of rehabilitation was needed for the eighteen patients with a large or massive tear. Iannotti et al.[30], in a prospective study of forty patients who had repair of the rotator cuff, found a significant association between functional outcome and the size of the tear at the time of the operation (p ≤ 0.002).

Several authors have recommended tendon débridement and decompression for the treatment of irreparable lesions of the rotator cuff. Rockwood et al.[44] reported a good or excellent result for forty-four (83 percent) of fifty-three patients who had open débridement and decompression. Gartsman[24] reported that twenty-six (79 percent) of thirty-three patients in his series believed that the condition of the shoulder had improved after operative débridement and subacromial decompression. Although there was a significant decrease in pain (p = 0.001) and a significant improvement in the range of motion (p = 0.038), strength was decreased. Overall, the results of débridement and decompression are inferior to those of decompression and repair of a torn rotator cuff[34,39]. It is difficult to compare the results of decompression and repair of large and massive tears of the rotator cuff in the present study with those of decompression and débridement alone for massive tears. It should be emphasized that in most studies the latter group consisted of patients who had a massive, irreparable tear, whereas in the present study all of the tears could be mobilized and repaired.

The results of the present study compare favorably with those of Bigliani et al.[8]. Those authors reported the long-term results of operative repair of a massive tear of the rotator cuff in sixty-one patients. Fifty-two (85 percent) of the patients had a satisfactory result, and fifty-six (92 percent) had satisfactory relief of pain. The mean improvement in the range of motion was 76 degrees in forward elevation and 30 degrees in external rotation. In the present study, twenty-three patients (77 percent) had a good or excellent result. There was a significant reduction in pain and significant improvements in function, range of motion, strength, and overall satisfaction of the patient. These results are also comparable with those of Ellman et al.[20], who evaluated patients with a much wider spectrum of tears. According to the University of California at Los Angeles shoulder score[20], forty-two (84 percent) of their fifty patients had a good or excellent result.

Careful selection of the patient is critical when the type of treatment is being chosen for a suspected large defect of the rotator cuff. Often, the size and reparability of a tear can be predicted on the basis of the preoperative history, physical examination, and imaging studies. When a patient reports an insidious onset of pain and loss of function, has substantial atrophy of the infraspinatus and supraspinatus muscles, and has a substantial loss of active motion and is unable to maintain a position of external rotation with the arm at the side, a sizable tear of the rotator cuff should be suspected. Furthermore, patients who have marked superior migration of the humeral head, as seen on plain anteroposterior radiographs, and atrophy and fatty replacement of the spinatus muscles, as seen on magnetic resonance imaging studies, do not have a reparable tear. Operative treatment is usually avoided for these patients unless there is substantial pain and poor function with associated arthritis, in which case hemiarthroplasty with preservation of the coracoacromial ligament can be considered. Gerber[25] reported good results with transfer of the latissimus dorsi for patients who did not have arthritis and who had preservation of a passive range of motion.

The present study group was a relatively homogeneous population of older individuals who had a chronic tear of the rotator cuff. No patient had substantial concomitant disease of the cervical spine or the acromioclavicular joint. Thus, these conditions were not suspected of playing an important role in the most recent functional outcome. Furthermore, no patient was involved in a Workers' Compensation claim or another form of litigation that could have influenced the subjective result. Nevertheless, a study of this kind has a number of limitations. It is difficult to differentiate true weakness from pain-related weakness with isokinetic strength-testing. This is an important consideration, as pain has been shown to adversely affect strength of the shoulder[5]. Furthermore, such testing represents only strength on maximum effort, not endurance, which may be more important in terms of functional recovery. Finally, no imaging studies were performed at the most recent follow-up examination, and thus the integrity of the rotator cuff and its effect on the postoperative outcome were not accurately determined. This is especially important with regard to the treatment of large or massive chronic tears of the rotator cuff, which have been shown to have a high prevalence of recurrence[28].

Another important point relates to treatment of the coracoacromial ligament. Some authors[23,38] have advocated preservation of the coracoacromial ligament in patients who have an irreparable tear of the rotator cuff, as resection leads to a loss of integrity of the coracoacromial arch and superior migration of the humeral head with a subsequent decrease in function of the shoulder. As the ligament was resected in all of the patients in the present study, it is possible that this could have adversely affected the overall results, especially in the patients in whom a recurrent defect of the cuff may have developed.

In summary, it is possible to obtain a satisfactory long-term outcome after repair of a large or massive chronic tear of the rotator cuff. A substantial decrease in pain as well as improved function, range of motion, and strength can be achieved. More than a year is needed for maximum recovery of strength after repair of a large or massive chronic tear of the rotator cuff, and the strength does not return to the level on the unaffected, contralateral side.

References

1. **Bakalim, G.,** and **Pasila, M.:** Surgical treatment of rupture of the rotator cuff tendon. *Acta Orthop. Scandinavica,* 46: 751-757, 1975.
2. **Bassett, R. W.,** and **Cofield, R. H.:** Acute tears of the rotator cuff. The timing of surgical repair. *Clin. Orthop.,* 175: 18-24, 1983.
3. **Bateman, J. E.:** The diagnosis and treatment of ruptures of the rotator cuff. *Surg. Clin. North America,* 43: 1523-1530, 1963.
4. **Bayne, O.,** and **Bateman, J. E.:** Long-term results of surgical repair of full-thickness rotator cuff tears. In *Surgery of the Shoulder,* pp. 167-171. Edited by J. E. Bateman and R. P. Walsh. Philadelphia, B. C. Decker, 1984.
5. **Ben-Yishay, A.; Zuckerman, J. D.; Gallagher, M.;** and **Cuomo, F.:** Pain inhibition of shoulder strength in patients with impingement syndrome. *Orthopedics,* 17: 685-688, 1994.
6. **Bigliani, L. U.,** and **McIlveen, S. J.:** Repair of massive rotator cuff tears. *Orthop. Trans.,* 9: 43, 1985.
7. **Bigliani, L. U.; McIlveen, S. J.; Cordasco, F. A.;** and **Musso, E. S.:** Operative management of failed rotator cuff repairs. *Orthop. Trans.,* 12: 674, 1988.
8. **Bigliani, L. U.; Cordasco, F. A.; McIlveen, S. J.;** and **Musso, E. S.:** Operative repairs of massive rotator cuff tears: long-term results. *J. Shoulder and Elbow Surg.,* 1: 120-130, 1992.
9. **Björkenheim, J.-M.; Paavolainen, P.; Ahouvo, J.;** and **Slätis, P.:** Surgical repair of the rotator cuff and surrounding tissues. Factors influencing the results. *Clin. Orthop.,* 236: 148-153, 1988.
10. **Burkhart, S. S.:** Arthroscopic treatment of massive rotator cuff tears. Clinical results and biomechanical rationale. *Clin. Orthop.,* 267: 45-56, 1991.
11. **Burkhart, S. S.:** Arthroscopic debridement and decompression for selected rotator cuff tears. Clinical results, pathomechanics, and patient selection based on biomechanical parameters. *Orthop. Clin. North America,* 24: 111-123, 1993.
12. **Burkhart, S. S.; Nottage, W. M.; Ogilvie-Harris, D. J.; Kohn, H. S.;** and **Pachelli, A.:** Partial repair of irreparable rotator cuff tears. *Arthroscopy,* 10: 363-370, 1994.
13. **Cofield, R. H.:** Tears of rotator cuff. In *Instructional Course Lectures, American Academy of Orthopaedic Surgeons.* Vol. 30, pp. 258-273. St. Louis, C. V. Mosby, 1981.
14. **Cofield, R. H.:** Subscapularis muscle transposition for repair of chronic rotator cuff tears. *Surg., Gynec. and Obstet.,* 154: 667-669, 1982.
15. **Cofield, R. H.:** Current concepts review. Rotator cuff disease of the shoulder. *J. Bone and Joint Surg.,* 67-A: 974-979, July 1985.
16. **Constant, C. R.:** Shoulder function after rotator cuff tears by operative and nonoperative means. In *Surgery of the Shoulder,* pp. 231-233. Edited by M. Post, B. F. Morrey, and R. J. Hawkins. St. Louis, Mosby-Year Book, 1990.
17. **Debeyre, J.; Patte, D.;** and **Elmelik, E.:** Repair of ruptures of the rotator cuff of the shoulder with a note on advancement of the supraspinatus muscle. *J. Bone and Joint Surg.,* 47-B(1): 36-42, 1965.
18. **DeOrio, J. K.,** and **Cofield, R. H.:** Results of a second attempt at surgical repair of a failed initial rotator-cuff repair. *J. Bone and Joint Surg.,* 66-A: 563-567, April 1984.
19. **Earnshaw, P.; Desjardins, D.; Sarkar, K.;** and **Uhthoff, H. K.:** Rotator cuff tears: the role of surgery. *Canadian J. Surg.,* 25: 60-63, 1982.
20. **Ellman, H.; Hanker, G.;** and **Bayer, M.:** Repair of the rotator cuff. End-result study of factors influencing reconstruction. *J. Bone and Joint Surg.,* 68-A: 1136-1144, Oct. 1986.
21. **Ellman, H.; Kay, S. R.;** and **Wirth, M.:** Arthroscopic treatment of full-thickness rotator cuff tears: 2- to 7-year follow-up study. *Arthroscopy,* 9: 195-200, 1993.
22. **Essman, J. A.; Bell, R. H.;** and **Askew, M.:** Full-thickness rotator-cuff tear. An analysis of results. *Clin. Orthop.,* 265: 170-177, 1991.
23. **Flatow, E. L.:** Coracoacromial ligament preservation in rotator cuff surgery. *J. Shoulder and Elbow Surg.,* 3: 573, 1994.
24. **Gartsman, G. M.:** Massive, irreparable tears of the rotator cuff. Results of operative débridement and subacromial decompression. *J. Bone and Joint Surg.,* 79-A: 715-721, May 1997.
25. **Gerber, C.:** Latissimus dorsi transfer for the treatment of irreparable tears of the rotator cuff. *Clin. Orthop.,* 275: 152-160, 1992.
26. **Godsil, R. D., Jr.,** and **Linscheid, R. L.:** Intratendinous defects of the rotator cuff. *Clin. Orthop.,* 69: 181-188, 1970.
27. **Gore, D. R.; Murray, M. P.; Sepic, S. B.;** and **Gardner, G. M.:** Shoulder-muscle strength and range of motion following surgical repair of full-thickness rotator-cuff tears. *J. Bone and Joint Surg.,* 68-A: 266-272, Feb. 1986.
28. **Harryman, D. T., II; Mack, L. A.; Wang, K. Y.; Jackins, S. E.; Richardson, M. L.;** and **Matsen, F. A., III:** Repairs of the rotator cuff. Correlation of functional results with integrity of the cuff. *J. Bone and Joint Surg.,* 73-A: 982-989, Aug. 1991.
29. **Hawkins, R. J.; Misamore, G. W.;** and **Hobeika, P. E.:** Surgery for full-thickness rotator-cuff tears. *J. Bone and Joint Surg.,* 67-A: 1349-1355, Dec. 1985.

30. **Iannotti, J. P.; Bernot, M. P.; Kuhlman, J. R.; Kelley, M. J.;** and **Williams, G. R.:** Postoperative assessment of shoulder function: a prospective study of full-thickness rotator cuff tears. *J. Shoulder and Elbow Surg.,* 5: 449-457, 1996.

31. **McLaughlin, H. L.:** Lesions of the musculotendinous cuff of the shoulder. I. The exposure and treatment of tears with retraction. *J. Bone and Joint Surg.,* 26: 31-51, Jan. 1944.

32. **McLaughlin, H. L.,** and **Asherman, E. G.:** Lesions of the musculotendinous cuff of the shoulder. IV. Some observations based upon the results of surgical repair. *J. Bone and Joint Surg.,* 33-A: 76-86, Jan. 1951.

33. **Matsen, F. A., III,** and **Arntz, C. T.:** Rotator cuff tendon failure. In *The Shoulder,* pp. 647-677. Edited by C. A. Rockwood and F. A. Matsen, III. Philadelphia, W. B. Saunders, 1990.

34. **Montgomery, T. J.; Yerger, B.;** and **Savoie, F. H.:** Management of rotator cuff tears: a comparison of arthroscopic debridement and surgical repair. *J. Shoulder and Elbow Surg.,* 3: 70-78, 1994.

35. **Neer, C. S., II,** and **Flatow, E. L.:** Tears of the rotator cuff. Long term results of anterior acromioplasty and repair. *Orthop. Trans.,* 12: 673-674, 1988.

36. **Neviaser, J. S.:** Ruptures of the rotator cuff of the shoulder. New concepts in the diagnosis and operative treatment of chronic ruptures. *Arch. Surg.,* 102: 483-485, 1971.

37. **Neviaser, J. S.; Neviaser, R. J.;** and **Neviaser, T. J.:** The repair of chronic massive ruptures of the rotator cuff of the shoulder by use of a freeze-dried rotator cuff. *J. Bone and Joint Surg.,* 60-A: 681-684, July 1978.

38. **Nirschl, R. P.:** Rotator cuff surgery. In *Instructional Course Lectures, American Academy of Orthopaedic Surgeons.* Vol. 38, pp. 447-462. Park Ridge, Illinois, American Academy of Orthopaedic Surgeons, 1989.

39. **Ogilvie-Harris, D. J.,** and **Demazière, A.:** Arthroscopic debridement versus open repair for rotator cuff tears. A prospective cohort study. *J. Bone and Joint Surg.,* 75-B(3): 416-420, 1993.

40. **Ozaki, J.; Fujimoto, S.; Masuhara, K.; Tamai, S.;** and **Yoishimoto, S.:** Reconstruction of chronic massive rotator cuff tears with synthetic materials. *Clin. Orthop.,* 202: 173-183, 1986.

41. **Packer, N. P.; Calvert, P. T.; Bayley, J. I. L.;** and **Kessel, L.:** Operative treatment of chronic ruptures of the rotator cuff of the shoulder. *J. Bone and Joint Surg.,* 65-B(2): 171-175, 1983.

42. **Post, M.; Silver, R.;** and **Singh, M.:** Rotator cuff tear. Diagnosis and treatment. *Clin. Orthop.,* 173: 78-91, 1983.

43. **Rabin, S. I.,** and **Post, M.:** A comparative study of clinical muscle testing and Cybex evaluation after shoulder operations. *Clin. Orthop.,* 258: 147-156, 1990.

44. **Rockwood, C. A., Jr.; Williams, G. R., Jr.;** and **Burkhead, W. Z., Jr.:** Débridement of degenerative, irreparable lesions of the rotator cuff. *J. Bone and Joint Surg.,* 77-A: 857-866, June 1995.

45. **Rokito, A. S.; Zuckerman, J. D.; Gallagher, M. A.;** and **Cuomo, F.:** Strength after surgical repair of the rotator cuff. *J. Shoulder and Elbow Surg.,* 5: 12-17, 1996.

46. **Uhthoff, H. K.; Sarkar, K.;** and **Lohr, J.:** Repair in rotator cuff tendons. In *Surgery of the Shoulder,* pp. 216-219. Edited by M. Post, B. F. Morrey, and R. J. Hawkins. St. Louis, Mosby-Year Book, 1990.

47. **Walker, S. W.; Couch, W. H.; Boester, G. A.;** and **Sprowl, D. W.:** Isokinetic strength of the shoulder after repair of a torn rotator cuff. *J. Bone and Joint Surg.,* 69-A: 1041-1044, Sept. 1987.

48. **Wolfgang, G. L.:** Surgical repair of tears of the rotator cuff of the shoulder. Factors influencing the result. *J. Bone and Joint Surg.,* 56-A: 14-26, Jan. 1974.

49. **Wolfgang, G. L.:** Rupture of the musculotendinous cuff of the shoulder. *Clin. Orthop.,* 134: 230-243, 1978.

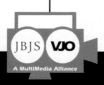

The Results of Repair of Massive Tears of the Rotator Cuff[*][†]

BY CHRISTIAN GERBER, M.D.‡, BRUNO FUCHS, M.D.‡, AND JUERG HODLER, M.D.‡

Investigation performed at the University of Zurich, Zurich, Switzerland

Abstract

Background: Massive tears of the tendons of the rotator cuff cause atrophy and fatty degeneration of the rotator cuff muscles and painful loss of function of the shoulder. Repair of massive rotator cuff tears is often followed by retears of the tendons, additional muscular degeneration, and a poor clinical outcome. The purposes of this study were to determine whether a new method of repair of rotator cuff tendons can yield a lower retear rate and a better clinical outcome than previously reported methods, to assess the muscular changes following repair of massive tears of the musculotendinous units, and to correlate findings on magnetic resonance imaging with the clinical results.

Methods: Twenty-nine massive rotator cuff tears involving complete detachment of at least two tendons were repaired operatively with use of a new laboratory-tested technique in a prospective study. At least two years (average, thirty-seven months; range, twenty-four to sixty-one months) postoperatively, twenty-seven patients were evaluated clinically and with magnetic resonance imaging to determine the clinical outcome, the integrity of the repair, and the condition of the rotator cuff muscles.

Results: The age and gender-adjusted Constant score improved from an average of 49 percent preoperatively to an average of 85 percent postoperatively, corresponding to a subjective shoulder value of 78 percent of that of a normal shoulder. Pain-free flexion improved from an average of 92 degrees to an average of 142 degrees, and abduction improved from an average of 82 degrees to an average of 137 degrees. Pain decreased and performance of activities of daily living improved significantly ($p < 0.05$). The seventeen patients who had a structurally successful repair all had an excellent clinical outcome. Muscle atrophy could not be reversed except in successfully repaired supraspinatus musculotendinous units. Fatty degeneration increased in all muscles.

Conclusions: The method of repair of massive rotator cuff tears that was used in this study yielded a comparatively low retear rate and good-to-excellent clinical results; however, the repair did not result in substantial reversal of muscular atrophy and fatty degeneration. Retears occurred more often in patients who had had a shorter interval between the onset of the symptoms and the operation ($p < 0.05$). Patients who had a retear had improvement of the shoulder compared with the preoperative state, but they had less improvement than did those who had a successful repair.

*No benefits in any form have been received or will be received from a commercial party related directly or indirectly to the subject of this article. No funds were received in support of this study.

†Recipient of the Neer Award of the American Shoulder and Elbow Surgeons, 1998.

‡Department of Orthopaedics (C. G. and B. F.) and Division of Diagnostic Radiology (J. H.), University of Zurich, Balgrist, Forchstrasse 340, 8008 Zurich, Switzerland. E-mail address for C. Gerber: cgerber@balgrist.unizh.ch.

The rotator cuff undergoes progressive degenerative changes with increasing age, which may lead to tears of rotator cuff tendons. Whereas small tears may be observed in elderly asymptomatic individuals, large or very large tears are symptomatic in younger people of working age[27,36]. These large or massive tears lead to weakness[25], are incompatible with manual labor[29,37], and may be associated with incapacitating, chronic pain and severe functional impairment. They also are often resistant to nonoperative treatment[8,10,33,40].

The term massive tear has been widely used to identify very large tears that are particularly difficult to repair and therefore are associated with an uncertain prognosis. Unfortunately, there is no universal agreement on the definition of a massive rotator cuff tear. In North America, Cofield's definition of a massive tear was a tear of greater than five centimeters in diameter[8]. Because of variations in the sizes of patients and the techniques of measurement, we believe that it is more appropriate to define the size of a tear in terms of the amount of tendon that has been detached from the tuberosities[32,33]. In the current study, rotator cuff tears were defined as massive if they involved the detachment of at least two entire tendons. Most massive tears involve the supraspinatus and the infraspinatus, but anterosuperior tears involving the supraspinatus and the subscapularis also occur moderately frequently[30,33].

Repairs of tears of the rotator cuff have been reported to be highly successful, yielding durable results that are superior to the natural history of the untreated disease[1,4,8,11,21,22,33]. The clinical outcome for patients who have a massive rotator cuff tear, however, is distinctly less satisfactory than that for patients who have a smaller tear[1,4,8,11,14,39], and repair may not always be warranted for massive tears.

Two important factors appear to explain the different outcomes associated with massive and smaller tears. First, the rate of retear after repair of massive tears, as

TABLE I
CLINICAL PARAMETERS IN RELATION TO WHICH ROTATOR CUFF TENDONS WERE TORN PREOPERATIVELY

	Tear of Supraspinatus and Infraspinatus (N = 17)			Tear of Supraspinatus and Subscapularis (N = 10)		
	Preop.*	Postop.*	P Value	Preop.*	Postop.*	P Value
Constant score						
Absolute[10] *(points)*	40	73.8	0.291	48.3	74.5	0.0011
Relative[9]† *(percent)*	60.6	89.3	0.123	58.3	90.5	0.0019
Pain‡ *(points)*	7.6	14.4	0.034	3.8	12.7	0.0001
Activities of daily living§ *(points)*	5.8	9.3	0.0084	4.9	9.8	0.0003
Functional use of arm# *(points)*	6.4	8.6	0.144	7.1	9.5	0.036
Active motion						
Flexion *(degrees)*	83	143	0.048	121	147	0.005
Abduction *(degrees)*	74	148	0.018	105	149	0.0043
External rotation *(degrees)*	41	29.3	0.74	58	52	0.54
Internal rotation§ *(points)*	6.8	8.6	0.122	5.6	7.6	0.05
Strength in abduction** *(kg)*	0.8	3.3	0.1002	3.1	3.9	0.039

*The values are given as the average.

†In relation to age and gender-matched normal values.

‡No pain = 15 points and intolerable pain = 0 points, according to a visual analog scale.

§According to the scoring system of Constant and Murley[10].

#Full overhead use = 10 points and elevation to less than waist level = 0 points.

**Measured with an electronic dynamometer with the arm in 90 degrees of abduction in the scapular plane, the elbow extended, resistance applied at the wrist, and the forearm pronated. (Patients with active abduction of less than 90 degrees have a strength of zero.)

assessed with imaging methods, has been reported to be between 50 and 70 percent[14,21,34,38], whereas it has been substantially lower after repair of smaller tears[1,11,14,22,34,39]. Although retear may not be associated with frank clinical failure, the clinical result of a shoulder with a structurally successful repair is significantly superior to that of a shoulder with a retear[21,38]. Second, repairs of massive rotator cuff tears are commonly associated with advanced atrophy and degeneration of the rotator cuff muscles[18,28,42]. These changes, demonstrated on imaging, reflect loss of the contractile elements and changes in the physiological properties of the remaining musculotendinous units[23].

These muscular changes may be irreversible. The development of a quantitative magnetic resonance imaging method for assessment of the rotator cuff muscles, and the availability of age and gender-related normal values[42], have made it possible to address this question with use of a noninvasive method.

The purposes of this study were to prospectively assess the results of a recently developed laboratory-tested technique[15,17] for the repair of massive tears of the rotator cuff, to determine whether or not the rotator cuff muscles recover after repair, and to correlate the structural results of magnetic resonance imaging studies with the clinical outcome.

Materials and Methods

We reviewed the results of twenty-nine operative repairs of massive tears of the rotator cuff that had been performed between 1992 and 1995. The criteria for operative repair included (1) failure of at least three months of nonoperative treatment, with the patient continuing to complain of subjectively unacceptable pain or disability, or both; (2) the desire or need of the patient to use the arm at or above the level of the head; (3) good motivation to comply with a postoperative treatment regimen; (4) an acromiohumeral distance of at least six millimeters, as seen on an anteroposterior radiograph of the shoulder, made with the patient standing, the arm in neutral rotation, and the muscles relaxed (shoulders with static superior subluxation of the humeral head were excluded from this series); and (5) the absence of moderate-to-marked osteoarthritis.

These criteria were met by twenty-nine (45 percent) of the sixty-four patients who were treated operatively for a massive tear during the period of the study. The other thirty-five patients were treated either with arthroscopic débridement or with repair including tendon transfers and therefore were not enrolled in the study. Two patients who had a complete clinical and magnetic resonance imaging examination at twelve and nineteen months after the operation refused additional imaging because the first examination had shown an intact cuff and the clinical result (a subjective shoulder value of 100 and 95 percent and a relative Constant score[9,10] of 108 and 110 percent) had remained unchanged subjectively.

The remaining twenty-seven patients were followed clinically and with magnetic resonance imaging for at least two years (average, thirty-seven months; range, twenty-four to sixty-one months). The ages of the eighteen men and nine women averaged fifty-six years (range, forty-one to seventy-two years). The dominant limb was involved in twenty-three patients. The preoperative symptoms had lasted for an average of twenty-two months (range, three to eighty-three months).

The final diagnosis of the lesion was made on the

TABLE II
CLINICAL PARAMETERS IN RELATION TO WHETHER THE TEAR INVOLVED TWO OR THREE TENDONS

	Tear Involving Two Tendons (N = 17)			Tear Involving Three Tendons (N = 10)		
	Preop.*	Postop.*	P Value	Preop.*	Postop.*	P Value
Constant score						
Absolute[10] (points)	47.6	74.2	0.0002	27	64.3	0.0034
Relative[9]† (percent)	59.1	90	0.0133	31.8	76.4	0.0024
Pain‡ (points)	5.2	13.4	0.0001	6.8	12.1	0.0077
Activities of daily living§ (points)	5.2	9.6	0.0001	3.4	8.8	0.001
Functional use of arm# (points)	6.9	9.1	0.0043	4.8	8.2	0.0263
Active motion						
Flexion (degrees)	107	145	0.0008	66	136	0.0019
Abduction (degrees)	94	149	0.002	59	117	0.0097
External rotation (degrees)	52	43	0.59	46	38	0.625
Internal rotation§ (points)	6	8	0.01	5.8	6.4	0.42
Strength in abduction** (kg)	2.3	3.6	0.011	0.2	2.6	0.42

*The values are given as the average.
†In relation to age and gender-matched normal values.
‡No pain = 15 points and intolerable pain = 0 points, according to a visual analog scale.
§According to the scoring system of Constant and Murley[10].
#Full overhead use = 10 points and elevation to less than waist level = 0 points.
**Measured with an electronic dynamometer with the arm in 90 degrees of abduction in the scapular plane, the elbow extended, resistance applied at the wrist, and the forearm pronated. (Patients with active abduction of less than 90 degrees have a strength of zero.)

basis of the intraoperative findings. If a very small muscular strand of the subscapularis was still attached to the most distal part of the crista of the lesser tuberosity, the subscapularis tear was considered complete. The infraspinatus insertion zone was identified by laying the two branches of the forceps over the scapular spine so that the forceps were in line with the fibers of the cuff. Fibers coming from a level inferior to the scapular spine are infraspinatus fibers. The teres minor insertion was identified by locating its insertion on the respective tubercle, which lies inferior and slightly medial to the infraspinatus insertion.

The clinical assessment was based on a structured interview and a detailed physical examination that was carried out in a standardized fashion (Tables I and II). The objective assessment of active pain-free flexion and abduction was carried out with the patient sitting. The range of pain-free flexion (in the sagittal plane) was measured as the angle between the humeral shaft and the midthoracic line (not the vertical). Abduction always was measured, with simultaneous maximal abduction of both arms, as the angle formed by the humeral shaft and the midthoracic line.

Functional external rotation was measured according to the method of Constant and Murley[10]. This method represents an attempt to measure the patient's ability to externally rotate the arm in the functional positions necessary in daily living. Two points are given for each of the following activities: bringing the hand actively behind the neck with the elbow above the acromion, bringing the elbow straight forward from that position, actively positioning the hand on top of the head with the elbow over the acromion, bringing the elbow straight forward from that position, and fully ele-

vating the arm from that position. The hand is not allowed to touch the head or neck during these functional movements.

The amount of active internal rotation was determined according to the spinous process that the patient could actively reach with the thumb without pain.

Abduction strength was assessed with use of an Isobex dynamometer (Cursor SA, Bern, Switzerland) with the patient standing and the arm abducted to 90 degrees in the scapular plane, the elbow extended, and the forearm pronated. The resistance was applied at the wrist. Three measurements of five seconds' duration (the B mode of the device) were averaged. One point was attributed to each pound (0.45 kilogram) of strength that was measured. If 90 degrees of abduction in the scapular plane was not reached, the abduction strength automatically was considered to be zero.

The total Constant score was recorded. In addition, the score for each patient was related to the age and gender-matched normal values that were established by Constant[9]. The patients also were asked to estimate the value of the shoulder as a percentage of the value of an entirely normal shoulder (subjective shoulder value).

Preoperatively, anteroposterior, lateral, and axial radiographs were made for each patient. All but one patient had either a magnetic resonance imaging study or an arthro-computerized tomographic scan.

An independent examiner reviewed the results for all twenty-seven patients at an average of thirty-seven months (range, twenty-four to sixty-one months) postoperatively. Twenty-five patients had a standardized magnetic resonance imaging scan; the two remaining patients refused to have magnetic resonance imaging because of claustrophobia and underwent ultrasonographic exami-

TABLE III
COMPARISON OF THE FINDINGS ON TWO FOLLOW-UP EXAMINATIONS*

	Intact Repair			Retear			Total		
	First Exam.	Second Exam.	P Value	First Exam.	Second Exam.	P Value	First Exam.	Second Exam.	P Value
Duration of follow-up *(mos.)*	16.5	39.8		16.5	39.6		16.5	39.7	
Subjective shoulder value *(percent)*	90	90.8	0.87	76.6	65.8	0.57	83.3	78.3	0.73
Relative Constant score[9] *(percent)*	95.6	95.5	0.87	63.1	69.6	0.52	79.4	82.6	0.69
Fatty degeneration[18,19] *(stage)*									
Supraspinatus	1.66	1.33	0.52	2.5	2.8	0.57	2.08	2.1	0.97
Infraspinatus	1.6	1.5	0.63	2.5	2.0	0.37	2.08	1.75	0.32
Subscapularis	0.53	0.5	0.06	1.33	1.16	0.93	1.13	0.83	0.15
Atrophy† *(mm²)*									
Supraspinatus	405	411	0.87	257	227	0.57	331	319	0.54
Infraspinatus	1033	1160	0.68	1028	913	0.68	1031	1036	0.72
Subscapularis	1228	1033	0.52	1192	949	0.17	1210	991	0.15

*The values are given as the average, for twelve patients.
†The values indicate the cross-sectional area of the muscle.

nation of the repaired cuff. Twelve patients had already undergone the same clinical and magnetic resonance imaging examinations between twelve and twenty-three months after the operation. Magnetic resonance imaging was performed with use of a 1.0-tesla scanner (Siemens, Erlangen, Germany). Parasagittal T1-weighted turbo-spin-echo magnetic resonance images (repetition time, 700 milliseconds; echo time, twelve milliseconds), made parallel to the glenohumeral joint, were obtained for qualitative and quantitative assessment of the rotator cuff muscles. The slice thickness was five millimeters, with an interslice gap of 1.5 millimeters. The sequence covered the rotator cuff from the humeral tuberosities to the medial third of the scapula. The field of view was eighteen centimeters, the image matrix was 210 by 256, and the echo train length was three. For quantitative assessment, the cross-sectional areas of the rotator cuff muscles and the fossa supraspinata were measured on the most lateral image on which the scapular spine was in contact with the remainder of the scapula. High intra-subject and interobserver reliability has been documented with use of this technique of magnetic resonance imaging interpretation[42] for cross-sectional areas of the supraspinatus, the subscapularis, and the infraspinatus and the teres minor combined. Intrasubject and interobserver reliability has been found to be substantially lower for the infraspinatus alone, but it has been found that it is more reasonable to report the values of the infraspinatus than those of the infraspinatus and the teres minor together, as the infraspinatus often is torn whereas the teres minor is not[42].

In addition to the quantitative assessment of cross-sectional areas of the muscles, intramuscular fatty degeneration was assessed with use of the criteria established by Goutallier et al. for determining the amount of fatty degeneration on computerized tomographic scans[18,19]. This classification was applied to parasagittal and axial T1-weighted turbo-spin-echo magnetic resonance images[12].

Retear of the tendon also was assessed with angled, coronal T2-weighted, proton-density-weighted, and short tau inversion recovery (STIR) sequences, according to established magnetic resonance imaging criteria[26,31].

Operative Technique

The patient was positioned in the beach-chair position. In seventeen patients with a tear involving mostly the supraspinatus and the infraspinatus, a superolateral approach was used, with elevation of the anterolateral deltoid origin with a bone chisel and splitting of the deltoid between the anterior and lateral portions along its fibers over a distance of less than six centimeters. In the other twelve patients, severe atrophy and retraction of the subscapularis were expected to require extensive dissection in the vicinity of the plexus in order to mobilize the subscapularis, so a deltopectoral approach was used. The lesions involved the supraspinatus and the infraspinatus in nine patients (31 percent), the supraspinatus and the subscapularis in ten patients (34 percent), and all three tendons in ten patients.

The infraspinatus and the supraspinatus then were mobilized with use of a subacromial spreader (Sulzer Medica AG, Baar, Switzerland) to subluxate or even dislocate the humeral head anteroinferiorly; the subscapularis was mobilized and repaired as described previously[16]. The musculotendinous units were mobilized to allow repair to their original area of insertion, with the arm abducted to no more than 30 to 45 degrees. The area of insertion was only cleaned of soft tissue; a deep osseous trough was not created.

To obtain optimal initial fixation strength and minimal gap formation upon postoperative movement, a transosseous repair technique that was validated *in vitro* and *in vivo*[15,17] was utilized. With this technique, the tendons are freed up extensively with release of the interval between the tendons to be repaired and capsulotomy performed between the capsule and the labrum from inside, with the joint distracted with use of a subacromial spreader. Number-3 braided polyester sutures and a modified Mason-Allen tendon stitch are used[15]; the latter improves the suture pullout strength by a factor of at least two. A thin titanium plate with seven round holes (Stratec Synthes SA, Waldenburg, Switzerland) was used as a cortical bone-augmentation device. Both strands of a single Mason-Allen stitch are brought through the tuberosity and through two holes of the plate. The suture then is tied under optimal tension over the bridge between the two holes of the plate. The plate and holes are designed not to cut the sutures, and the titanium does not interfere with magnetic resonance assessment of the affected shoulder.

A resection of the acromioclavicular joint also was performed if the joint was painful (fourteen patients). An anterior acromioplasty was avoided if the likelihood of postoperative anterosuperior subluxation seemed high due to difficulty in obtaining an optimal closure of the rotator interval (ten patients).

Postoperative Regimen

Postoperatively, the patients wore a sling if the subscapularis had been the most retracted musculotendinous unit and the supraspinatus and the infraspinatus were not under relevant tension in the adducted position (ten patients), and they wore an abduction splint for six weeks if the surgeon thought that the supraspinatus and the infraspinatus were under relevant tension with the arm in adduction (nineteen patients). Immediately postoperatively, passive range-of-motion exercises were begun within the range that had been found to be safe intraoperatively. Active range-of-motion exercises were started after six weeks.

Results

Preoperative Findings

Patients who had a tear involving all three tendons were much more disabled functionally, with poorer performance of the activities of daily living; decreased flexion, abduction, and strength in abduction; and a poorer overall shoulder score according to the criteria of Constant and Murley[10] (Table II). Interestingly, tears involving all three tendons tended to be less painful than those involving two tendons, and they were clearly less painful than the anterosuperior variant of the two-tendon tears.

Of the two-tendon tears, those that were posterosuperior caused a distinctly greater functional handicap in terms of decreased abduction, external rotation, and abduction strength. However, the anterosuperior tears tended to be more painful, so they were not associated with significantly better overall shoulder scores (Table I).

TABLE IV

INTEGRITY OF THE ROTATOR CUFF
AS SEEN ON MAGNETIC RESONANCE IMAGING*

	Supraspinatus and Infraspinatus	Supraspinatus and Subscapularis	All Three Tendons
Preop. tear	7	10	10
Postop.			
Intact	4	8	5
Retear			
<1.5 cm	0	0	1
1.5-3.0 cm	2	1	2
3.1-5.0 cm	1	1	2
>5.0 cm	0	0	0

*The values are given as the number of patients.

Neither atrophy, measured as cross-sectional area, nor fatty degeneration of the subscapularis and the infraspinatus was much more advanced if the subscapularis and infraspinatus musculotendinous units were torn than if they were intact (Tables IV and VII). The areas of muscle were, however, always smaller than those of an age and gender-matched healthy population[42].

Complications

There were no relevant complications in this series of patients. Specifically, we did not observe hematoma, wound dehiscence or infection, stiffness requiring manipulation, deltoid dehiscence, or nerve injury. No complications related to the titanium plate were observed.

Clinical Outcome

In the entire series, the relative Constant score increased from 49 percent of that of a normal shoulder preoperatively to 85 percent postoperatively. The postoperative value corresponded well with a subjective shoulder value of 78 percent. Pain-free flexion improved from an average of 92 degrees to an average of 142 degrees, and abduction improved from an average of 82 degrees to an average of 137 degrees.

All of the clinical parameters that were studied, with the exception of active internal and external rotation and strength in abduction, improved significantly after the operations for both the two and the three-tendon tears (Tables I and II). Except for pain, the parameters showed greater improvement in the shoulders with a three-tendon tear than in those with a two-tendon tear. Postoperatively, the shoulders with a three-tendon tear had, on the average, increases of 45 percent in the relative Constant score ($p = 0.0024$), 5.3 points on the 15-point visual analog assessment of pain ($p = 0.0077$), 70 degrees of flexion ($p = 0.0019$), and 2.3 kilograms of abduction strength ($p = 0.42$), whereas the increases for the shoulders with a two-tendon tear were 31 percent ($p = 0.0133$), 8.2 points ($p = 0.0001$), 38 degrees ($p = 0.0008$), and 1.3 kilograms ($p = 0.011$), respectively (Table II). Nonetheless, the subjective shoulder value (the subjective value as a percentage of that of a normal shoulder), the relative Constant score, the pain score,

TABLE V
CLINICAL RESULTS AS A FUNCTION OF THE INTEGRITY OF THE ROTATOR CUFF

	Preop. Two-Tendon Tear			Preop. Three-Tendon Tear		
	Intact Repair* (N = 12)	Retear* (N = 5)	P Value†	Intact Repair* (N = 5)	Retear* (N = 5)	P Value†
Subjective shoulder value (percent)	84.2	74	0.08	91	56	0.022
Constant score						
Absolute[10] (points)	76.9	67.8	0.37	77.2	51.4	0.0088
Relative[9] (percent)	94.4	79.4	0.126	91	61.8	0.016
Pain (points)	13.1	14.2	0.67	14.2	10	0.094
Flexion (degrees)	149.5	135	0.75	158	113	0.012
Strength in abduction (kg)	4.3	2.0	0.05	4.4	0.7	0.011

*The values are given as the average.
†According to the Mann-Whitney U test, with the level of significance set at $p < 0.05$.

and abduction remained better in the shoulders with a two-tendon tear. The differences between function associated with anterosuperior two-tendon tears and that associated with posterosuperior two-tendon tears disappeared after operative repair (Table I).

Seventeen (63 percent) of the twenty-seven shoulders, as well as the two that were evaluated at less than twenty-four months, had an unequivocally intact rotator cuff at the time of the latest follow-up. It is notable that the results of the follow-up examination at more than two years were no different from those between one and two years and, specifically, that neither healing of a retear nor the presence of an additional retear were observed during this interval (Table III). In the group of patients who had an intact repair at the time of the latest follow-up examination, the results for those who had had a two-tendon tear were as excellent as the results for those who had had a three-tendon tear. The patients who had had a two-tendon tear had an average relative Constant score of 94 percent, an average pain score of 13 points, an average flexion of 150 degrees, and an average abduction strength of 4.3 kilograms, whereas those who had had a three-tendon tear had average values of 91 percent, 14 points, 158 degrees, and 4.4 kilograms, respectively (Table V). Thus, successful repair restored almost normal shoulder function in these patients and, notably, also restored good abduction strength.

There were ten retears: five in the two-tendon-tear group and five in the three-tendon-tear group (Table IV). When the patients who had a subsequent retear were compared with those who had an intact repair, they differed significantly with regard to only one preoperative variable: the duration of shoulder pain and dysfunction before the operation had been significantly shorter (eleven compared with twenty-eight months; p = 0.021) for the patients who had a retear. In addition, the onset of the symptoms in those patients often had been associated with a minor traumatic event. The clinical status of the patients who had a subsequent retear was worse preoperatively with regard to all other vari-

ables that were studied, but these differences did not reach significance (Table VIII).

Compared with the patients who had a retear, the patients who had a successful repair had significantly better results in terms of strength, active range of motion, the Constant score, and the subjective shoulder value (Table V). Although these patients also did better in terms of pain, this difference did not reach significance.

Neither the intraoperative state of the tendon of the long head of the biceps (normal versus dislocated, hypertrophic, or torn) nor its treatment (tenodesis versus relocation) influenced the outcome.

Structural Results

The structure of the repaired tendons, as judged on magnetic resonance imaging, was never normal. The supraspinatus tendon and infraspinatus tendon especially showed a scarlike signal. The overall rate of retears of the cuff was 34 percent (ten of twenty-nine). Three of the nine patients who had had a posterosuperior two-tendon tear, two of the ten who had had an anterosuperior two-tendon tear, and five of the ten who had had a three-tendon tear had a retear. Four retears were the same size as the original tear, and six were distinctly smaller; none were larger than the initial tear. The clinical results for the patients who had a retear were significantly inferior to those for the patients who had an intact cuff. Interestingly, the clinical results for the six patients who had a small retear were not better than those for the four in whom the retear was as big as the initial tear; the crucial finding was the presence or absence of a retear and not its size. Regardless of the type of tear, all groups of patients, including the four who had a massive retear, had a substantial improvement postoperatively compared with the preoperative state. In the group with a massive retear, the relative Constant score improved from an average of 31 to 70 percent; flexion, from an average of 34 to 116 degrees; and the pain score, from an average of 6.3 to 13.5 points. Only abduction strength did not improve in this group of patients.

TABLE VI
POSTOPERATIVE MUSCLE ATROPHY AS A FUNCTION OF THE
PREOPERATIVE AND POSTOPERATIVE INTEGRITY OF THE TENDONS

	Preop. Cross-Sectional Area (mm²)	Postop. Cross-Sectional Area (mm²)			P Value for Difference Between Preop. and Postop. Values in Entire Series*
		Intact Preop.	Torn Preop.	Entire Series	
Supraspinatus†					
Entire series	382	—	374	—	0.841
Intact repair	—	—	435	—	—
Failure	382	—	247	—	0.1002
P value for difference between intact repair and failure*	—	—	0.008	—	—
Subscapularis					
Entire series	1516	1913	1416	1516	0.1949
Intact repair	1913	2135	1240	1496	0.1109
Failure	1416	1692	1107	1705	0.1893
P value for difference between intact repair and failure*	0.2963	—	0.655	0.83	—
Infraspinatus					
Entire series	919	1193	1044	1163	0.0662
Intact repair	843	1168	1316	1219	0.0549
Failure	1046	1307	909	1092	0.698
P value for difference between intact repair and failure*	0.584	0.34	0.071	0.547	—

*According to the Mann-Whitney U test, with the level of significance set at p < 0.05.

†In the group that had an intact repair of the supraspinatus, the preoperative cross-sectional area had been 364 square millimeters and the postoperative cross-sectional area was 434 square millimeters (p = 0.234). In the group that had a failure of the repair of the supraspinatus, the preoperative cross-sectional area had been 408 square millimeters and the postoperative cross-sectional area was 247 square millimeters (p = 0.174). The p value for the difference between the preoperative cross-sectional areas of the two groups (intact repair and failure of the repair) was 0.99, and that for the difference between the postoperative cross-sectional areas was 0.0088.

The postoperative degree of muscular atrophy of the infraspinatus and the subscapularis did not depend on the integrity of the repair of the tendon (Table VI); however, the square area of the supraspinatus did depend on this factor insofar as atrophy increased if the repair of the supraspinatus failed and the cross-sectional area increased if the repair was successful. Overall, the preoperative muscular atrophy was not reversed postoperatively, but in the patients who had a successful repair the increase in the cross-sectional area of the supraspinatus almost reached significance (p = 0.054).

Fatty degeneration increased postoperatively in all three muscles that were studied. It increased significantly more if the tendon of the respective muscle was found to be torn intraoperatively than if it was found to be intact. It was only for the supraspinatus that we could document statistically that a successful repair had a beneficial effect on fatty degeneration because the repaired musculotendinous units showed significantly less progression of fatty degeneration than the failed repairs (Table VII).

Discussion

The optimal form of treatment of massive rotator cuff tears is controversial. Whereas operative repair has yielded good-to-excellent clinical results in many studies[4,6,20,21,24], some authors have thought that repairs of massive tears of the rotator cuff fail so often that it may be preferable to treat patients with such tears nonoperatively, with rotator cuff débridement, or with other operative procedures[2,3,7,13].

The differences in the reported results and opinions may be due to various reasons. First, differences in the definition of the tear size make it difficult to compare the results from different institutions[1,4,8,11,13]. The maximum diameter[8] is possibly not the best indication of the size of a tear. If, at the time of measurement, the humerus is pushed proximally, the diameter of the tear increases, and it decreases if the head is pulled distally. The measured size of the tear also may be affected by rotation of the humerus. In addition, most published reports do not state whether the size of the tear was measured before or after resection of nonviable edges of the tendinous stump. Finally, with the wide variation in the sizes and heights of patients, a given diameter may have very different relevance for different individuals. We believe that the amount of tendon tissue that has become detached from the humerus is a much more repro-

TABLE VII
FATTY MUSCLE DEGENERATION AS A FUNCTION OF THE
PREOPERATIVE AND POSTOPERATIVE INTEGRITY OF THE TENDONS

		Postop. Stage[18,19]				
	Preop. Stage[18,19]	Intact Preop.	Torn Preop.	P Value for Difference Between Intact and Torn Preop.*	Entire Series	P Value for Difference Between Preop. and Postop. Stage in Entire Series*
Supraspinatus						
Entire series	1.50	—	2.04		2.037	0.062
Intact repair	—	—	1.79		1.79	
Failure	1.50	—	2.63		2.63	0.0062
P value for difference between intact repair and failure*			0.017		0.017	
Subscapularis						
Entire series	1.14	0.83	2.07	0.0084	1.79	0.052
Intact repair	1.125	0.83	2.03	0.007	1.71	0.477
Failure	1.143	—	2.25		2.25	0.0495
P value for difference between intact repair and failure*	0.957		0.68		0.337	
Infraspinatus						
Entire series	1.735	1.70	2.47	0.027	2.093	0.1229
Intact repair	1.375	1.70	2.46	0.033	2.06	0.056
Failure	2.056	—	2.5		2.5	0.41
P value for difference between intact repair and failure*	0.1124		0.999		0.517	

*According to the Mann-Whitney U test, with the level of significance set at $p < 0.05$.

ducible and relevant indicator of tear size[32,33]; therefore, we defined a massive tear as one with complete detachment of at least two cuff tendons. This anatomical description of the lesion corresponds generally to a tear size of more than five centimeters, so the current study included only tears that met previously used criteria. Among shoulders with a massive tear, those with static superior subluxation (an acromiohumeral distance of less than six millimeters) appear to have a poorer prognosis after direct repair than do those with a centered head[39,41]. Indeed, we tend not to use direct repair for patients with documented static superior subluxation of the humeral head, and in the present study we included only shoulders with an acromiohumeral distance of at least six millimeters as seen on an anteroposterior radiograph made in neutral rotation[6].

Second, the techniques of repair vary greatly, as shown by the results of an inquiry of leading shoulder surgeons in America and Europe[15]. It has been shown that currently recommended standard techniques are mechanically suboptimal and can be improved substantially[15,17]. In the current study, we used only a laboratory-tested method of repair with number-3 braided polyester sutures, a special tendon-grasping technique, and augmentation of the osteoporotic cortical bone to allow secure fixation of the transosseous sutures[15]. With this method, the retear rate remained high (37 percent [ten of twenty-seven], or 34 percent [ten of twenty-nine] if the two shoulders with less than two years of follow-up are

included), but it was distinctly lower than the 50 to 70 percent failure rate that has been reported after other methods of repair of comparable tears[14,21,34,38]. The retear was the same size as the preoperative tear in four patients, and it was smaller than the original tear in six[27]. The clinical results of the patients who had a small retear were similar to those of the patients who had a large retear but were unlike those of the patients who had a successful repair. This finding raises questions about the concept of partial repair of the rotator cuff[7]. Conversely, it reemphasizes that every effort to promote healing of the repaired tendons is justified. The present study does not answer the question regarding the necessity of postoperative protection because an abduction splint was not used by patients with a tear predominantly involving the subscapularis. We think that our experimental data[17,23] sufficiently support the use of an abduction splint when it allows a reduction in the tension on the repair, as in a shoulder with a supraspinatus tear.

The structural results of rotator cuff repairs have been analyzed only rarely[14,21,34,38]. In the current study, the integrity of the repairs and the presence of retears were determined with magnetic resonance imaging; however, this modality is demanding as well as labor-intensive, and it may become even more difficult to use due to legal and monetary constraints. Several authors[14,21,38] have documented the structural quality of their repairs and have shown that patients who have a successful repair do better than those who have a failed repair. The find-

TABLE VIII
ANALYSIS OF FAILURES

	Preop.			Postop.			P Value for Difference Between Preop. and Postop. Values†	
	Failure*	Intact Repair*	P Value†	Failure*	Intact Repair*	P Value†	Failure	Intact Repair
Age *(yrs.)*	56.8	56.2	0.51					
Durat. of symptoms preop. *(mos.)*	11	28.1	0.021					
Durat. of follow-up *(mos.)*				36.9	37.1	0.404		
Constant score								
Absolute[10] *(points)*	34.6	43.8	0.35	59.6	77	0.0112	0.0099	0.0001
Relative[9] *(percent)*	40.1	54.1	0.26	70.6	93.4	0.0077	0.037	0.0001
Pain *(points)*	4.4	6.3	0.34	12.1	13.4	0.64	0.0087	0.0004
Activities of daily living *(points)*	4.5	4.28	0.758	8.4	9.8	0.075	0.0045	0.0001
Functional use of arm *(points)*	5.3	6.6	0.261	7.6	9.47	0.108	0.109	0.001
Flexion *(degrees)*	80	98.9	0.246	124	152.1	0.0038	0.012	0.0001
Abduction *(degrees)*	72.6	86.8	0.53	119	147.4	0.157	0.032	0.0001
External rotation *(degrees)*	45.6	52.1	0.707	32.5	45.8	0.16	0.53	0.47
Internal rotation *(points)*	5.3	6.28	0.339	7.2	7.5	0.911	0.056	0.122

*The values are given as the average and represent the integrity of the repair on follow-up magnetic resonance imaging.
†According to the Mann-Whitney U test, with the level of significance set at p < 0.05.

ings in the present study reemphasize that fact and document a markedly significant superiority in the results of patients with a successful repair compared with those of patients who did not have a successful repair. The fact that no new retears were observed after two years in the twelve patients who had already had complete documentation at one to two years is consistent with the experimental finding that retears occur very early[17] and also with the clinical finding that the results of rotator cuff repair are durable[4,8]. We believe that the significantly shorter preoperative duration of the symptoms in the shoulders that could not be successfully repaired was most likely due to a traumatic extension of a large preexisting tear, leading to very poor function and often to pseudoparalysis. Whether immediate repair or preoperative rehabilitation is preferable after such a traumatic event is currently not known. Despite the findings in this study, it is our experience that a long-standing pseudoparalysis can almost never be reversed with operative cuff repair, whereas the regaining of useful overhead function after an acute loss of overhead elevation is a reasonable expectation; therefore, we continue to recommend early repair if pseudoparalysis has suddenly developed.

In our entire series, abduction strength improved compared with the preoperative value, but not significantly. However, when the successfully repaired shoulders were evaluated separately, abduction strength was found to have increased very significantly (from 1.55 to 4.4 kilograms). These findings are consistent with the observation of Thomazeau et al. that an intact cuff is mandatory if abduction strength of more than four kilograms is to be achieved[38].

Fatty degeneration and atrophy occur in association with chronic rotator cuff tears in both animals[5] and humans[18,28,38]. Clinical experience suggests that advanced muscular atrophy may not be reversible and that weakness after rotator cuff repair is a certainty[25]. The present study shows that, at least within two years, muscular atrophy is at least stopped and may be reversed in successfully repaired supraspinatus musculotendinous units whereas atrophy increases after an unsuccessful repair. This finding is in agreement with the data of Thomazeau et al., who also reported a reversal of supraspinatus atrophy in half of the successfully repaired cuffs but in none that had a failed repair[38]. In the other muscles that were studied, however, atrophy tended to increase, especially after a failed repair. Due to the large variation in the size and musculature of patients, it may be necessary to study larger patient populations to clarify the apparent reversibility of supraspinatus atrophy and the absence of reversibility in the other two muscles, since in our study only the supraspinatus tendon was preoperatively torn in all patients.

Fatty degeneration is not reversible as assessed with our methodology. It increased in the supraspinatus more rapidly when a tendon repair failed than when it did not. An increase in fatty degeneration was seen predominantly in the musculotendinous units that were noted to be torn intraoperatively and therefore were repaired, suggesting that operative repair may damage the musculotendinous units and thereby result in progression of fatty degeneration. We have always palpated the supraspinatus and infraspinatus and have never found any clinical evidence of neurological damage, which poten-

tially can be caused by the extensive mobilization of the cuff[43]. However, we cannot exclude the possibility that the tension created by the repair causes damage due to fatty degeneration. In light of the potential effects of postoperative tension, it seems logical to try to minimize tension by optimal protection of the repair[5,23] in order to avoid iatrogenic damage to the musculotendinous unit.

References

1. **Adamson, G. J.,** and **Tibone, J. E.:** Ten-year assessment of primary rotator cuff repairs. *J. Shoulder and Elbow Surg.,* 2: 57-63, 1993.
2. **Augereau, B.,** and **Apoil, A.:** La réparation des grandes ruptures de la coiffe des rotateurs de l'épaule. *Rev. chir. orthop.,* 74 (Supplement 2): 59-62, 1988.
3. **Augereau, B.; Koechlin, P.; Moinet, P.; Apoil, A.; Bonnet, J. C.;** and **Doursounian, L.:** L'arthrolyse antéro-supérieure de l'épaule pour lésions trophiques de la coiffe des rotateurs, sur tête centrée. *Rev. chir. orthop.,* 74: 292-296, 1988.
4. **Bigliani, L. U.; McIlveen, S. J.; Cordasco, F.;** and **Musso, E.:** Operative repair of massive rotator cuff tears: long term results. *J. Shoulder and Elbow Surg.,* 1: 120-130, 1992.
5. **Bjorkenheim, J.-M.:** Structure and function of the rabbit's supraspinatus muscle after resection of its tendon. *Acta Orthop. Scandinavica,* 60: 461-463, 1989.
6. **Bonnin, M.:** La radiographie simple dans les ruptures de coiffe. *Journées Lyonnaises l'épaule,* pp. 14-19, 1993.
7. **Burkhart, S. S.; Nottage, W. M.; Ogilvie-Harris, D. J.; Kohn, H. S.;** and **Pachelli, A.:** Partial repair of irreparable rotator cuff tears. *Arthroscopy,* 10: 363-370, 1994.
8. **Cofield, R. H.:** Current concepts review. Rotator cuff disease of the shoulder. *J. Bone and Joint Surg.,* 67-A: 974-979, July 1985.
9. **Constant, C. R.:** Age related recovery of shoulder function after injury. Thesis, University College, Cork, Ireland, 1986.
10. **Constant, C. R.,** and **Murley, A. H.:** A clinical method of functional assessment of the shoulder. *Clin. Orthop.,* 214: 160-164, 1987.
11. **Ellman, H.; Hanker, G.;** and **Bayer, M.:** Repair of the rotator cuff. End-result study of factors influencing reconstruction. *J. Bone and Joint Surg.,* 68-A: 1136-1144, Oct. 1986.
12. **Fuchs, B.; Weishaupt, D.; Zanetti, M.; Hodler, J.;** and **Gerber, C.:** Fatty degeneration of the muscles of the rotator cuff: assessment by computed tomography versus magnetic resonance imaging. *J. Shoulder and Elbow Surg.,* 8: 599-605, 1999.
13. **Gartsman, G. M.:** Massive, irreparable tears of the rotator cuff. Results of operative débridement and subacromial decompression. *J. Bone and Joint Surg.,* 79-A: 715-721, May 1997.
14. **Gazielly, D. F.; Gleyze, P.;** and **Montagnon, C.:** Functional and anatomical results after rotator cuff repair. *Clin. Orthop.,* 304: 43-53, 1994.
15. **Gerber, C.; Schneeberger, A. G.; Beck, M.;** and **Schlegel, U.:** Mechanical strength of repairs of the rotator cuff. *J. Bone and Joint Surg.,* 76-B(3): 371-380, 1994.
16. **Gerber, C.; Hersche, O.;** and **Farron, A.:** Isolated rupture of the subscapularis tendon. Results of operative repair. *J. Bone and Joint Surg.,* 78-A: 1015-1023, July 1996.
17. **Gerber, C.; Schneeberger, A. G.; Perren, S. M.;** and **Nyffeler, R. W.:** Experimental rotator cuff repair. A preliminary study. *J. Bone and Joint Surg.,* 81-A: 1281-1290, Sept. 1999.
18. **Goutallier, D.; Bernageau, J.;** and **Patte, D.:** L'évaluation par le scanner de la trophicité des muscles des coiffes des rotateurs ayant une rupture tendineuse. *Rev. chir. orthop.,* 75 (Supplement I): 126-127, 1989.
19. **Goutallier, D.; Postel, J.-M.; Bernageau, J.; Lavau, L.;** and **Voisin, M.-C.:** Fatty muscle degeneration in cuff ruptures. Pre- and postoperative evaluation by CT scan. *Clin. Orthop.,* 304: 78-83, 1994.
20. **Grana, W. A.; Teague, B.; King, M.;** and **Reeves, R. B.:** An analysis of rotator cuff repair. *Am. J. Sports Med.,* 22: 585-588, 1994.
21. **Harryman, D. T., II; Mack, L. A.; Wang, K. Y.; Jackins, S. E.; Richardson, M. L.;** and **Matsen, F. A., III:** Repairs of the rotator cuff. Correlation of functional results with integrity of the cuff. *J. Bone and Joint Surg.,* 73-A: 982-989, Aug. 1991.
22. **Hawkins, R. J.; Misamore, G. W.;** and **Hobeika, P. E.:** Surgery for full-thickness rotator-cuff tears. *J. Bone and Joint Surg.,* 67-A: 1349-1355, Dec. 1985.
23. **Hersche, O.,** and **Gerber, C.:** Passive tension in the supraspinatus musculotendinous unit after long-standing rupture of its tendon: a preliminary report. *J. Shoulder and Elbow Surg.,* 7: 393-396, 1998.
24. **Iannotti, J. P.; Bernot, M. P.; Kuhlman, J. R.; Kelley, M. J.;** and **Williams, G. R.:** Postoperative assessment of shoulder function: a prospective study of full-thickness rotator cuff tears. *J. Shoulder and Elbow Surg.,* 5: 449-457, 1996.
25. **Itoi, E.; Minagawa, H.; Sato, T.; Sato, K.;** and **Tabata, S.:** Isokinetic strength after tears of the supraspinatus tendon. *J. Bone and Joint Surg.,* 79-B(1): 77-82, 1997.
26. **Magee, T. H.; Gaenslen, E. S.; Seitz, R.; Hinson, G. A.;** and **Wetzel, L. H.:** MR imaging of the shoulder after surgery. *AJR: Am. J. Roentgenol.,* 168: 925-928, 1997.
27. **Milgrom, C.; Schaffler, M.; Gilbert, S.;** and **van Holsbeeck, M.:** Rotator-cuff changes in asymptomatic adults. The effect of age, hand dominance and gender. *J. Bone and Joint Surg.,* 77-B(2): 296-298, 1995.
28. **Nakagaki, K.; Ozaki, J.; Tomita, Y.;** and **Tamai, S.:** Alterations in the supraspinatus muscle belly with rotator cuff tearing: evaluation with magnetic resonance imaging. *J. Shoulder and Elbow Surg.,* 3: 88-93, 1994.
29. **Noël, E.:** Les ruptures de la coiffe des rotateurs avec tête humérale centrée. Résultats du traitement conservateur. A propos de 171 épaules. *Journées Lyonnaises l'épaule,* pp. 283-297, 1993.
30. **Nové-Josserand, L.; Gerber, C.;** and **Walch, G.:** Lesions of the antero-superior rotator cuff. In *Complex and Revision Problems in Shoulder Surgery,* pp. 165-176. Edited by J. J. P. Warner, J. P. Iannotti, and C. Gerber. Philadelphia, Lippincott-Raven, 1997.
31. **Owen, R. S.; Iannotti, J. P.; Kneeland, J. B.; Dalinka, M. K.; Deren, J. A.;** and **Oleaga, L.:** Shoulder after surgery: MR imaging with surgical validation. *Radiology,* 186: 443-447, 1993.
32. **Patte, D.; Goutallier, D.; Monpierre, H.;** and **Debeyre, J.:** Etude des lésions étendues. *Rev. chir. orthop.,* 74: 314-318, 1983.
33. **Patte, D.,** and **Debeyre, J.:** Essai comparatif de deux séries de ruptures de coiffes opérées et non opérées. *Rev. chir. orthop.,* 74: 327-328, 1988.

34. **Postel, J. M.; Goutallier, D.; Lavau, L.;** and **Bernageau, J.:** Anatomical results of rotator cuff repairs: study of 57 cases controlled by arthrography. *J. Shoulder and Elbow Surg.,* 3: S20, 1994.

35. **Rockwood, C. A., Jr.; Williams, G. R., Jr.;** and **Burkhead, W. Z., Jr.:** Débridement of degenerative, irreparable lesions of the rotator cuff. *J. Bone and Joint Surg.,* 77-A: 857-866, June 1995.

36. **Sher, J. S.; Uribe, J. W.; Posada, A.; Murphy, B. J.;** and **Zlatkin, M. B.:** Abnormal findings on magnetic resonance images of asymptomatic shoulders. *J. Bone and Joint Surg.,* 77-A: 10-15, Jan. 1995.

37. **Takagishi, N.:** Conservative treatment of the ruptures of the rotator cuff. *J. Japanese Orthop. Assn.,* 52: 781-787, 1978.

38. **Thomazeau, H.; Boukobza, E.; Morcet, N.; Chaperon, J.;** and **Langlais, F.:** Prediction of rotator cuff repair results by magnetic resonance imaging. *Clin. Orthop.,* 344: 275-283, 1997.

39. **Walch, G.; Maréchal, E.; Maupas, J.;** and **Liotard, J. P.:** Traitement chirurgical des ruptures de la coiffe des rotateurs. Facteurs de pronostic. *Rev. chir. orthop.,* 78: 379-388, 1992.

40. **Wallace, W. A.,** and **Wiley, A. M.:** The long-term results of conservative management of full-thickness tears of the rotator cuff. In Proceedings of the British Orthopaedic Association. *J. Bone and Joint Surg.,* 68-B(1): 162, 1986.

41. **Weiner, D. S.,** and **Macnab, I.:** Superior migration of the humeral head. A radiological aid in the diagnosis of tears of the rotator cuff. *J. Bone and Joint Surg.,* 52-B(3): 524-527, 1970.

42. **Zanetti, M.; Gerber, C.;** and **Hodler, J.:** Quantitative assessment of the muscles of the rotator cuff with magnetic resonance imaging. *Invest. Radiol.,* 33: 163-170, 1998.

43. **Zanotti, R. M.; Carpenter, J. E.; Blasier, R. B.; Greenfield, M. L.; Adler, R. S.;** and **Bromberg, M. B.:** The low incidence of suprascapular nerve injury after primary repair of massive rotator cuff tears. *J. Shoulder and Elbow Surg.,* 6: 258-264, 1997.

Continuous Passive Motion after Repair of the Rotator Cuff

A PROSPECTIVE OUTCOME STUDY*

BY PAUL C. LASTAYO, P.T., C.H.T.†, THOMAS WRIGHT, M.D.‡, RACHEL JAFFE, O.T.R., C.H.T.‡,
AND JONATHAN HARTZEL, M.STAT.‡, GAINESVILLE, FLORIDA

Investigation performed at the Department of Orthopaedics, University of Florida, Gainesville

ABSTRACT: Despite the apparent success of continuous passive motion after soft-tissue procedures or joint replacements, its effect after repair of the rotator cuff is still unknown. The purpose of this prospective, randomized outcome study was to compare the results of continuous passive motion with those of manual passive range-of-motion exercises after repair of the rotator cuff.

Thirty-one patients (thirty-two rotator cuffs) were randomly assigned to one of two types of postoperative management: continuous passive motion (seventeen patients) or manual passive range-of-motion exercises (fifteen patients). There were seventeen women and fourteen men, and the mean age was sixty-three years (range, thirty to eighty years). The patients were followed for a mean of twenty-two months (range, six to forty-five months). Five tears of the rotator cuff were small, eighteen were medium, and nine were large.

All of the operations were performed by one surgeon. The patients who were managed with continuous passive motion used the device for the first four weeks postoperatively. The patients who were managed with manual passive range-of-motion exercises were assisted by a trained relative, friend, or home-care nurse. After the four-week period, the two groups were managed similarly for two to five months.

According to the Shoulder Pain and Disability Index, a valid and reliable self-administered questionnaire, the treatment was extremely successful in both groups. The overall score was excellent for twenty-seven shoulders (84 per cent), good for two (6 per cent), fair for two (7 per cent), and poor for one (3 per cent). With the numbers available, we could detect no significant differences (p > 0.05) between the two groups with respect to the score according to the Index, pain (according to a visual-analog scale), range of motion, or isometric strength.

Manual passive range-of-motion exercises were more cost-effective than continuous passive motion. The limited number of physical-therapy visits associated with the manual passive range-of-motion exercises in the present study appeared to be more cost-effective than a traditional physical-therapy schedule of three visits per week.

Postoperative therapy with continuous passive motion or manual passive range-of-motion exercises appears to yield favorable results after repair of a small, medium, or large tear of the rotator cuff.

The functional outcome after repair of the rotator cuff depends on many variables. Appropriate postoperative management is critical for maximizing function in a timely and efficient manner. Typically, the postoperative care is individualized to the patient and depends on the status of the deltoid muscle, the size of the tear, the ability to move the shoulder without injuring the tissues, and the patient's postoperative support system[15]. Other factors that have an effect on therapy and the final outcome are the duration between the original injury and the operation, the age of the patient, and the limitation of the active range of motion preoperatively. Supervised therapeutic exercises, starting with passive motion, are generally begun soon after the repair and are continued for approximately three months[16].

The use of early passive range-of-motion exercises is no longer controversial, as the exercises can be performed with protection of the repair and prevention of deleterious adhesions that can limit function[2,18]. Continuous passive motion, performed in a reciprocal fashion by a mechanical device, is one form of passive motion that facilitates beneficial changes in articular cartilage, synovial membrane, joint capsule, ligament, and tendon[12,25,26]. Although much of the clinical research on continuous passive motion has focused on patients who have had an operative procedure on the knee[3,4], its use after procedures on the upper extremity is becoming more frequent[12]. Better healing of repaired flexor tendons of the hand after continuous passive motion compared with that after intermittent passive motion[1,9], and the successful outcome associated with its use at other joints[3,12,26], have prompted clinicians to use this mode of

*No benefits in any form have been received or will be received from a commercial party related directly or indirectly to the subject of this article. No funds were received in support of this study.

†DeRosa Physical Therapy, 77 West Forest Avenue, Suite 303, Flagstaff, Arizona 86001.

‡Departments of Orthopaedics (T. W. and R. J.) and Statistics (J. H.), University of Florida, Gainesville, Florida 32610.

TABLE I
PATIENT DEMOGRAPHICS

Variable	Continuous Passive Motion (N = 17)	Manual Passive Range-of-Motion Exercises (N = 15)
Gender†		
Male	8	6
Female	9	9
Side of operation†		
Dominant	10	12
Non-dominant	7	3
Size of tear†		
Small	2	3
Medium	10	8
Large	5	4
Duration of follow-up *(mos.)*		
Mean	23.1	20.3
Range	(12-42)	(6-45)
Age *(yrs.)*		
Mean	62.9	63.7
Range	(30-80)	(45-75)

†The values are given as the number of patients.

therapy in an attempt to improve the biological response after repair of the rotator cuff. Continuous passive motion has been used after repair of the rotator cuff when no other mode of passive motion was available, and it also has been used to assist in the relief of pain, to improve healing, and to restore a passive range of motion[5,18]. However, we are not aware of any prospective study documenting its effectiveness in a well defined population of patients who had a repair of the rotator cuff. The purpose of the present prospective, randomized study was to compare the functional outcome of continuous passive motion with that of a more traditional program of manual passive range-of-motion exercises for patients who had a repair of the rotator cuff.

Materials and Methods

Patients

The study included thirty-one patients (seventeen women and fourteen men) who had had repair of a total of thirty-two tears of the rotator cuff between 1991 and 1994. Nine of the tears were large (greater than three but less than five centimeters), eighteen were medium (one to three centimeters), and five were small (less than one centimeter). One patient had bilateral repair; the tear on the dominant side was repaired first, after which the patient was randomly assigned to management with continuous passive motion, and the repair on the non-dominant side was performed six months later, after which she was randomly assigned to management with manual passive range-of-motion exercises. The mean age at the time of the repair was sixty-three years (range, thirty to eighty years) (Table I). The third-party payer was Medicare or a private insurance company, or both, for twenty-nine patients; the remaining

two patients were receiving Workers' Compensation. Patients who had a massive (greater than five-centimeter) or irreparable tear of the rotator cuff; preoperative evidence of pathological instability of the shoulder, a rheumatological disorder, reflex sympathetic dystrophy, fracture, or glenohumeral arthritis; or concomitant adhesive capsulitis were excluded from the study. Those who had had a previous operation on the shoulder were excluded as well. The study was approved by the Institutional Review Board at the University of Florida, and informed consent was obtained from all patients. Randomization was carried out with use of a table of random numbers.

Operative Technique

All repairs were performed in an open fashion by one of us (T. W.). The attachment of the deltoid to the anterior and lateral aspects of the acromion was exposed with use of a saber incision. The deltoid was split for two centimeters between its anterior and lateral heads, and the two portions were elevated as fascial-periosteal sleeves off of the anterior aspect of the acromion. An anterior-inferior acromioplasty was performed, and the bursa was debrided. The rotator cuff was mobilized by first placing stay sutures in the torn ends and then applying traction to the torn ends to retract the cuff. The subacromial and subdeltoid bursae were excised. All scar tissue between the torn tendon and the overlying acromion was released by blunt dissection with use of Darrach retractors or, when scar tissue was thick, by sharp dissection with Mayo scissors. Once this had been done, the cuff could be stretched to its original insertion, where it was repaired back to bone with use of osseous tunnels. (No suture anchors were used.) The subscapularis was not transposed in any patient. Patients who were found to have a massive defect were eliminated from the study. The fascial-periosteal sleeves of the deltoid then were carefully repaired to themselves. (Drill-holes through the acromion for attachment of the deltoid were not used routinely.)

Postoperative Management

All patients were managed initially with a sling. Pain was managed with the parenteral administration of morphine (two to four milligrams every three to four hours) as needed for one day, and then Vicodin (hydrocodone bitartrate and acetaminophen; one or two tablets every four hours) was taken orally as needed. No specific protocol for pain medication was followed postoperatively, but all patients had stopped taking narcotics by two to four weeks postoperatively.

While hospitalized, each patient was managed with passive range-of-motion exercises once a day for a mean of two days (one, two, or three days). The patient was discharged from the hospital when he or she was comfortable enough to return home and initiate the home-exercise program. Each patient was instructed to remove the sling three or four times a day to perform gentle passive pendulum exercises. Before the patients were discharged from the hospital, they were randomly assigned to management with continuous passive motion or management with manual passive range-of-motion exercises. Continuous passive motion was not started while the patient was in the hospital because it would have been difficult to arrange for and set up a bed-mounted continuous-passive-motion device, the hospital stay was relatively short, and the availability of bed-mounted continuous-passive-motion devices was limited. The patients were instructed in the proper use of a home continuous-passive-motion device (Thera-kinetics, Mount Laurel, New Jersey) for elevation and external rotation of the shoulder. The patients were told to use the device for four hours a day (three or four periods of continuous motion, each lasting for one to one and a half hours). The actual duration of continuous passive motion averaged three hours a day according to the patients' reports in a diary. The patients were instructed to progressively increase the range of the continuous passive motion but to maintain a comfortable arc.

Manual passive range-of-motion exercises were carried out by a relative, friend, or home-care nurse who was trained to perform them. Elevation and external rotation exercises — three sets of ten to fifteen repetitions — were performed individually three times a day. The total duration of the exercises averaged forty-five minutes a day according to the patients' reports. If the trained assistant was not available for a session, the passive external-rotation exercises were performed with the use of a cane or a pendulum. For the exercises with the cane, the patient lay supine, with the involved shoulder supported by a towel roll to prevent hyperextension of the shoulder; held the cane in the hand on the involved side; and moved the cane with the other hand so as to externally rotate the involved shoulder.

After the first four postoperative weeks, use of the continuous-passive-motion device was stopped and both groups were managed similarly: passive external-rotation exercises were performed with a cane, and passive elevation exercises were performed by an assistant or with the use of pulleys. Active rotation of the shoulder was initiated at six weeks; active-assisted elevation, at eight weeks; active elevation, at ten to twelve weeks; resistive rotation, at ten to twelve weeks; and resistive elevation, at twelve to fourteen weeks. Functional use and progressive strengthening began during the third or fourth postoperative month and were encouraged for as long as one year.

Evaluation of the Patients

The data were collected by three occupational therapists (two of whom were certified hand therapists), one physical therapist who was a certified hand therapist, and one occupational-therapy assistant. These examiners were not blinded with regard to the treatment groups, and there was crossover in terms of which therapist examined a patient at a given time-point.

Outcome Measures: Pain, Impairment, and Disability

During the first four weeks postoperatively, the patients assessed the pain with use of a visual-analog scale[19] once a week and recorded the amount of time for which the passive exercises were performed each day. Active and passive external rotation and elevation were measured with a goniometer (North Coast Medical, San Jose, California) at two weeks (except for active elevation), six weeks, and twelve weeks; at six and twelve months; and at the most recent follow-up evaluation. Isometric strength in external rotation and in elevation were measured with a handheld dynamometer (Spark Instruments and Academics, Coralville, Iowa) at six months, at twelve months, and at the most recent follow-up evaluation. The patient completed the Shoulder Pain and Disability Index[23] at the most recent follow-up evaluation. The range of motion and strength at each time-point were measured three times, and the mean was determined. The mean duration of follow-up (and standard deviation) was 22 ± 9.8 months (range, six to forty-five months).

A pilot study was performed on twelve normal shoulders to assess the within-examiner and the between-examiner reliability of the measurements of range of motion with the goniometer and the measurement of strength with the handheld dynamometer. Intraclass correlation coefficients (model 3,1[27]) were calculated to assess the within-examiner and between-examiner reliability for the five therapists who examined the patients. The within-examiner reliability was relatively good, with the intraclass correlation coefficients ranging from 0.72 to 0.97 for the measurements of range of motion and strength. The intraclass correlation coefficients for the between-examiner reliability, however, were fairly low (range, 0.11 to 0.56). Still, the between-examiner reliability and the error square root of the mean square, estimates of the standard deviation in the unit of measurement, may be clinically acceptable (range, 4.5 to 9.7), with the possible exceptions of the between-examiner reliability of the measurement of active external rotation (13.0), active elevation (18.3), and strength in external rotation (30.1).

Statistical Methods

The range-of-motion profiles for the patients were found to be relatively linear when considered on a logarithmic time scale and a logarithmic range-of-motion scale. Linear regression[24] was thus used to estimate these slopes, which were inversely related to the rate at which the range-of-motion profile leveled off over time. Therefore, a smaller slope for the range of motion would level off sooner than a larger slope.

Because the scores according to the Shoulder Pain and Disability Index[23] were excessively skewed in both

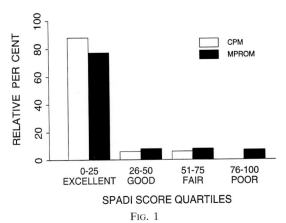

FIG. 1

Frequency distribution histogram showing the scores, divided into quartiles, according to the Shoulder Pain and Disability Index (SPADI)[23] for the two groups. CPM = continuous passive motion and MPROM = manual passive range-of-motion exercises.

groups, the scores for the two groups were compared with use of the non-parametric Fisher exact test and the Wilcoxon rank-sum test[24].

The t test for independent samples[24] and the Wilcoxon rank-sum test were used to compare the two groups with respect to the simple mean values and the rank sums, respectively, of all other dependent variables.

Analysis of covariance[6] also was used to compare the mean values (except for the score according to the Index[23]) in the two groups while controlling separately for the baseline range of motion (the passive range of motion at two weeks and the active range of motion at twelve weeks), isometric strength (at four months), and the score on the visual-analog scale (at one week). In addition, analysis of covariance was used to compare the mean values for the two groups, controlling separately for gender, age (less than sixty-five years or more than sixty-five years), and size of the tear (small or medium [one group] or large).

A retrospective power analysis was performed with use of the given variability and sample sizes to determine detectable differences between the two groups. Detectable differences were reported as the per cent difference in the mean response between the two groups. The reported percentages were calculated with use of a power of 80 per cent and a type-I error rate of 5 per cent.

Results

Clinically, both groups did well across all outcome measures. Overall, there were no significant differences, before or after adjustments for baseline levels, between the two groups with respect to the simple mean values for active and passive motion or strength. The patients who were managed with continuous passive motion had much less pain during the first postoperative week.

Pain and Disability

The scores according to the Shoulder Pain and Disability Index[23] were analyzed in two different ways.

First, the total score was arbitrarily divided into quartiles: 0 to 25 points indicated an excellent result, 26 to 50 points indicated a good result, 51 to 75 points indicated a fair result, and 76 to 100 points indicated a poor result. There were fifteen excellent results, one good result, one fair result, and no poor results in the group that had been managed with continuous passive motion, and there were twelve excellent results, one good result, one fair result, and one poor result in the group that had been managed with manual passive range-of-motion exercises (Fig. 1). With the numbers available for study, we could not detect a significant difference between the two groups with respect to the scores ($p = 0.853$, Fisher exact test). The raw scores also were analyzed statistically and, again, we could detect no significant difference between the two groups ($p = 0.16$, Wilcoxon rank-sum test).

Pain

The data from the visual-analog scales indicated that pain had decreased in both groups from the first to the fourth week postoperatively. With the numbers available, we could detect no difference between the two groups with respect to the slopes for the scores with use of the Wilcoxon rank-sum test ($p = 0.22$) or the t test ($p = 0.15$). In addition, analysis of covariance demonstrated no significant difference between the slopes for the mean scores in the two groups ($p = 0.92$). However, the group that was managed with continuous passive motion had significantly less pain during the first post-

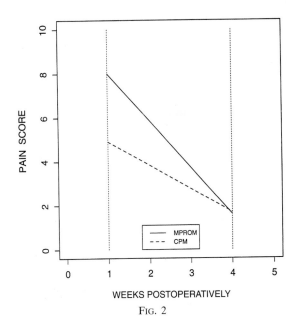

FIG. 2

Graph showing the scores for pain, during the first four weeks postoperatively, as indicated on the visual-analog scale by the patients managed with manual passive range-of-motion exercises (MPROM) and those managed with continuous passive motion (CPM). The group that was managed with continuous passive motion had significantly less pain than the group that was managed with manual passive range-of-motion exercises ($p = 0.046$, Wilcoxon rank-sum test).

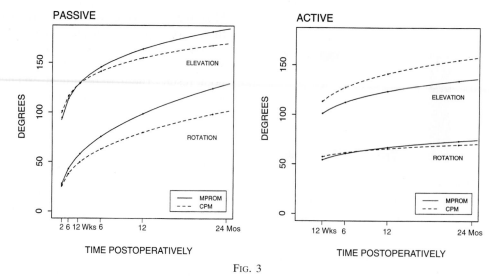

FIG. 3

Graphs showing the slopes predicting the return of passive and active motion in both groups. No significant differences were detected between the two groups. MPROM = manual passive range-of-motion exercises and CPM = continuous passive motion.

operative week than the group that was managed with manual passive range-of-motion exercises (p = 0.046, Wilcoxon rank-sum test) (Fig. 2).

Range of Motion

Predicted time-courses for the change in the range of motion were derived with use of analysis of covariance, which controls for the initial (baseline) measurement. The time-points thereafter were the actual time-points for the respective patients in the group, and a line was drawn that best fit the data. The line is interpolated and is not an extrapolation of the actual data, and it allows for interpretation of the progress over time. With the numbers available, we could detect no significant difference between the two groups with respect to the baseline measurements of external rotation and elevation (p > 0.20, t test) (Fig. 3). We also could detect

no difference between the passive external rotation or elevation in the two groups at twelve or twenty-four months, after adjusting for the baseline passive range of motion at two weeks (p > 0.15, analysis of covariance). Similarly, we found no differences in the active range of motion in the two groups at twelve and twenty-four months, after adjusting for the baseline values at twelve weeks (p > 0.20, analysis of covariance).

With use of the logarithmically transformed slopes for the range of motion, the rates at which the two groups regained passive and active external rotation and elevation were compared. With the numbers available, we could detect no differences between the two rates when they were compared parametrically with use of the t test and non-parametrically with use of the Wilcoxon rank-sum test (p > 0.20). Adjusting for the baseline range of motion yielded the same results (p >

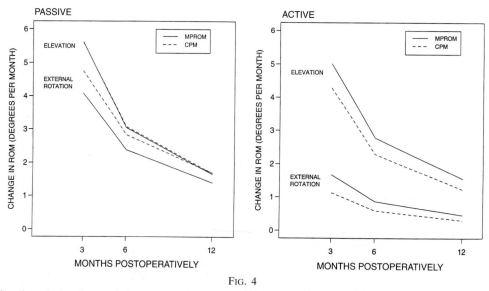

FIG. 4

Graphs showing the calculated rate of change in the passive and active ranges of motion (ROM) for the two groups. No significant differences were detected between the groups. MPROM = manual passive range-of-motion exercises and CPM = continuous passive motion.

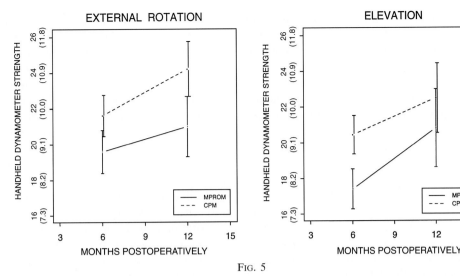

FIG. 5

Graphs showing the mean isometric strength (in pounds with kilograms in parentheses) of the involved extremity, as measured with a handheld dynamometer. No significant differences were detected between the two groups. MPROM = manual passive range-of-motion exercises and CPM = continuous passive motion. The I-bars indicate the standard error of the mean.

0.15, analysis of covariance). The median rate of recovery (expressed as degrees per month) was similar for the two groups at three, six, and twelve months (Fig. 4). The similarities in the medians at each time-point demonstrated that the patients in both groups regained motion at the same rate. The decreasing pattern also demonstrated that the recovery of motion leveled off with time in both groups. The power analysis denoted that, given the variability in the data, a 115 per cent increase compared with the mean rate of recovery of active external rotation in the group managed with manual passive range-of-motion exercises could have been detected with 80 per cent power. Similarly, a 124 per cent increase compared with the mean rate of recovery of active elevation in that group could have been detected with 80 per cent power.

Strength

The isometric strength was measured with the handheld dynamometer during external rotation and elevation in scaption[16]. We compared the two groups with respect to the values at six months, the values at twelve months, and the difference between the six and twelve-month values. The comparisons were made after adjusting for the baseline strength at four months. With the numbers available for study, we could detect no significant difference between the two groups with respect to the strength in external rotation (p ≥ 0.20, analysis of covariance). An 18 per cent increase compared with the mean response in the group managed with manual passive range-of-motion exercises could have been detected with 80 per cent power. There was a marginal difference between the two groups with respect to the strength in elevation at six months (p = 0.06, analysis of covariance), but we detected no difference in the values for the two groups at twelve months or between the differences between the values at six and twelve months.

A plot of the adjusted mean values for each group showed that strength continued to improve for one year (Fig. 5).

Age, Gender, and Size of Tear

The data were further subdivided and analyzed for the potential effect of age. With the numbers available, we could detect no significant differences (p = 0.07 to 0.89), across all dependent variables, between the two groups when controlling for age (less than sixty-five years old [fifteen patients] and more than sixty-five years old [seventeen patients]). We also could detect no significant difference (p = 0.08 to 0.97) between the two groups when controlling for gender, with one exception: women indicated significantly less pain (p = 0.029) on the visual-analog scale at one week than men did. We could detect no significant differences (p = 0.07 to 0.92) between the two groups when controlling for the size of the tear (small or medium and large).

Outpatient Visits for Postoperative Therapy

During the first three months postoperatively, the group that was managed with continuous passive motion had a median of nine outpatient visits for physical therapy and the group that was managed with manual passive range-of-motion exercises had a median of ten visits. During the visits, the therapist measured the range of motion and the strength and advanced the postoperative program as dictated by the protocol or modified the program depending on the clinical progress of the patient. Three of the visits during the three-month period were mandatory to allow for the collection of data and to continue instruction in the exercise program. Any visits other than the three mandatory ones were considered clinically necessary by the therapist to monitor the patient more closely, to adjust the program, or to reinforce the patient's home-exercise program. By the third or fourth postoperative month, all patients were using the arm on the involved side for functional activities and were performing progressive strengthening exercises at home. Any outpatient visits after four months were for follow-up and for modification of the exercise or strengthening program. No patient was seen regularly on an outpatient basis for formal therapy after four months.

Complications

One patient who was managed with continuous passive motion had an infection four months postoperatively; the clinical result was excellent after débridement and repeat repair of the cuff. One patient who was managed with manual passive range-of-motion exercises had reflex sympathetic dystrophy, and one had occult glenohumeral instability; the latter patient had a fair result at the time of the latest follow-up.

Discussion

To our knowledge, this is the first prospective, randomized study to compare the functional outcome after continuous passive motion with that after a program of manual passive range-of-motion exercises for patients who had had repair of the rotator cuff. Our primary finding is that continuous passive motion is a safe technique that results in little disability and an excellent or good outcome after a repair of a small, medium, or large tear of the rotator cuff. Continuous passive motion does not, however, provide a better outcome than a program of manual passive range-of-motion exercises, which is more cost-effective.

It appears, from the results of the present study, that forty-five minutes of manual passive range-of-motion exercises a day, performed outside of the clinical setting, is adequate for a good functional outcome after repair of a small, medium, or large tear of the rotator cuff. The two groups had very similar improvements in the range of motion and strength. For example, the improvements in the active and passive ranges of motion were greater at earlier time-points (three and six months) than at later time-points (twelve months) in both groups; however, we could detect no significant differences between the groups with the numbers available. We adjusted the data for the first (baseline) measurement (at two weeks for the passive range of motion and at twelve weeks for the active range of motion) as a covariate to eliminate the effect of the amount of motion that the patient had before the operation, as this can vary tremendously and may confound the results. We did consider the influence, either beneficial or detrimental, that passive range-of-motion exercises may have on active range of motion and strength, but, again, we could detect no significant differences with respect to any measurement (with the possible exception of strength in elevation at six months, which approached significance [p = 0.06]) between the two groups at any time postoperatively. The group that

was managed with continuous passive motion had significantly less pain during the first postoperative week (p = 0.046), but we detected no differences thereafter.

We were concerned that the between-examiner reliability was poor for the measurement of the active range of motion and of strength in external rotation. In an attempt to overcome the influence of any problems with between-examiner reliability, we made an effort to have the same therapist perform all of the measurements for a given patient. (The within-examiner reliability was very good.) However, this could not be strictly controlled. Given the power to detect only very large differences between groups with regard to active external rotation and elevation, the non-significant results in the present study need to be verified. However, there was good power to detect a fairly small difference in the strength in external rotation in the two groups, which supports the conclusion of the study. The measurement of pain and disability (the Shoulder Pain and Disability Index[23]) had good reliability.

More importantly, there was little functional limitation or disability in either group, regardless of age, gender, or size of the tear. The three complications subsequently resolved or had little effect on function. The one poor result, in a patient who was managed with manual passive range-of-motion exercises, was thought be due to limited function of the deltoid both before and after the operation.

The scores according to the Shoulder Pain and Disability Index were equally good for the two groups. We chose this scale because it is a unique shoulder-specific index that has demonstrated consistency, test-retest reliability, and criterion and construct validity, primarily in a population of older men[22,23]. Therefore, it might be safer to generalize the results of this study to male patients who are beyond the fourth or fifth decade of life than to female patients.

As both groups had good results, we were interested in determining which postoperative protocol was the most cost-effective. After repair of the rotator cuff, the greatest investment in terms of both time and dollars is during the first three months. Although there was only a small difference between the two groups with respect to the number of outpatient visits, the cost to the third-party payer for continuous-passive-motion therapy would have been substantially higher if the patients had been charged for the device. This additional cost may not be warranted after repair of a small, medium, or large tear in a patient who is forty years old or more and has a relative, friend, or home-care nurse who can be trained to perform manual passive range-of-motion exercises.

Before initiating the study, we arbitrarily chose four weeks as the duration of continuous passive motion, as the first four postoperative weeks is the period when passive motion is the focus of therapy and active motion is encouraged. (Passive range-of-motion exercises are continued after the four-week period on an as-needed basis.) We believe that, although the repair should be protected throughout this period, passive motion is needed to prevent the formation of restrictive adhesions, which can occur during the biologically active fibroblastic proliferation phase of wound-healing[13]. We were surprised to find that the passive range of motion was better (although not significantly so) in the group that was managed with manual passive range-of-motion exercises, even though the exercises with the continuous-passive-motion device were performed for a longer period each day than the manual exercises were. Another reason that we chose a duration of four weeks for continuous passive motion was to try to facilitate greater tendinous force capabilities, which have been noted in healing tendons that are subjected to prolonged periods of motion[17,28]. The long-term use of continuous passive motion may have contributed to a trend (although not a significant one) toward improvements in active elevation and strength in the group treated with that method.

When no one is available to perform manual passive range-of-motion exercises for the patient, it is possible that other types of passive range-of-motion exercises, performed at the same frequency and for the same duration as were used in the present study, could yield similar results. Performance of passive external-rotation and elevation exercises with use of a cane or with use of the uninvolved extremity in a gravity-minimized plane has been shown to result in little activity of the shoulder muscles. Any exercises that require the arm to move against gravity, such as those done with pulleys, will result in more muscle activity[14]. Despite the anecdotal evidence that exercises with pulleys are safe and effective, the question still remains as to how much muscle activity facilitates a successful outcome. When passive range-of-motion exercises cannot be performed in an appropriate manner, more frequent visits for physical therapy or the use of a continuous-passive-motion device, or both, may be warranted. Although the efficacy of continuous passive motion has not been proved, we would seriously consider its use, with an arc of motion that protects the repair, when the passive range-of-motion exercises must be performed for a long duration. This is the case when a patient has a preexisting frozen shoulder or when restrictive adhesions are likely to form, such as after a repair of a massive tear or after a repeat repair. We excluded patients who had a massive tear or adhesive capsulitis, or both, in order to better represent the typical patient who has a non-complicated tear of the rotator cuff. Future studies are needed to assess the effectiveness of continuous passive motion for a patient who has a more complex tear.

It is difficult to compare the findings of the present study with those of previous reports, as we know of no other prospective analyses of postoperative protocols after repair of the rotator cuff. Still, we believe that the results in both of our groups compare favorably with those in other outcome studies[7,10,11]. In a review in which the results were presented as the average of the percentages derived from several series, Cofield reported an 85 per cent rate of excellent or good results; 87 per cent of the patients had relief of pain, and 77 per cent were satisfied with the outcome. We did not measure our patients' satisfaction with the results, but the scores according to the Shoulder Pain and Disability Index[23] suggest that function was more than adequate for the patients' needs.

Other investigators[1,9] have found that the outcome after repair of digital tendons was better when continuous passive motion had been used. The quicker healing and greater strength of repaired tendons and ligaments associated with continuous passive motion has been attributed to increased blood flow and metabolic activities of cells[8,26]. The healing capability of the rotator cuff, specifically that of the supraspinatus, may be enhanced by continuous passive motion, as the supraspinatus tendon has a tenuous blood supply[21]. However, this potential for improved vascular and cellular activity resulted in no significant clinical advantage in our study. Craig conducted a preliminary study comparing immediate continuous passive motion for two to three days with immobilization for three to four days after operative reconstruction of the shoulder and found no adverse effects, a shorter hospital stay, and less postoperative pain for the patients who were managed with continuous passive motion. It is difficult to compare the results of our study with those of Craig's investigation. We compared two therapeutic modes of early passive range-of-motion exercises in a well defined group of patients who had had repair of the rotator cuff. In contrast, Craig compared continuous passive motion with immobilization in a series of patients who had had repair of the rotator cuff, acromioplasty, excision of the coracoacromial ligament, or total shoulder replacement. Even though Craig found a beneficial response after forty-eight to seventy-two hours, we chose a four-week period of continuous passive motion, as we sought to influence the remodeling phase of the wound-healing process. In both the study by Craig and the present study, continuous passive motion was more effective in diminishing pain during the first postoperative week and, empirically (in our study), it seemed to help minimize involuntary co-contractions during the exercises. This effect during the first week may be clinically relevant in terms of decreased use of narcotics or increased independence, or both, during this time, but those data were not collected. In our study, however, continuous passive motion had no significant influence on the range of motion, strength, or disability. We would, however, consider its use if pain and co-contractions interfered with the rehabilitation process. Reyes et al., who reported retrospectively the results of continuous passive motion after repair of the rotator cuff, found no important differences in the duration of the hospital stay, the intake of pain medication, and the days on which range-of-motion landmarks were achieved between patients who had and those who had not been managed with continuous passive motion. The patients who were managed with continuous passive motion in that study had fewer visits for physical therapy, but the total cost for the therapy was greater[21].

It seems unlikely that the functional outcome after a repair of the rotator cuff could be much better than it was in the present study. However, future studies that document the results of more visits for therapy or the use of continuous passive motion by patients who have had a repeat repair or a repair of a massive tear may be worthwhile. Conversely, the assessment of the outcomes of repairs of the rotator cuff in patients who had even fewer visits for outpatient therapy than the patients in the present study may reveal an even more cost-effective postoperative approach.

Although no significant differences in the clinical outcome were noted between the two groups in our study, as stated we would still consider the use of continuous passive motion when restrictive adhesions are a concern, as when a patient has had a repeat repair of the rotator cuff, concomitant adhesive capsulitis, or a repair of a massive tear. Continuous passive motion also may be beneficial for a patient who lives alone and does not have a relative, friend, or home-care nurse who can be trained to perform manual passive range-of-motion exercises. In addition, continuous passive motion may be helpful for patients who have severe postoperative pain or problems with muscular co-contractions during passive range-of-motion exercises.

Limitations of the Study

It is difficult to assess the effects of two different interventions during the first four weeks after repair of the rotator cuff and then to analyze the effects of those treatments at twenty months. Many variables can influence the outcome, such as the consistency of range-of-motion and strengthening exercises performed at home after formal therapeutic visits have been discontinued. There was no formal documentation of the compliance of the patients or of modifications to the program after the first four weeks. These variables may have confounded our results.

In conclusion, continuous passive motion and manual passive range-of-motion exercises contributed positively to the range of motion, strength, function, and relief of pain; however, we could detect no significant difference in the clinical outcome between the two groups.

References

1. **Bunker, T. D.; Potter, B.;** and **Barton, N. J.:** Continuous passive motion following flexor tendon repair. *J. Hand Surg.,* 14-B: 406-411, 1989.
2. **Cofield, R. H.:** Current concepts review. Rotator cuff disease of the shoulder. *J. Bone and Joint Surg.,* 67-A: 974-979, July 1985.
3. **Coutts, R. D.; Toth, C.;** and **Kaita, J. H.:** The role of continuous passive motion in the rehabilitation of the total knee patient. In *Total Knee Arthroplasty: A Comprehensive Approach,* pp. 126-132. Edited by D. S. Hungerford, K. A. Krackow, and R. V. Kenna. Baltimore, Williams and Wilkins, 1984.
4. **Coutts, R. D.; Craig, E. V.; Mooney, V.; Osterman, A. L.;** and **Salter, R. B.:** Symposium: the use of continuous passive motion in the rehabilitation of orthopaedic problems. *Contemp. Orthop.,* 16: 75-106, 1988.
5. **Craig, E. V.:** Continuous passive motion in the rehabilitation of the surgically reconstructed shoulder. A preliminary report. *Orthop. Trans.,* 10: 219, 1986.
6. **Fleiss, J. L.:** *The Design and Analysis of Clinical Experiments.* New York, Wiley, 1986.
7. **Gazielly, D. F.; Gleyze, P.;** and **Montagnon, C.:** Functional and anatomical results after rotator cuff repair. *Clin. Orthop.,* 304: 43-53, 1994.
8. **Gelberman, R. H.; Amiel, D.; Gonsalves, M.; Woo, S.;** and **Akeson, W. H.:** The influence of protected passive mobilization of flexor tendons: a biochemical and microangiographic study. *Hand,* 13: 120-128, 1981.
9. **Gelberman, R. H.; Nunley, J. A., II; Osterman, A. L.; Breen, T. F.; Dimick, M. P.;** and **Woo, S. L-Y.:** Influences of the protected passive mobilization interval on flexor tendon healing. A prospective randomized clinical study. *Clin. Orthop.,* 264: 189-196, 1991.
10. **Grana, W. A.; Teague, B.; King, M.;** and **Reeves, R. B.:** An analysis of rotator cuff repair. *Am. J. Sports Med.,* 22: 585-588, 1994.
11. **Harryman, D. T., II; Mack, L. A.; Wang, K. Y.; Jackins, S. E.; Richardson, M. L.;** and **Matsen, F. A., III:** Repairs of the rotator cuff. Correlation of functional results with integrity of the cuff. *J. Bone and Joint Surg.,* 73-A: 982-989, Aug. 1991.
12. **LaStayo, P. C.:** Continuous passive motion for the upper extremity. In *Rehabilitation of the Hand: Surgery and Therapy,* edited by J. M. Hunter, E. J. Mackin, and A. D. Callahan. Ed. 4, vol. 2, pp. 1545-1560. St. Louis, C. V. Mosby, 1995.
13. **Liu, S. L.; Sen Yang, R.-S.; Al-Shaikh, R.;** and **Lane, J. M.:** Collagen in tendon, ligament, and bone healing. A current review. *Clin. Orthop.,* 318: 265-278, 1995.
14. **McCann, P. D.; Wootten, M. E.; Kadaba, M. P.;** and **Bigliani, L. U.:** A kinematic and electromyographic study of shoulder rehabilitation exercises. *Clin. Orthop.,* 288: 179-188, 1993.
15. **Marks, P. H.; Warner, M. J.;** and **Irrgang, J. J.:** Rotator cuff disorders of the shoulder. *J. Hand Ther.,* 7: 90-98, 1994.
16. **Matsen, F. A., III,** and **Arntz, C. T.:** Rotator cuff tendon failure. In *The Shoulder,* edited by C. A. Rockwood, Jr., and F. A. Matsen, III. Vol. 2, pp. 647-677. Philadelphia, W. B. Saunders, 1990.
17. **Michna, H.,** and **Hartmann, G.:** Adaptation of tendon collagen to exercise. *Internat. Orthop.,* 13: 161-165, 1989.
18. **Gristina, A. G.; Craig, E. V.; Neviaser, R. J.;** and **Norris, T. R.:** Symposium: management of rotator cuff problems. *Contemp. Orthop.,* 20: 621-646, 1990.
19. **Price, D. D.,** and **Harkins, S. W.:** Combined use of experimental pain and visual analogue scales in producing standardized measurement of clinical pain. *Clin. J. Pain,* 3: 1-8, 1987.
20. **Rathbun, J. B.,** and **Macnab, I.:** The microvascular pattern of the rotator cuff. *J. Bone and Joint Surg.,* 52-B(3): 540-553, 1970.
21. **Reyes, A. M.; Pati, A. B.;** and **Gartsman, G. M.:** Effects of shoulder CPM vs no CPM on rotator cuff repair rehabilitation [abstract]. *Phys. Ther.,* 72 (Supplement): S99, 1992.

22. **Richards, R. R.,** and **Beaton, D. E.:** Measuring shoulder function: a cross-sectional comparison of five different questionnaires [abstract]. *J. Shoulder and Elbow Surg.,* 4-1(Part 2): S61, 1995.

23. **Roach, K. E.; Budiman-Mak, E.; Songsiridej, N.;** and **Lertratanakul, Y.:** Development of a Shoulder Pain and Disability Index. *Arthrit. Care and Res.,* 4: 143-149, 1991.

24. **Rosner, B.:** *Fundamentals of Biostatistics.* Ed. 3. Boston, PWS-Kent, 1990.

25. **Salter, R. B.:** *Continuous Passive Motion (CPM): A Biological Concept for the Healing and Regeneration of Articular Cartilage, Ligaments and Tendons: From Its Origination to Research to Clinical Applications.* Baltimore, Williams and Wilkins, 1993.

26. **Salter, R. B.; Hamilton, H. W.; Wedge, J. H.; Tile, M.; Torode, I. P.; O'Driscoll, S. W.; Murnaghan, J. J.;** and **Saringer, J. H.:** Clinical application of basic research on continuous passive motion for disorders and injuries of synovial joints: a preliminary report of a feasibility study. *J. Orthop. Res.,* 1: 325-342, 1984.

27. **Shrout, P. E.,** and **Fleiss, J. L.:** Intraclass correlations: uses in assessing rater reliability. *Psychol. Bull.,* 86: 420-428, 1979.

28. **Woo, S. L.; Gomez, M. A.; Woo, Y. K.;** and **Akeson, W. H.:** Mechanical properties of tendons and ligaments. II. The relationships of immobilization and exercise on tissue remodeling. *Biorheology,* 19: 397-408, 1982.

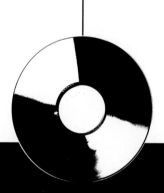

JBJS
The Journal of Bone & Joint Surgery

JAAOS
Journal of the American Academy of Orthopaedic

section four

Specific Conditions

Frozen Shoulder: Diagnosis and Management

Jon J. P. Warner, MD

Abstract

"Frozen shoulder" comprises a group of conditions caused by different process-es. Effective treatment depends on recognition of the underlying pathologic dis-order in each individual case. Idiopathic adhesive capsulitis usually responds to nonoperative therapy or closed manipulation, but shoulder stiffness due to trau-ma or surgery may necessitate either an arthroscopic or an open-release proce-dure. Both of these technically demanding techniques are effective in restoring motion in cases of frozen shoulder refractory to nonoperative treatment.

J Am Acad Orthop Surg 1997;5:130-140

Although many researchers have considered the etiology of frozen shoulder,[1-4] few have presented an organized treatment approach based on the underlying diagnosis as well as on variations in natural history related to the specific diag-nosis. The purpose of this article is to present an organized overview of the various causes of motion loss in the shoulder and the treatment options available for each.

Epidemiology and Natural History

"Frozen shoulder" is a general term denoting all causes of motion loss in the shoulder. The condition is one in which there is both active and passive limitation of motion due to soft-tissue contracture that results in a mechanical block. This soft-tissue contracture can occur in combination with other conditions, such as rotator cuff tear and degen-erative arthritis. In the latter, joint incongruity may also limit motion. In all cases, the soft-tissue contrac-tures must be treated concurrently with the other underlying or asso-ciated disorders. This article will address all causes of motion loss that involve soft-tissue contracture and scarring about the region of the glenohumeral joint.

When discussing the idiopathic form of motion loss in the shoul-der, the term "primary adhesive capsulitis" is preferable to "frozen shoulder," as it more precisely describes the pathologic changes in the joint capsule. The pathogenesis of this idiopathic condition remains a subject of debate. Possible causes include immunologic, inflammato-ry, biochemical, and endocrine alterations.[1,3] Systemic disorders, such as diabetes mellitus, cardio-vascular disease, and neurologic conditions, can also be contributing causes. In particular, patients with diabetes are at greater risk of adhe-sive capsulitis than the general population; the condition is often bilateral and resistant to all forms of treatment.[1,5]

Regardless of the biologic cause, adhesive capsulitis is characterized by thickening and contracture of the joint capsule,[6] which results in decreased intra-articular volume and capsular compliance so that glenohumeral motion is limited in all planes. The natural history of primary adhesive capsulitis is well described and has been termed benign because it tends to resolve over the course of 1 to 3 years.[3,7] Despite this favorable natural his-tory, some patients are unwilling to endure the painful limitation of motion while they wait for resolu-tion of the condition. Most patients will have some residual loss of motion even after many years, although the literature suggests that most do not have serious func-tional limitations or pain.[7]

Secondary, or acquired, shoul-der stiffness develops when there is a known intrinsic, extrinsic, or sys-temic cause.[8-11] Examples include postsurgical and posttraumatic stiffness, which can occur with or without an associated fracture. Both types of shoulder stiffness usually occur in association with prolonged immobilization. While the management of primary adhe-

Dr. Warner is Director, Shoulder Service, University of Pittsburgh Medical Center, and Associate Professor of Orthopaedic Surgery, University of Pittsburgh School of Medicine.

Reprint requests: Dr. Warner, Shoulder Service, Center for Sports Medicine, 4601 Baum Boulevard, Pittsburgh, PA 15213.

sive capsulitis is usually conservative with physical therapy, most surgeons believe that acquired stiffness of the shoulder after surgical procedures for instability merits more aggressive treatment because of the potential unfavorable consequences.[1,8-14] For example, if an excessively tight anterior soft-tissue repair for instability causes an internal rotation contracture, it may result in chronic posterior subluxation of the humeral head, leading to incongruity of the joint and rapid deterioration of articular cartilage.[8,9] In the case of motion loss after immobilization of a traumatized shoulder, a supervised therapy program might be successful in restoring motion.

Normal Anatomy and Pathology

The inherently loose articulation of the normal shoulder joint is a necessary anatomic feature that permits the large range of multiplanar motion required for normal shoulder function. In this nonconstrained articulation, the larger humeral head has a nearly perfect congruity with the smaller osseous glenoid. The surface area of the articulation is enlarged by the fibrous glenoid labrum attached around its periphery. The stability of this joint is largely maintained by rotator cuff muscle action, which creates compression of the convex humeral head into the matched concave articular glenoid fossa. The glenohumeral ligaments and capsule, which are normally lax or under minimal tension during most shoulder rotations, function mainly at the extreme positions of rotation and translation to statically constrain the joint against excessive movement of the humeral head on the glenoid.[15]

During motion of the normal shoulder, the tightening and loosening of the glenohumeral ligaments and capsule encircling the humeral head are accompanied by lengthening and shortening of the rotator cuff and deltoid tendons and muscles.[16] Loss of motion in the shoulder can be the result of any condition that directly affects these structures or their ability to glide relative to one another during shoulder movements. A coexisting joint incongruity, such as arthritis or an osseous block due to a malunited or displaced greater tuberosity fracture, may be present. Both arthritis and fractures are also commonly associated with capsular contracture and scarring between soft-tissue planes.

The etiology of shoulder stiffness includes contracture or shortening of the capsule and glenohumeral ligaments, contracture or shortening of the extra-articular tissues, and scarring between the tissue planes of the shoulder (Fig. 1). The exact cause can usually be predicted with some degree of accuracy. For example, in primary adhesive capsulitis, the soft tissue principally affected is the joint capsule, while the rotator cuff and soft-tissue planes remain normal (Fig. 1, A). In cases of postsurgical stiffness, the specific disorder is related to the nature of the antecedent surgical procedure. When surgical treatment was for instability, capsular contracture and/or extra-articular constraint may be the cause of the motion loss. For example, when a capsular shift or a Bankart procedure for recurrent dislocation results in excessive loss of external rotation, the main cause of motion loss is capsular scarring rather than extra-articular constraint. In most instances, arthroscopic treatment can improve motion, although subscapularis shortening can sometimes be

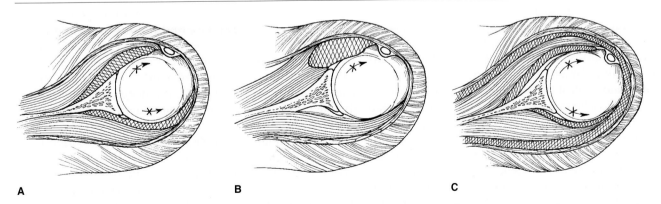

A   **B**   **C**

Fig. 1 Etiology of shoulder stiffness. **A,** Contracture of the capsule (cross-hatched areas) results in loss of all rotation (arrows). **B,** Extra-articular entrapment of the subscapularis (cross-hatched area) results in loss of external rotation (arrow). **C,** Scarring between tissue planes (cross-hatched areas) results in loss of all rotation (arrows).

a factor. In contrast, if stiffness after a Bristow procedure is due in part to entrapment of the subscapularis, an open procedure is necessary for definitive treatment (Fig. 1, B).[9,17]

If the shoulder has been immobilized for a prolonged period of time after a traumatic event or surgical procedure, associated scarring between tissue planes may concurrently restrict motion. For example, the motion loss that follows a fracture and prolonged immobilization is usually characterized by marked scarring in the tissue planes between the deltoid and the humerus, as well as in the deeper layers of the rotator cuff and capsule (Fig. 1, C).

Clinical Evaluation

Assessment of Motion

Shoulder motion must be assessed and documented carefully and consistently to obtain an accurate and ongoing measure of the efficacy of a given treatment. Both active and passive motion losses must be recorded and compared, since concomitant conditions, such as a rotator cuff tear, can result in loss of active motion in a shoulder that is also stiff due to adhesions. In patients with glenohumeral stiffness, there may often be the appearance of relatively good motion due to increased scapulothoracic motion or trunk lean. The examiner must be careful to identify and control these compensatory motions in order to measure only pure glenohumeral motion. Active shoulder flexion is measured anterior to the scapular plane, with the patient seated, and is referenced to the patient's thorax, not to a line vertical to the floor. This avoids measurement of any associated trunk tilt or increased scapulothoracic contribu-

tion to overall motion. Active pain-free motion is recorded. Active external and internal rotation are measured with the shoulder in adduction as well.

In some situations, pain inhibition may result in poor active motion. For example, in the case of a subacromial disorder, an injection of 1% lidocaine into this region will reveal the true active motion possible when pain is eliminated. Recording the increase in motion after injection helps differentiate motion loss due to pain from that due to a soft-tissue contracture. I perform this test on patients with painful flexion through an arc of at least 90 degrees. An individual with limited motion due to painful flexion from rotator cuff disease will have relief of pain with improved motion; an individual with a soft-tissue contracture will continue to have limited motion.

Passive motion should be evaluated with the patient supine, which restricts excessive scapulothoracic movement, therefore providing a more accurate assessment of pure glenohumeral rotation. Passive flexion, external rotation in adduction (arm at the side), external and internal rotation in abduction (arm to 90 degrees abduction), and cross-chest adduction must be measured.

Patterns of Motion Loss

Primary adhesive capsulitis is usually associated with global motion loss, whereas postsurgical or posttraumatic shoulder stiffness may present with global loss of motion in all planes or with a more discrete limitation of motion affecting some planes while relatively sparing others. Recognition of these different patterns of motion loss is important in planning surgical treatment when shoulder stiffness is refractory to nonoperative

care. Motion loss often correlates with the location of a capsular contracture. For example, limitation of external rotation of the adducted shoulder is associated with contracture in the anterosuperior capsular region and the rotator interval; release of this area will usually improve the arc of motion.[12-14,18] Limitation of external rotation when the shoulder is abducted is usually associated with scarring in the anteroinferior region of the capsule. Limitation of internal rotation in adduction and abduction is associated with scarring of the posterior capsule, which is also reflected in loss of horizontal or cross-chest adduction.[15]

Even though these observations are useful guidelines for surgical treatment, it should be remembered that any capsular contracture will limit motion in more than one plane. Extra-articular contractures, such as subscapularis entrapment and scarring between tissue planes, may also contribute to global motion loss.

Secondary Findings

Both postsurgical and posttraumatic shoulder stiffness are characterized by the presence of some intrinsic shoulder disorder, such as rotator cuff disease, postsurgical scarring, or trauma to the soft tissues with or without fracture. The key finding in this setting is passive motion loss. Therefore, the physical examination should carefully document motion loss in all planes. Prolonged immobilization of the shoulder may also be a factor.

Some patients with postsurgical or posttraumatic shoulder stiffness, as well as those with primary adhesive capsulitis, will have pain patterns that suggest impingement or rotator cuff disease or another concomitant condition, even though there is no objective evidence. The plain radiographs (specifically, the supraspinatus outlet view) may show a flat acromion (Bigliani type I),[19] but the magnetic resonance imaging study may be normal.

The biomechanical consequences of soft-tissue contractures may be "nonoutlet"-type impingement, in which the capsular contracture causes excessive translation of the humeral head on the glenoid during attempted shoulder rotation. Both anterior and posterior capsular contractures have been shown experimentally to cause increased superior translation of the humeral head during attempted flexion.[15,18] This abnormal superior movement of the humeral head has the effect of compressing the rotator cuff and subacromial bursa between the coracoacromial arch and the humeral head, thus causing the impingement-type symptoms. Some patients have partial pain relief with a subacromial injection of lidocaine. Experimental work by Harryman et al[18] has shown that capsular release eliminates abnormal translation and restores normal ball-and-socket kinematics (concentric rotation) to the glenohumeral joint.

Loss of glenohumeral motion will not only profoundly restrict overall upper extremity function but also alter the normal kinematic relationship of the glenohumeral and scapulothoracic joints. A compensatory increase in scapulothoracic motion can create additional symptoms, described by the patient as discomfort medial to the scapula.

Radiologic Studies

Plain Radiography

In most cases, but particularly in instances of primary adhesive capsulitis, radiographic studies do not help to clarify the causation of stiffness of the shoulder, but they do confirm the presence of a normal glenohumeral joint by identifying fractures, arthritis, or metallic implants that may be contributing to motion loss. Disuse osteoporosis may occasionally be evident, especially in patients who have the clinical features of reflex sympathetic dystrophy.

Arthrography

Many authors have asserted that arthrographic confirmation of decreased joint capacity, defined as the inability of the joint to accept more than 5 to 10 mL of contrast medium, is essential to a definitive diagnosis of adhesive capsulitis.[3,5,20] However, it has been shown that there is no direct correlation between arthrographic findings and motion loss.[20] Therefore, I do not use this test unless I want to rule out the possibility of a concomitant full-thickness rotator cuff tear.

Magnetic Resonance Imaging and Computed Tomography

Magnetic resonance imaging can be of use in selected cases in which there is a question of an associated disorder, such as a rotator cuff tear. Contrast medium–enhanced computed tomography can also provide information about articular injury and placement of hardware about the joint that might be impinging on the articular surface.

Physical Therapy

For most patients, a supervised physical therapy program will be successful in treating primary adhesive capsulitis,[1,2,4,7] but there has never been a careful study of the cost-effectiveness of this approach. Some orthopaedic surgeons do not believe that super-vised therapy is important for these patients, and instead prefer a home program. In cases of idiopathic adhesive capsulitis, I combine a home program with supervised physical therapy three times a week for an initial 6-week trial. If the patient is making progress, the combined program is continued for an additional 6 weeks, followed by a home program.

In contrast to primary adhesive capsulitis, postsurgical or posttraumatic shoulder stiffness is often more resistant to a conservative approach.[1,8-11] The likely natural history can be predicted from an understanding of the pathologic features and the potential for future articular injury, such as that associated with a fixed subluxation of the joint. Although the literature clearly shows that limitation of external rotation to less than neutral can be associated with the development of arthritis, the minimal acceptable external rotation loss remains unclarified.[8,9,11] It is my impression that after instability surgery, limitation of external rotation to less than 60% of that of the contralateral shoulder should be treated aggressively to avoid development of arthritis from eccentric articular contact. A supervised physical therapy program is tried first, but my experience has been that even an aggressive stretching program by a knowledgeable shoulder therapist is often ineffective when there is a history of surgery or trauma. The length of time for which the supervised physical therapy program is continued depends on the cause of the motion loss and the patient's response to this treatment. If after 12 to 16 weeks the patient is getting progressively worse or there has been no improvement, an operative intervention is recommended. The risks and benefits of the operative approach have been carefully described and may include fracture, neurovascular injury, residual stiffness, instability, and infection.

Selection of Operative Treatment

It is important to emphasize that treatment of primary adhesive capsulitis should not be considered while the patient is experiencing severe pain in addition to motion loss because this may represent the inflammatory phase of the disease. Neviaser and Neviaser[3] have pointed out that any surgical treatment in this stage will likely exacerbate the patient's motion loss by increasing capsular injury. It is important to wait until pain is present only at the end of the range of motion, indicating that the active inflammatory process has resolved.

When an operative approach is contemplated, it is also important to reemphasize that the diagnosis can be used to predict the likelihood of extra-articular scarring as well as capsular contracture. The surgical treatment must be tailored to address all of these factors. In all cases of refractory primary adhesive capsulitis, closed manipulation should be the initial approach. This approach is also used in relatively acute cases of motion loss after surgery or trauma when therapy has failed to restore motion. However, when there is a suspected or known extra-articular contracture (e.g., after a Bristow or Putti-Platt procedure), an open approach is usually required, and closed manipulation should not be attempted.

Closed Manipulation

Closed manipulation is performed with the patient under general anesthesia with drug-induced complete muscle relaxation. However, if the patient has marked osteopenia or underwent an antecedent surgical repair within the previous 3 months, this approach is contraindicated because of the risk of fracture, disruption of the soft-tissue repair, nerve injuries, and postmanipulation instability.[1,3-5]

The anesthetic technique is an extremely important aspect of the overall treatment. There must be complete muscle paralysis during the procedure. In my experience, while general anesthesia is an adequate method, patients often have subsequent pain that interferes with their therapy in the immediate postoperative period. It is therefore recommended that an interscalene block with a long-acting agent (bupivacaine) be used. The block is administered either as a single percutaneous injection or by placement of an indwelling interscalene catheter.[21-23] If a simple block is performed, it is repeated in the morning on the first and second postoperative days. Use of 0.5% bupivacaine will provide about 12 hours of analgesia, which will markedly reduce the patient's requirement for narcotics while increasing tolerance to physical therapy. If an interscalene catheter is used, a continuous slow drip of bupivacaine is administered.

The method of closed manipulation has been described by Neviaser and Neviaser[3] and Harryman.[1] The scapula is stabilized by one hand while the humerus is grasped with the other hand just above the elbow. The forearm should not be used as a lever in this manipulation. An attempt is first made to recover external rotation with the arm at the side. As firm pressure is gradually exerted, palpable and audible yielding of soft tissue occurs and motion improves. Although there may be some concern about fracture with this initial rotatory force, I attempt this motion first because it is easier to recover flexion and abduction if the greater tuberosity can be rotated out from under the acromion. If external rotation cannot be recovered, flexion is attempted, followed by abduction and then external and internal rotation. Finally, the arm is brought back into adduction and internally rotated. Motion is usually restored in all planes.

Arthroscopic Release

Although most patients with primary adhesive capsulitis respond to physical therapy, some will require closed manipulation to achieve and maintain sufficient improvement in motion. A small percentage of those patients will continue to have motion loss that is refractory even to manipulation of the shoulder under anesthesia. I have found the technique of arthroscopic capsular release very helpful in this situation. Similarly, in cases of postsurgical or posttraumatic shoulder stiffness in which closed manipulation fails, arthroscopic release can also be attempted, provided there is no extra-articular component to the motion loss.[9-14]

This approach continues to be controversial, however. Some surgeons suggest that arthroscopy is of little diagnostic and therapeutic value in treating patients with adhesive capsulitis of the shoulder.[3] Others suggest that the arthroscope may be helpful in delineating pathologic changes, documenting the results of closed manipulation, and treating concomitant intra-articular and subacromial disorders.[23,24] Over the past 4 years, I have used arthroscopic release in selected cases in which motion loss appeared to be principally due to capsular contracture that was unresponsive despite closed manipulation. This technique has the advantage of allowing the detection of coexisting disorders, as well as permitting a controlled and precise capsular release. It also allows concurrent treatment of concomitant subacromial disease, as documented by preoperative temporary relief from local anesthetic injection and the intraoperative finding of an inflamed subacromial bursa. Furthermore, in cases of both idiopathic and postsurgical motion loss, I have found that the force of manual manipulation required to regain motion is greatly reduced by arthroscopically releasing the capsule before manipulating the shoulder. The arthroscopic technique also has the advantage over an open release of avoiding the morbidity associated with an

extensive open surgical dissection. If motion loss remains unchanged intraoperatively after attempted arthroscopic release and manipulation, conversion to an open release is possible.

Anesthetic technique is an important component of the surgical plan for arthroscopic capsular release. The method of obtaining complete muscle paralysis with an interscalene block, as already described for closed manipulation, is recommended for both anterior and posterior release procedures.

Anterior Release

Anterior capsular release (Fig. 2) is performed with the patient seated in the "beach chair" position.[25] With use of this position, arm traction is unnecessary, although some surgeons prefer the added joint distraction produced when traction is applied with the patient in a lateral decubitus position. It is always dif-

ficult to insert the arthroscope into a stiff shoulder because of the capsular contracture and decreased joint volume, and articular injury from forceful insertion of the arthroscope is a concern. Chondral damage can be avoided by gently inserting the arthroscope over the humeral head. Although some surgeons[24] recommend use of a smaller arthroscope (3.9-mm diameter), such as that used for small-joint arthroscopy in the wrist, I have used the standard 30-degree arthroscope (5.5-mm diameter) without difficulty.

The biceps tendon is the first anatomic landmark that should be identified. It marks the upper edge of the "rotator interval region," which is formed by the anterior edge of the supraspinatus tendon and the cranial border of the subscapularis tendon.[18] This region is usually composed of a thick band of scar tissue, which obscures the

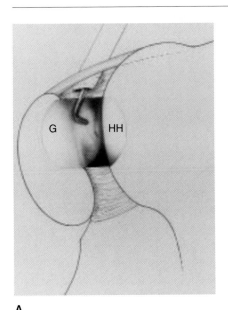
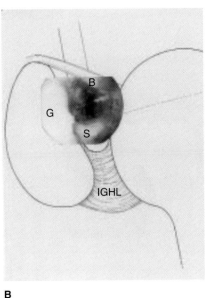
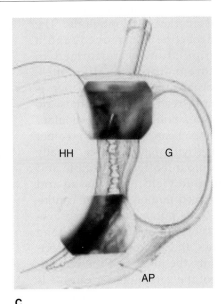

A   **B**   **C**

Fig. 2 Anterior arthroscopic capsular release is performed through an anterosuperior portal (G = glenoid; HH = humeral head). **A,** Left shoulder as viewed through a posterior portal. An arthroscopic probe is placed onto the thick wall of scarred capsule in the anterosuperior (rotator interval) region of the capsule. **B,** An arthroscopic electrocautery device has divided the anterosuperior region of the capsule, and the subscapularis tendon (S) and the remaining thickened inferior glenohumeral ligament (IGHL) are visible. B = biceps tendon. **C,** If necessary, the anteroinferior capsule is released down to the bottom of the glenoid, but not through the axillary pouch (AP).

normally visible upper edge of the subscapularis tendon. A varying amount of synovitis may also be present.

An arthroscopic cannula is inserted just beneath the biceps tendon, and the capsular scar tissue is divided with the use of an electrocautery device and a motorized shaver (Fig. 2, A). The capsular division begins superiorly from just anterior and inferior to the biceps tendon and continues inferiorly until the discrete upper edge of the subscapularis tendon is encountered (Fig. 2, B). This is a surgical release of the rotator-interval region of the capsule.[18] Both Ozaki et al[14] and Neer et al[12] have shown that such a release performed through an open approach is successful in restoring external rotation in shoulders with refractory adhesive capsulitis.

After release of this region of the capsule, the humeral head moves inferiorly and laterally, allowing more space in the joint for the arthroscope to be moved both anteriorly and inferiorly. The arthroscope is removed, and a manipulation is performed to restore motion in all planes. External rotation in adduction is usually restored with almost no manipulation force. The shoulder can then be manipulated into other planes with minimal force, usually accompanied by an audible and palpable yielding of tissue and improved motion. If there continues to be minimal or no improvement of motion in the remaining planes, the arthroscope is reinserted into the joint, and the remainder of the anteroinferior capsule is released. The capsular release is performed in the midcapsular region, extending down to the five-o'clock position for the right glenoid and down to the seven-o'clock position for the left glenoid (Fig. 2, C).

Some surgeons have expressed concern about risk to the axillary nerve with a capsular release in this region,[23] but I have not encountered any neurologic complications. The subscapularis is interposed between the anteroinferior capsule and the axillary nerve when the arm is adducted. It should be reemphasized that the axillary pouch should not be released with this technique. Release of the anteroinferior capsule will usually restore external rotation in abduction, but some patients will still lack internal rotation in abduction after release of the entire anterior capsule; if that is the case, the posterior capsule must be released as well.

When the capsular release is begun in the rotator interval region, it is extremely important to identify a discrete subscapularis tendon. If this structure cannot be identified, the procedure must be converted to an open release. Failure to curtail the arthroscopic release in this situation can result in division of the subscapularis tendon as well as the anterior capsule. When such a conversion has been necessary, distortion and scarring of the subscapularis and extra-articular scarring were identified, all of which were successfully managed with open release.

Posterior Release

In those few instances in which there is continued loss of internal rotation and flexion after an anterior release, arthroscopic release of the posterior capsule is also necessary to accomplish a global capsular release (Fig. 3). This technique is indicated when the loss of internal rotation in abduction exceeds 40 degrees compared with the contralateral side.

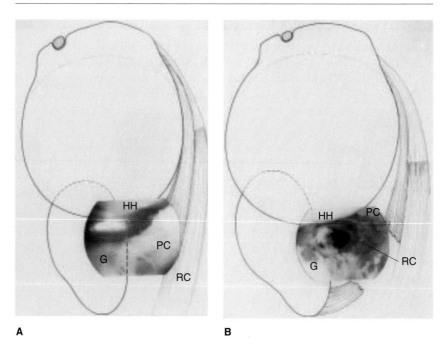

A   **B**

Fig. 3 Technique of arthroscopic posterior capsular release, depicted in a right shoulder viewed through an anterosuperior portal (G = glenoid; HH = humeral head; PC = posterior capsule; RC = rotator cuff). **A,** An arthroscopic shaver has been placed through the thickened posterior capsule. **B,** After release of the posterior capsule, the rotator cuff muscle can be seen.

A small subset of patients may have an isolated posterior capsular contracture characterized by motion loss primarily limited to internal rotation, cross-chest (horizontal) adduction, and flexion with relative preservation of external rotation. These patients often have impingement-type pain and in some cases have undergone acromioplasty or other surgery without relief. Their capsular contracture may result in a form of nonoutlet-type impingement by causing increased obligate anterosuperior translation during shoulder flexion and internal rotation. This condition is treated with a posterior capsular release to restore lost motion and normal kinematics.

I typically perform posterior release with the patient in the beach-chair position, although lateral decubitus positioning may be used alternatively. The arthroscope is placed through a cannula in an anterosuperior portal, while the arthroscopic sheath in the posterior portal is removed over a switching stick and is replaced with an operative cannula. An electrocautery device and a motor-ized shaver are then used to release the posterior capsule from just posterior to the biceps tendon origin down to the posteroinferior rim of the glenoid. The posterior capsule is always observed to be markedly thickened and without the redundancy seen in a normal shoulder, in which it is no more than 1 mm thick and is redundant when the arm is adducted and in neutral rotation (Fig. 3, A).

The arthroscopic release of the posterior capsule must be just at the glenoid rim. Because the muscle of the infraspinatus is superficial at this point, this is taken as the endpoint for capsular division (Fig. 3, B). If the capsular division is performed more laterally, there is a risk of dividing the infraspinatus tendon, because it conjoins with the capsule lateral to the joint line; this would potentially weaken external rotation by creating a tear in the infraspinatus tendon.

Open Release

In cases in which arthroscopic release is contraindicated or fails to restore motion, an open release can be performed.[8-13] Since arthroscopy is performed with the patient in a seated position, immediate conversion to an open approach is feasible.

As with closed manipulation and arthroscopic release, use of an interscalene block is the preferred anesthetic technique. A deltopectoral incision is used. Extensive scarring through all layers of the dissection is often identified. The deltopectoral interval is gently dissected, and the adhesions between the deltoid and the humerus are sharply released (Fig. 4, A). This must be done with care, as the axillary nerve may be at risk. The axillary nerve can often be palpated on the deep surface of the deltoid muscle approximately 3 to 5 cm below the lateral border of the acromion. The dissection is easier if the shoulder is abducted (Fig. 4, B), which allows the deltoid to become lax and more easily retracted. Internal rotation of the arm while gently retracting the deltoid muscle will allow anterior-to-posterior release of subdeltoid

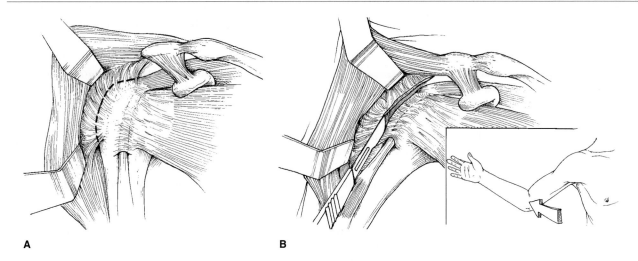

A   **B**

Fig. 4   Release of subdeltoid scar. **A,** Scar obliterates the plane between the deltoid and the proximal humerus and rotator cuff. **B,** Abduction of the shoulder allows the deltoid to relax and makes release of scar tissue easier.

adhesions until the deltoid can move freely over the proximal humerus when the arm is rotated.

The dissection then proceeds medially into the subacromial space. After the coracoacromial ligament is excised, the subacromial space may be found to be filled with dense scar adhesions between the rotator cuff and the acromion, which should be sharply released. Care must be taken with deltoid retraction, as overzealous retraction can either tear the muscle or avulse it from its origin or insertion. The conjoined tendon is then separated from the scarred area joining it to the underlying subscapularis and retracted medially. This can usually be accomplished with a combination of blunt and sharp dissection. The surgeon should be mindful of the musculocutaneous nerve; it is essential to keep the dissection lateral to the base of the coracoid process to prevent injury to neurovascular structures.

The superior border of the subscapularis tendon is identified, and the rotator interval is released, extending from the humerus to the coracoid.[12-14] As the dissection proceeds from superficial to deep between tissue layers, the shoulder should be gently manipulated to regain motion. If there is still marked limitation of external rotation due to scarring in the interval between the subscapularis and the capsule, the subscapularis is split between its fibers, and an elevator is used to release adhesions between its tendon and the underlying capsule. If there is still limitation of external rotation, a coronal Z-plasty lengthening of the subscapularis and capsule is performed (Fig. 5). This is done by dividing the scarred capsule and subscapularis tendon in the coronal plane so that the superficial half of the tendon remains attached

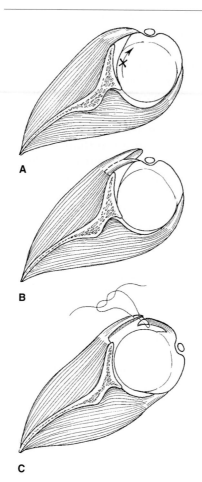

Fig. 5 Coronal Z-plasty lengthening of subscapularis and capsule. **A,** Entrapment of the subscapularis causes loss of external rotation (arrow). **B,** The subscapularis and capsule are divided in the coronal plane, beginning laterally at their insertion and developing a superficial layer. **C,** The capsule (deep layer) is then divided at the glenoid, and the arm is externally rotated for completion of the Z-plasty lengthening procedure.

to the muscle; the remaining deep half is divided at the glenoid and remains attached to the lesser tuberosity. The orientation of this coronal dissection can be guided by determining the thickness of the scarred tendon and capsular tissue once the rotator interval region is opened. The surgeon can usually both see and palpate the thickness of the anterior tissues through this interval.

When the anterior capsule and subscapularis have been dissected, the subscapularis is usually found to be entrapped in scar tissue. To achieve full mobility, it may be necessary to visualize and dissect the axillary nerve (Fig. 6, A and B). A vessel loupe is placed around the axillary nerve, and the subscapularis is released globally on its superior, inferior, deep, and superficial surfaces.

If abduction and internal rotation are still limited, the inferior and posterior capsule can be released through the joint. To do this, I place a humeral head retractor to displace the humeral head posteriorly and also put a blunt retractor beneath the inferior capsule to protect the axillary nerve (Fig. 6, C). The capsule is then released from inferior to posterior and superior under direct vision. The retractors are removed, and the shoulder is placed through the range of motion to evaluate motion gains. The arm is positioned in the maximum external rotation that will allow secure closure of the Z-plasty of the anterior capsule and subscapularis tendon with the use of large, nonabsorbable, braided suture. The patient usually gains at least 40 degrees of external rotation; however, this depends on the quality of the tendon and capsular tissue. Range of motion is assessed again to determine where there is tension on the soft-tissue repair and thus define a "safe zone" for early passive range-of-motion activity.

Postoperative Treatment

On the morning of the first postoperative day, either a repeat interscalene block is instituted or the interscalene catheter infusion is continued. Therapy is performed twice a day, in the morning and the

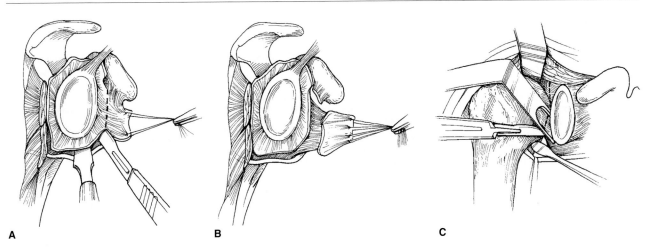

Fig. 6 Subscapularis mobilization in a left shoulder (humeral head omitted from drawing for better visualization). **A,** Sutures are placed into the contracted and shortened subscapularis tendon. An elevator protects the axillary nerve as the inferior and anterior capsules are divided. The coracohumeral ligament (dotted line) is also divided. **B,** After the capsular release and coracohumeral ligament division, the subscapularis is mobilized. **C,** An inferior and posterior capsular release can be performed if the axillary nerve is carefully mobilized and protected (shown elevated with a vessel loupe around it and an elevator beneath it).

afternoon. The patient is discharged after the second therapy session on the second postoperative day. Narcotic analgesia is used as necessary to supplement the interscalene analgesia. Therapy consists of an aggressive stretching program in all planes, and the patient is instructed in self-assisted stretching exercises as well. As the interscalene block usually results in only partial muscle paralysis, the patient can perform some stretching independently.

When a soft-tissue repair has been performed, as with a Z-plasty lengthening in the front of the shoulder, motion should be only passive for 4 weeks. The positions at which resistance is felt and the repair is observed to be under tension should be noted at the time of surgery and specified for the treating therapist as the limits of passive motion. After 4 weeks, an aggressive active-motion program with therapist-assisted stretching is begun.

The patient who has undergone an arthroscopic capsular re-

lease is discharged on the afternoon of the second postoperative day. The patient is encouraged to use the surgically treated arm for activities of daily living, and a sling is not worn. The patient continues a home program with self-assisted stretching and a pulley device, as well as supervised physical therapy on an outpatient basis five times per week for the first 2 weeks and then three times per week for the next 2 weeks.

After 4 weeks, the patient's progress is assessed, and the need for additional therapy is individualized. I do not recommend use of a continuous passive motion machine, as it has been my experience that this device is not reliable for maintaining motion gains. Whether the patient was treated arthroscopically or with open release, the strengthening phase of the postoperative therapy program is delayed until a nearly full pain-free arc of motion has been achieved. This usually takes about 3 months.

Summary

Proper treatment of motion loss in the shoulder depends on an initial recognition of the causative disorder and its natural history. Although a nonoperative approach of supervised or unsupervised therapy is usually successful in treating adhesive capsulitis, it may fail in patients whose stiffness is due to surgery or trauma. Closed manipulation restores motion in most cases of idiopathic adhesive capsulitis, but is often ineffective in the treatment of postsurgical motion loss. An arthroscopic release technique allows precise and controlled release of capsular contractures in cases of both idiopathic adhesive capsulitis and postsurgical motion loss. When there is an extra-articular component to the soft-tissue contracture, an open approach will improve motion. Postoperative treatment must emphasize pain control and maintenance of motion gains achieved at the time of manipulation or surgery.

References

1. Harryman DT II: Shoulders: Frozen and stiff. *Instr Course Lect* 1993;42:247-257.
2. Murnaghan JP: Frozen shoulder, in Rockwood CA Jr, Matsen FA III (eds): *The Shoulder*. Philadelphia: WB Saunders, 1990, pp 837-862.
3. Neviaser RJ, Neviaser TJ: The frozen shoulder: Diagnosis and management. *Clin Orthop* 1987;223:59-64.
4. Zuckerman JD, Cuomo F: Frozen shoulder, in Matsen FA III, Fu FH, Hawkins RJ (eds): *The Shoulder: A Balance of Mobility and Stability*. Rosemont, Ill: American Academy of Orthopaedic Surgeons, 1992, pp 253-267.
5. Janda DH, Hawkins RJ: Shoulder manipulation in patients with adhesive capsulitis and diabetes mellitus: A clinical note. *J Shoulder Elbow Surg* 1993;2:36-38.
6. Neviaser JS: Adhesive capsulitis of the shoulder: A study of pathological findings in periarthritis of the shoulder. *J Bone Joint Surg* 1945;27:211-222.
7. Shaffer B, Tibone JE, Kerlan RK: Frozen shoulder: A long-term follow-up. *J Bone Joint Surg Am* 1992;74:738-746.
8. Hawkins RJ, Angelo RL: Glenohumeral osteoarthritis: A late complication of the Putti-Platt repair. *J Bone Joint Surg Am* 1990;72:1193-1197.
9. Lusardi DA, Wirth MA, Wurtz D, et al: Loss of external rotation following anterior capsulorrhaphy of the shoulder. *J Bone Joint Surg Am* 1993;75:1185-1192.
10. Kieras DM, Matsen FA III: Open release in the management of refractory frozen shoulder. *Orthop Trans* 1991;15:801-802.
11. MacDonald PB, Hawkins RJ, Fowler PJ, et al: Release of the subscapularis for internal rotation contracture and pain after anterior repair for recurrent anterior dislocation of the shoulder. *J Bone Joint Surg Am* 1992;74:734-737.
12. Neer CS, Satterlee CC, Dalsey R, et al: The anatomy and potential effects of contracture of the coracohumeral ligament. *Clin Orthop* 1992;280:182-185.
13. Neer CS II: Frozen shoulder, in Neer CS II (ed): *Shoulder Reconstruction*. Philadelphia: WB Saunders, 1990, pp 422-427.
14. Ozaki J, Nakagawa Y, Sakurai G, et al: Recalcitrant chronic adhesive capsulitis of the shoulder: Role of contracture of the coracohumeral ligament and rotator interval in pathogenesis and treatment. *J Bone Joint Surg Am* 1989;71:1511-1515.
15. Harryman DT II, Sidles JA, Clark JM, et al: Translation of the humeral head on the glenoid with passive glenohumeral motion. *J Bone Joint Surg Am* 1990;72:1334-1343.
16. Warner JJP, Caborn DNM, Berger R, et al: Dynamic capsuloligamentous anatomy of the glenohumeral joint. *J Shoulder Elbow Surg* 1993;2:115-133.
17. Young DC, Rockwood CA Jr: Complications of a failed Bristow procedure and their management. *J Bone Joint Surg Am* 1991;73:969-981.
18. Harryman DT II, Sidles JA, Harris SL, et al: The role of the rotator interval capsule in passive motion and stability of the shoulder. *J Bone Joint Surg Am* 1992;74:53-66.
19. Bigliani LU, Morrison DS, April AW: The morphology of the acromion and its relation to the rotator cuff tear. *Orthop Trans* 1986;10:228.
20. Itoi E, Tabata S: Range of motion and arthrography in frozen shoulders. *J Shoulder Elbow Surg* 1992;1:106-112.
21. Brown AR, Weiss R, Greenberg C, et al: Interscalene block for shoulder arthroscopy: Comparison with general anesthesia. *Arthroscopy* 1993;9:295-300.
22. Kinnard P, Truchon R, St-Pierre A, et al: Interscalene block for pain relief after shoulder surgery: A prospective randomized study. *Clin Orthop* 1994;304:22-24.
23. Pollock RG, Duralde XA, Flatow EL, et al: The use of arthroscopy in the treatment of resistant frozen shoulder. *Clin Orthop* 1994;304:30-36.
24. Wiley AM: Arthroscopic appearance of frozen shoulder. *Arthroscopy* 1991;7:138-143.
25. Warner JJP: Shoulder arthroscopy in the beach-chair position: Basic set-up. *Operative Techniques Orthop* 1991;1:147-154.

Calcific Tendinopathy of the Rotator Cuff: Pathogenesis, Diagnosis, and Management

Hans K. Uhthoff, MD, FRCSC, and Joachim W. Loehr, MD, FRCSC

Abstract

Calcific tendinopathy, or calcifying tendinitis, is a disease characterized by multifocal, cell-mediated calcification of living tissue. After spontaneous disappearance of the calcific deposits or, less frequently, surgical removal, the tendon reconstitutes itself. Attention to the clinical presentation and the radiologic, morphologic, and gross characteristics of the calcium deposit will facilitate differentiation between the formative phase and the resorptive phase, which is of paramount importance in the management of this disease. Should conservative treatment fail, surgical removal may be indicated during the formative phase, but only under exceptional circumstances during the resorptive phase. Aspiration and lavage of the deposit should be performed only during the latter phase.

J Am Acad Orthop Surg 1997;5:183-191

Calcific tendinopathy, or calcifying tendinitis, of the rotator cuff, is a common disorder of unknown etiology in which multifocal, cell-mediated calcification of a living tendon is usually followed by spontaneous phagocytic resorption.[1] After resorption or surgical removal of the deposit, the tendon reconstitutes itself. During the deposition of calcium, the patient may be free of pain or may suffer only a mild to moderate degree of discomfort. The disease becomes acutely painful only when the calcium undergoes resorption.

Calcifying tendinitis must be distinguished from degenerative or dystrophic calcifications, which occur at the insertion into bone but not in the midsubstance of the tendon. Radiologic signs of degenerative processes are extremely rare in calcific tendinopathies.

Pathogenesis

The etiology of calcifying tendinitis is still a matter of controversy. Circumscribed tissue hypoxia and localized pressure have been invoked as causative factors. Two fundamentally different processes leading to formation of calcium deposits in the cuff have been proposed: degenerative calcification and reactive calcification.

Degenerative Calcification

Codman[2] proposed that degeneration of the tendon fibers precedes calcification. The fibers become necrotic, and dystrophic calcification follows. Degeneration of the fibers of the rotator cuff tendons is usually attributed to a wear-and-tear effect as well as to aging. Obviously, these two causes are interrelated. The glenohumeral joint is not only a universal joint but is also probably the most used joint in the body, and studies performed in Sweden indicate that the stress and strain induced by work involving the arm can lead to supraspinatus tendinitis.[3] However, there is no evidence that even a worker engaged in heavy manual labor will necessarily develop calcifying tendinitis in time, and Olsson[4] has shown that the cuff tendons from the dominant arm show no more evidence of degeneration than those from the contralateral arm.

Aging is considered to be the foremost cause of degeneration in cuff tendons. Brewer[5] believes that with aging there is a general diminution in the vascularity of the supraspinatus tendon along with fiber changes. The most conspicuous age-related changes are seen in the fascicles, the well-delineated bundles of collagen that constitute the distinctive architecture of the

Dr. Uhthoff is Professor Emeritus, Department of Surgery, University of Ottawa, Ottawa, Ontario, Canada. Dr. Loehr is Associate Professor and Chief, Department of Orthopaedic Surgery, Schulthess Klinik, Zurich, Switzerland.

Reprint requests: Dr. Uhthoff, University of Ottawa, 5004-501 Smyth Road, Ottawa, Ontario, Canada K1H 8L6.

tendon.[4] Beginning at the end of the fourth or during the fifth decade, most of the fascicles undergo thinning and fibrillation, both of which are defined as degenerative processes. The thinned fascicles show irregular cellular arrangement, and the fragmented fibers are often hypocellular. The volume of the connective tissue that carries the blood vessels between the fascicles may appear increased when compared with the volume of the fascicles.

Inasmuch as calcifying tendinitis seldom affects persons before the fourth decade, it can be argued that primary degeneration of tendon fibers is responsible for the subsequent deposition of calcium. Codman[2] proposed the degenerative nature of calcifying tendinitis, and many investigators have supported this concept. According to McLaughlin,[6] the earliest lesion is focal hyalinization of fibers, which eventually become fibrillated and detach from the surrounding normal tendon. Continued motion of the tendon grinds the detached, curled-up fibers into a wenlike substance consisting of necrotic debris, which becomes calcified.

Mohr and Bilger[7] believe that the process of calcification starts with necrosis of the tenocytes, with concomitant intracellular accumulation of calcium, often in form of microspheroliths, or psammomas. We have never observed psammomas during the early phases of formation but have noted them regularly during the phase of resorption. Our electron-microscopic examinations confirm that the electron-dense material is intracellular. It is unfortunate that Mohr and Bilger failed to distinguish between calcifications at the insertion and intratendinous calcifications, nor did they describe morphologic features characteristic of either formation or resorption.

In general, supporters of the theory of degenerative calcification fail to take into consideration the typical age distribution of affected persons, the course of the disease, and the morphologic aspects of calcific tendinopathy. The incidence of calcification increases with age in cases of degenerative calcification, whereas it peaks during the fifth decade in cases of calcifying tendinitis. Moreover, degenerative diseases never exhibit a potential for self-healing. Furthermore, the histologic and ultrastructural features of degenerative calcification and calcifying tendinosis are quite different.

Reactive Calcification

We concur with other investigators that the process of calcification is actively mediated by cells in a viable environment,[8-11] and there cannot be the slightest doubt that formation of the calcium deposit must precede its resorption. Consequently, we propose that the evolution of the disease can be divided into three distinct stages: precalcific, calcific, and postcalcific (Fig. 1).

Precalcific Stage

In the precalcific stage, the site of predilection for calcification undergoes fibrocartilaginous transformation. This metaplasia of tenocytes into chondrocytes is accompanied by metachromasia, indicative of the elaboration of proteoglycan.

Calcific Stage

The calcific stage is subdivided into the formative phase, the resting phase, and the resorptive phase.[11] Our "formative phase" seems to be identical to the "early phase of increment" of Lippmann,[12] and his "late phase of increment" is analogous to our "resorptive phase."

During the formative phase, calcium crystals are deposited primarily in matrix vesicles, which coalesce to form large foci of calcifi-

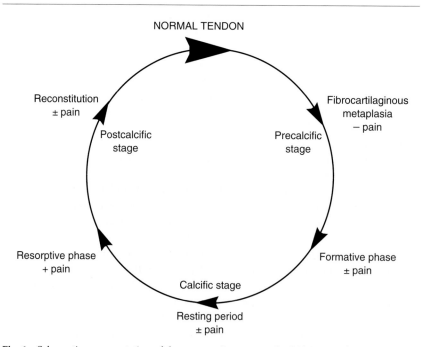

Fig. 1 Schematic representation of the progressive stages of calcifying tendinitis.

cation.[10] If the patient undergoes surgery during this stage, the deposit appears chalklike and must be scooped out. The fibrocartilaginous septa between the foci of calcification are generally devoid of vascular channels. They do not consistently stain positively for type II collagen, which is known to be a component of fibrocartilage. These fibrocartilaginous septa are gradually eroded by the enlarging deposits.

During the resting phase, fibrocollagenous tissue borders the foci of calcification. The presence of this tissue indicates that deposition of calcium at that site is terminated.

During the resorptive phase, after a variable period of inactivity of the disease process, spontaneous resorption of calcium is heralded by the appearance of thin-walled vascular channels at the periphery of the deposit. Soon thereafter, the deposit is surrounded by macrophages and multinucleated giant cells that phagocytose and remove the calcium. If an operation is performed during this stage, the calcific deposit contains a thick, creamy or toothpastelike material that is often under pressure.

Postcalcific Stage

Simultaneously with the resorption of calcium, granulation tissue containing young fibroblasts and new vascular channels begins to remodel the space occupied by calcium. These sites stain positively for type III collagen. As the scar matures, fibroblasts and collagen eventually align along the longitudinal axis of the tendon. During this remodeling process, type III collagen is replaced by type I collagen.

Although the pathogenesis of the calcifying process can be reasonably constructed from morphologic studies, it is difficult to establish what triggers the fibrocartilagi-

nous transformation in the first place. Codman[2] suggested tissue hypoxia as the primary etiologic factor. This still remains an attractive hypothesis because of the peculiarity of the blood supply of the tendon and the mechanics of the shoulder. We have found an increased frequency of HLA-A1 in patients with calcifying tendinitis, indicating that they may be genetically susceptible to the condition.[13] Factors that trigger the onset of resorption also remain unknown.

Pathoanatomy

The calcium deposits are usually not in contact with the bone insertion; rather, they are at least 1.5 to 2.0 cm away from it. Only in isolated reports has the presence of calcific deposits in subchondral bone been described. It is important to note that not all foci of calcification in a given patient are in the same phase of evolution. In general, however, one phase predominates. The morphologic aspect of an individual deposit can vary from fibrocollagenous tissue to foreign body–like granulomatous tissue.

Precalcific Stage

We believe the disease starts with fibrocartilaginous metaplasia of tendinous tissue. The fibrocartilaginous areas are generally avascular. The intercellular substance is metachromatic, and glycosaminoglycan-rich pericellular halos around rounded cells are prominent.[14] Surprisingly, Archer et al[14] found that monoclonal collagen staining did not reveal the presence of type II collagen. In our studies performed with the use of type II collagen monoclonal antibodies, we could occasionally document its presence (Fig. 2, A). The different outcomes may be due to differences in tissue preparation, source

of monoclonal antibodies, and/or staining technique.

Calcific Stage

Formative Phase

Under the light microscope, the calcific deposits appear multifocal, separated by fibrocollagenous tissue or fibrocartilage (Fig. 2, B). The latter consists of easily distinguishable chondrocytes (described by Archer et al[14] as chondrocytelike cells) within a matrix showing various degrees of metachromasia. The appearance of chondrocytes within the tendon substance near calcification has been documented by many authors since 1912. The ultrastructure of these chondrocytes shows that the cells often have a fair amount of cytoplasm containing a well-developed endoplasmic reticulum, a moderate number of mitochondria, one or more vacuoles, and numerous cell processes.[10] The margin of the nucleus is indented. The cells are surrounded by a distinct band of pericellular matrix with or without an intervening lacuna.

The first evidence of calcium deposition is the presence of loosely granular material that stains positive with the von Kossa method (Fig. 2, C) and coalesces to form clumps. On transmission electron microscopy, aggregates of rounded structures containing crystalline material are found in a matrix of amorphous debris or irregularly fragmented collagen fibers. Irregularly rectangular crystals are sometimes found within membrane-bound structures resembling matrix vesicles, or calcifying globules. Infrequently, crystalline densities seem to be embedded between collagen fibers. High-resolution transmission electron microscopy has revealed that the crystals are much larger than the classic apatite crystals and have a different configuration.[11]

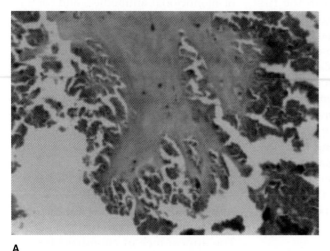

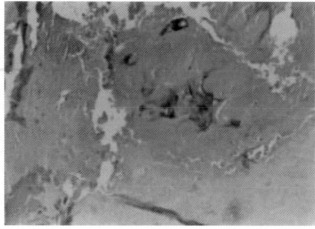

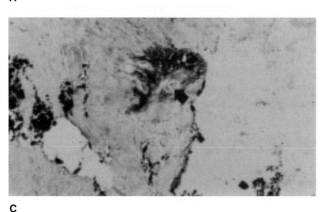

Fig. 2 Formative phase. **B,** Some septa contain type II collagen (immunohistochemical monoclonal staining for type II collagen, ×50). **A,** Septa of fibrocartilaginous tissue are seen between calcium deposits (Masson's trichrome, ×50). **C,** Note early calcifications around living chondrocytes (arrow) (von Kossa, ×50).

Resting Phase

During the formative phase, inflammation and vessels are notably absent. Other foci are surrounded by tendinous tissue without evidence of inflammation. These areas seem to correspond to the resting phase.

Resorptive Phase

Other foci show the presence of young mesenchymal cells, epithelioid cells, leukocytes, lymphocytes, and occasionally giant cells. The presence of these cells is indicative of resorptive activity. Indeed, the marked cellular reaction around calcific deposits, often called a calcium granuloma, is considered to constitute a charac-teristic lesion of calcifying tendinitis. The granulomatous appearance is imparted by the presence of multinucleated giant cells (Fig. 3, A) and macrophages. Archer et al[14] interpreted the presence of the latter two cell types as a resorption phenomenon. The cellular reaction is often accompanied by capillaries or thin-walled vascular channels around the deposits (Fig. 3, B). Phagocytosed material within macrophages or multinucleated giant cells can be easily discerned.

Ultrastructural examination of these cells shows electron-dense crystalline particles in cytoplasmic vacuoles, but the crystals are somewhat different in appearance from those in the extracellular deposits.[10] Some of the intracellular accumulations have a rounded aspect and are known as microspheroliths, or psammomas (Fig. 3, C).

Postcalcific Stage

Small areas representing the process of repair can be found in the general vicinity of calcification, showing considerable variation in appearance. Granulation tissue with young fibroblasts and newly formed capillaries (Fig. 4) contrasts with well-formed scars with vascular channels and maturing fibroblasts that are in the process of alignment with the long axis of the tendon fibers. Using monoclonal antibodies against type III collagen,

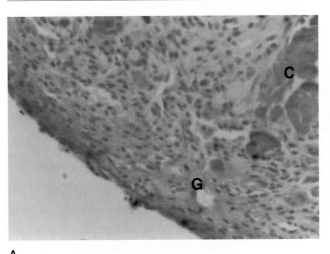

A

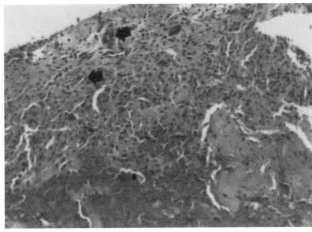

B

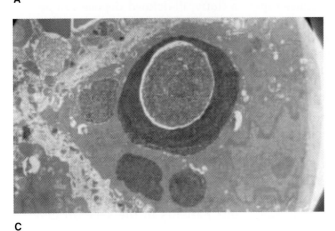

C

Fig. 3 Resorptive phase. **A,** Note the presence of giant cells (G) around calcium deposits (C) (Masson's trichrome, ×100). **B,** Many thin-walled vascular channels (arrows) are seen in the vicinity of calcium deposits undergoing phagocytic resorption (hematoxylin-eosin, ×50). **C,** A psammoma inside a macrophage and three smaller accumulations of electron-dense material. The multilayered structure of the psammoma is quite evident (uranyl acetate and lead citrate, ×14,500).

we were able to confirm collagen neoformation, which was most pronounced around vascular channels.

The subacromial bursa is rarely the site of a reaction. Should the size of the calcific deposit provoke a subacromial impingement, a localized bursal reaction may be present.

Radiologic Evaluation

Calcium deposits in calcifying tendinitis are most often localized in the supraspinatus tendon. Radiographs must be obtained whenever calcification of the cuff is suspected. Radiographic evaluation is also important during follow-up examinations because it permits assessment of changes in density and extent of calcification.

Initial radiographs should include anteroposterior views with the shoulder in the neutral position and in internal and external rotation. Deposits in the supraspinatus are readily visible on films obtained in neutral rotation, whereas deposits in the infraspinatus and teres minor are best seen on internal-rotation films. Calcifications in the subscapularis occur only in rare instances; a radiograph obtained with external rotation will show them well. Axillary views are rarely indicated. Scapular views,

however, will help to determine whether a calcification is causing impingement.

Calcium deposits are often barely visible on radiographs, particularly in the acute or resorptive phase. We suspect that computed tomography may show them. Magnetic resonance imaging may be indicated in rare circumstances. On T1-weighted images, calcifications appear as areas of decreased signal intensity. T2-weighted images frequently show a perifocal band of increased signal intensity compatible with edema.

We have not found bursography to be of great value. Arthrograms show a distinct delineation between

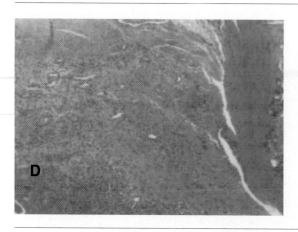

Fig. 4 Postcalcific stage. In the immediate vicinity of the calcific deposit (D) there is still evidence of phagocytic resorption. Farther away, fibroblasts elaborate new collagen (hematoxylin-eosin, ×25).

deposit and joint cavity. We believe they are indicated only in exceptional instances, as when a tear is suspected.

Radiographs not only allow confirmation of the absence or presence of calcium deposits, but also permit assessment of their extent, delineation, and density. DePalma and Kruper[15] described two radiographic types. Type I has a fluffy, fleecy appearance, with a poorly defined periphery. It is usually encountered in patients with acute pain. An overlying crescentic streak indicates rupture of the deposit into the bursa, which occurs only in this type. Type II is characterized by discrete, homogeneous deposits with uniform density and a well-defined periphery. This type is seen in subacute and chronic cases. DePalma and Kruper reported that in 52% of their patients, the calcification was seen as a single lesion.

Our observations confirm those of DePalma and Kruper.[15] During the formative phase, when pain is chronic or even absent, the deposit is dense, well defined, and homogeneous (Fig. 5, A). During the resorptive phase, which is characterized by acute pain, the deposit is fluffy, cloudlike, ill defined, and irregular in density (Fig. 5, B). Rupture of the calcific deposit into the bursa can occur only during the resorptive phase, because of the toothpastelike or creamy consistency. Radiographs show a crescentic radiodensity overlying the deposit (Fig. 5, C). In longitudinal studies, a change from a dense, well-delineated deposit into a fluffy, ill-defined deposit can be observed, but the contrary is never seen.

Most authors agree that radiographic evidence of degenerative joint disease is usually lacking in patients with calcific tendinopathies. This is true of patients in the fourth and fifth decades of life, when calcifying tendinitis peaks. It is not surprising, however, that acromioclavicular osteophytes were observed in three of our patients in the seventh decade.

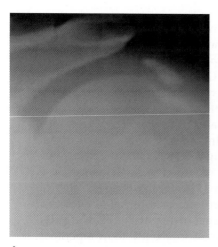

A

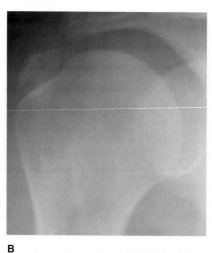

B

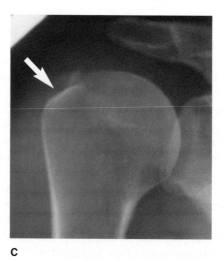

C

Fig. 5 **A,** In the formative phase, the deposit is dense, well circumscribed, and homogeneous. In the resorptive phase, the deposit is fluffy and ill defined **(B),** and the calcium that has ruptured into the subacromial bursa is seen as a crescentic shadow (arrow) overlying the intratendinous deposit **(C).**

Calcifications seen in arthropathies have a quite different appearance. They are stippled and overlie the bone insertion and are always accompanied by degenerative osseous or articular changes. These calcium deposits must be clearly distinguished from reactive intratendinous calcifications.

In a study of 217 patients, Hartig and Huth[16] found sonography more sensitive than radiography in detecting calcium deposits. The deposit was visualized sonographically (as well as histologically) in 100% of cases but was depicted radiographically in only 90%. In addition, sonography permits more exact localization of the deposit without subjecting the patient to radiation.

Management

Distinguishing between the formative phase and the resorptive phase is important for proper management. During the formative phase, the pain is chronic or even absent. On radiographs, the deposit appears as a well-delineated, dense, and homogeneous calcification with a chalklike consistency. Histologic examination shows calcification around living chondrocytes. During the resorptive phase, the pain is acute; the deposit has a fluffy, ill-defined radiographic appearance; the consistency is creamy or toothpastelike; and the histologic features are compatible with phagocytic resorption.

Conservative Measures

The patient is instructed to do a daily program of exercises to avoid loss of mobility of the glenohumeral joint and to keep the arm in abduction as much as possible. The latter can be achieved by placing the arm on

the backrest of a chair or, when lying down, by putting a pillow in the axilla. Application of moist heat is suggested when the symptoms are subacute. Although ultrasound is occasionally used in our physiotherapy department and some patients have commented on its beneficial effect, we have not seen any evidence that this accelerates the disappearance of calcium.

During the formative phase, when the symptoms are chronic, intrabursal injections of corticosteroids are appropriate only in the presence of an impingement syndrome. Needling of dense, homogeneous deposits has never been attempted by our group, nor has lavage been successful, presumably because of the chalklike consistency of the calcification.

During the resorptive phase, when the symptoms are acute or subacute and when radiographs indicate ongoing resorption, we attempt lavage of the deposit with the use of two large-bore needles and 2% lidocaine. The site of lavage is determined radiologically and clinically. In the outflow, liquid calcium particles can be recognized easily. Even when the lavage is negative, the multiple perforations of the site of deposition will decrease the intratendinous pressure and thus the pain. In a few instances, the lavage must be repeated.

Although we prescribe nonsteroidal anti-inflammatory drugs for 1 week, we have no proof of their beneficial action, nor could we find a relevant publication to support their use. The symptoms usually decrease after 1 week, at which point the patient is referred to the physiotherapy department. Patients are assessed clinically and radiographically every 4 weeks. We have never used ultrasound during this phase, nor do we recommend radiotherapy.

Extracorporeal Shock-Wave Therapy

Extracorporeal shock-wave therapy, which is now commonly employed for lithotripsy in urology, has recently been used for treating calcific deposits. Rompe et al[17] reported on a series of 40 patients who received 1,500 impulses to the shoulder area under regional anesthesia during a single therapy session. Fifteen patients had no improvement, but in 25 a partial or complete disappearance of the calcific deposit was observed. A similar experience was reported by Loew et al.[18] Of 20 patients with "chronic, symptomatic calcifying tendinitis," 14 experienced symptomatic improvement at the time of follow-up 12 weeks after the procedure. Local hematomas developed in 14 patients after this therapy. Thirty percent of the patients had an improvement of the Constant-Murley score; in 7, the deposit had disappeared completely.

This technique is still under investigation. Longer follow-up studies, a larger patient population, and reports from other centers are needed before it can be recommended.

Surgical Indications

Should conservative therapy fail during the formative phase, surgery may become necessary. During the resorptive phase, when natural mechanisms usually succeed in removing the deposit, surgery is very rarely indicated. De Sèze and Welfling[19] have stated that during the hyperalgic phase, the disease usually heals with the use of only supportive measures.

Gschwend et al[20] formulated three indications for surgery: (1) progression of symptoms, (2) constant pain interfering with activities of daily living, and (3) absence of improvement of symptoms after conservative therapy. Surgery, whether performed arthroscopically or as an open procedure, should be done on an outpatient basis.

Arthroscopy

Ark et al[21] cited a number of advantages of arthroscopic surgery in treating calcifying tendinitis. These include a shorter rehabilitation time, the possibility of a better functional result, and a better cosmetic appearance than after open surgery.

The recommended arthroscopic technique is as follows: The patient is placed in a beach-chair position for surgery under general endotracheal anesthesia. Interscalene regional anesthesia is also instituted for postoperative pain relief. Posterior, anterolateral, and, if necessary, posterolateral portals are used.

Initially, the glenohumeral joint is explored through the posterior portal with a 4.5-mm 30-degree tilt arthroscope. A vascular injection pattern can sometimes be seen on the articular surface of the rotator cuff tendons, indicating an inflammatory response to the calcific deposit; this should be marked with a suture.

The scope is then introduced into the subacromial space. A working cannula is placed through the anterolateral portal, and the surface of the rotator cuff is palpated. The acromion is then inspected, as well as the coracoacromial ligament and the undersurface of the acromioclavicular joint. The rotator cuff is palpated for any hardening indicative of a calcific deposit. Needling can then be performed; during the resorptive stage, an 18-gauge spinal needle will usually fill with the calcific material when withdrawn from the tendon. Depending on the consistency of the deposit, the calcium might be extruded as a hard paste, or small flakes will be seen. The latter are present when the deposits are sharply demarcated radiographically, which is an ideal indication for arthroscopic surgery.

Once the deposit has been identified, we prefer to make a longitudinal incision in line with the direction of the fibers, avoiding deep penetrating cuts. In general, the use of a hook will best facilitate removal of the calcific material. Large curettes, knives, or tissue cutters should not be used, because of the risk of creating a rotator cuff defect.

Careful irrigation of the subacromial space is then performed, as the calcific debris can act as an irritating agent in the subacromial bursa. Subacromial decompression is performed only if there is an associated lesion, such as an obvious acromial beak or signs of subacromial impingement. There is no compelling published evidence that routine acromioplasty improves the surgical result. Once the subacromial space has been drained, a suction drain is inserted into the subacromial space.

The drain is removed 24 hours postoperatively, and range-of-motion exercises are begun, starting with pendulum exercises, followed by active assisted exercises after the third day, and progressing to active exercises as tolerated. An arm sling is usually not necessary except for patient comfort at night.

Open Procedures

It should be stressed that surgical removal is the exception and that it is indicated only when conservative measures have failed and symptoms interfere with work or activities of daily living.

Calcium deposits are removed under general anesthesia. The patient is in a supine position, and a sandbag is placed under the affected shoulder. We make sure that the side of the patient to be operated on is as close to the edge of the table as possible. The arm is draped free to permit full mobilization during surgery.

We use the skin incision recommended by Neer,[22] going from the acromion to the coracoid process. The deltoid fibers are bluntly separated. The deltoid muscle is not detached from the acromion. The bursa is then opened, the edges are retracted, and the bursal wall is inspected. The narrowness of the interval between the rotator cuff and the ligament is then tested, usually using the little finger, the introduction of which is made easier by longitudinal traction of the arm. While the finger is in place, the arm is rotated and lifted in a position between flexion and abduction. The undersurface of the acromion is also palpated. If the space between the ligament and the rotator cuff is tight, it is usually necessary to proceed with an anterior acromioplasty, although this is definitely the exception. External and internal rotation of the arm will permit inspection of the entire rotator cuff. If a bursal reaction is present, it is usually limited to a hyperemic reaction around the calcific deposit.

The tendon is incised in the direction of its fibers, and the calcific mass is removed by curettage. We then proceed with a limited resection of the frayed tendon edges, which are usually sites of calcium encrustation. Sometimes more than one deposit is present, necessitating separate tendon incisions. If no calcium can be seen during inspection, small incisions are made at the site of calcifications suspected on the preoperative radiographs.

After removal of the deposit, a copious lavage is performed. The shoulder is then moved through its full range of motion, and the tendon edges are approximated if necessary. A sling is applied after surgery. The sling must be removed at least four times a day for pendulum and gentle passive range-of-motion exercises. The sling is discontinued entirely after 3 days, and active exercises are started. We encourage patients to keep the arm in abduction as much as possible. We have never used postoperative corticosteroid injections.

Summary

For optimal treatment results, it is not sufficient to diagnose calcifying tendinitis; one must also determine the stage of the disease. Chronic calcific tendinitis and acute calcific tendinitis, rather than being separate entities, are actually two phases of the same disease. If conservative management fails, surgery may become necessary, preferably in the formative phase of the disease.

References

1. Uhthoff HK, Sarkar K: Calcifying tendinitis, in Rockwood CA Jr, Matsen FA III (eds): *The Shoulder*. Philadelphia: WB Saunders, 1990, vol 2, pp 774-790.

2. Codman EA: *The Shoulder: Rupture of the Supraspinatus Tendon and Other Lesions in or About the Subacromial Bursa*. Boston: Thomas Todd, 1934, pp 178-215.

3. Herberts P, Kadefors R, Högfors C, Sigholm G: Shoulder pain and heavy manual labor. *Clin Orthop* 1984;191: 166-178.

4. Olsson O: Degenerative changes of the shoulder joint and their connection with shoulder pain: A morphological and clinical investigation with special attention to the cuff and biceps tendon. *Acta Chir Scand Suppl* 1953;181: 5-130.

5. Brewer BJ: Aging of the rotator cuff. *Am J Sports Med* 1979;7:102-110.

6. McLaughlin HL: Lesions of the musculotendinous cuff of the shoulder: III. Observations on the pathology, course and treatment of calcific deposits. *Ann Surg* 1946;124:354-362.

7. Mohr W, Bilger S: Morphologische Grundstrukturen der kalzifizierten Tendopathie und ihre Bedeutung für die Pathogenese. *Z Rheumatol* 1990;49: 346-355.

8. Perugia L, Postacchini F: The pathology of the rotator cuff of the shoulder. *Ital J Orthop Traumatol* 1985;11:93-105.

9. Remberger K, Faust H, Keyl W: Tendinitis calcarea: Klinik, Morphologie, Pathogenese und Differential diagnose. *Pathologe* 1985;6:196-203.

10. Sarkar K, Uhthoff HK: Ultrastructural localization of calcium in calcifying tendinitis. *Arch Pathol Lab Med* 1978; 102:266-269.

11. Uhthoff HK, Sarkar K, Maynard JA: Calcifying tendinitis: A new concept of its pathogenesis. *Clin Orthop* 1976;118: 164-168.

12. Lippmann RK: Observations concerning the calcific cuff deposit. *Clin Orthop* 1961;20:49-60.

13. Sengar DPS, McKendry RJ, Uhthoff HK: Increased frequency of HLA-A1 in calcifying tendinitis. *Tissue Antigens* 1987;29:173-174.

14. Archer RS, Bayley JIL, Archer CW, Ali SY: Cell and matrix changes associated with pathological calcification of the human rotator cuff tendons. *J Anat* 1993;182:1-12.

15. DePalma AF, Kruper JS: Long-term study of shoulder joints afflicted with and treated for calcific tendinitis. *Clin Orthop* 1961;20:61-72.

16. Hartig A, Huth F: Neue Aspekte zur Morphologie und Therapie der Tendinosis calcarea der Schultergelenke. *Arthroskopie* 1995;8:117-122.

17. Rompe JD, Rumler F, Hopf C, Nafe B, Heine J: Extracorporal shock wave therapy for calcifying tendinitis of the shoulder. *Clin Orthop* 1995;321: 196-201.

18. Loew M, Jurgowski W, Mau HC, Thomsen M: Treatment of calcifying tendinitis of rotator cuff by extracorporeal shock waves: A preliminary report. *J Shoulder Elbow Surg* 1995;4: 101-106.

19. de Sèze S, Welfling J: Tendinites calcifiantes. *Rhumatologie* 1970;22:45-50.

20. Gschwend N, Scherer M, Löhr J: Die Tendinitis calcarea des Schultergelenks (T. c.). *Orthopade* 1981;10:196-205.

21. Ark JW, Flock TJ, Flatow EL, Bigliani LU: Arthroscopic treatment of calcific tendinitis of the shoulder. *Arthroscopy* 1992;8:183-188.

22. Neer CS II: Impingement lesions. *Clin Orthop* 1983;173:70-77.

Current Concepts Review

Rotator Cuff Tear Arthropathy*

BY KIRK L. JENSEN, M.D.†, OAKLAND, CALIFORNIA, GERALD R. WILLIAMS, JR., M.D.‡, PHILADELPHIA, PENNSYLVANIA,
I. J. RUSSELL, M.D.§, AND CHARLES A. ROCKWOOD, JR., M.D.§, SAN ANTONIO, TEXAS

The association between massive tears of rotator cuff tendons and severe glenohumeral degenerative arthritis is complex and poorly understood. The theories that have been proposed to account for rotator cuff tear arthropathy of the shoulder joint include severe, localized rheumatoid arthritis[1,2]; hemorrhagic arthritis[27]; microcrystalline-induced arthritis[67]; and arthritis due to chronic attrition, leading to a massive tear of the rotator cuff tendons[19,75]. The confusion concerning the etiology of rotator cuff tear arthropathy is in part due to the fact that different authors have described its clinical characteristics in general terms and have given it various names, such as l'arthropathie destructrice rapide de l'épaule[58], apatite-associated destructive arthritis[30], Milwaukee shoulder[40,45,67], and cuff tear arthropathy[75].

Historical Review

Adams[1,2] and Smith[90,91] provided the earliest description of the pathoanatomical features of rotator cuff tear arthropathy, in the nineteenth century. Adams, who was the Regius Professor of Surgery at the University of Dublin, described two types of chronic rheumatoid arthritis: a generalized form resembling rheumatoid arthritis and a localized form involving the shoulder, which had the morphological characteristics of what is now known as rotator cuff tear arthropathy[2]. In his 1934 monograph, Codman[19] reported the case of a fifty-one-year-old woman who had what he termed a subacromial space hygroma. He described recurrent swelling of the shoulder, absence of the rotator cuff, cartilaginous bodies attached to the synovial tissue, and severe destructive glenohumeral arthritis. These clinical descriptions of the entity now known as rotator cuff tear arthropathy were made without the benefit of modern diagnostic tests, such as serological analysis or synovial crystal analysis.

L'épaule sénile hémorragique (the hemorrhagic

shoulder of the elderly) was described by DeSeze[27] in 1968. This clinical entity, which was seen in three elderly women who did not have a history of trauma, consisted of recurrent, blood-streaked effusions of the shoulder and radiographic findings of severe degenerative glenohumeral arthritis and a chronic tear of the rotator cuff. DeSeze also cited previous reports in the literature by Galmiche and Deshayes[39], Burman et al.[12], Banna and Hume[6], Shepard[89], and Snook[92], which documented a total of thirty cases of spontaneous hemarthrosis of the glenohumeral joint in elderly patients.

Apart from a single case report by Bauduin and Famaey[7] in 1969, the hemorrhagic shoulder of the elderly was not mentioned again in the literature until 1977[56]. The report published at that time described nine elderly women who had painful spontaneous effusions of the glenohumeral joint and identified an association between rotator cuff tear arthropathy and arthritis of the knee joint.

The term Milwaukee shoulder was introduced in 1981 to describe the condition in four elderly women who had recurrent bilateral shoulder effusions, severe radiographic destructive changes of the glenohumeral joints, and massive tears of the rotator cuff[40,45,67]. In 1982, spontaneous large glenohumeral effusions, mild pain, and tears of the rotator cuff were reported in six elderly women, and the condition was described as l'arthropathie destructrice rapide de l'épaule (rapid destructive arthritis of the shoulder)[58]. Neer et al.[75] introduced the term cuff tear arthropathy to describe glenohumeral degenerative arthritis and a rotator cuff tear in twenty-six patients who had a total shoulder replacement. Two other terms, apatite-associated destructive arthritis and idiopathic destructive arthritis[14], were introduced by Dieppe et al.[30] in 1984 to describe rotator cuff tear arthropathy of the shoulder.

Etiology

Crystalline-Induced Arthritis of the Shoulder

An association between rotator cuff tear arthropathy and the intra-articular presence of basic calcium-phosphate crystals was identified in 1981[40,45,67]. These three reports on the Milwaukee shoulder included clinical aspects and studies of synovial fluid as well as morphological and biochemical studies of excised synovial tissue from four patients, three of whom had bilateral disease. McCarty et al.[67] identified collagenolytic and neutral protease activity in synovial fluid with use of

*No benefits in any form have been received or will be received from a commercial party related directly or indirectly to the subject of this article. No funds were received in support of this study.

†Peralta Orthopaedics, 3100 Telegraph Avenue, Suite 100, Oakland, California 94563.

‡Department of Orthopaedic Surgery, University of Pennsylvania, Silverstein Pavilion, Second Floor, 3400 Spruce Street, Philadelphia, Pennsylvania 19140.

§Departments of Medicine (I. J. R.) and Orthopaedic Surgery (C. A. R., Jr.), University of Texas Health Science Center, 7703 Floyd Curl Drive, San Antonio, Texas 78284-7774.

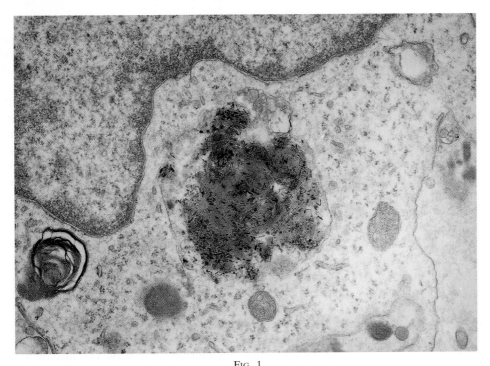

FIG. 1

Transmission electron photomicrograph showing basic calcium-phosphate crystals (black material) in the synovial tissue ($\times$ 26,000).

assays measuring the release of soluble enzymatic products. Electron microscopic analysis of synovial tissue from the glenohumeral joints of patients who had rotator cuff tear arthropathy revealed microspheroids of basic calcium-phosphate crystals, suggesting phagocytosis of these crystals by cells in the synovial tissue (Fig. 1). Histological study revealed foci of calcific deposits in synovial microvilli and the subsynovial layers.

The theory that has been proposed to explain the Milwaukee shoulder begins with the concept that a hydroxyapatite-mineral phase develops in the altered capsule, synovial tissue, or degenerative articular cartilage and releases basic calcium-phosphate crystals into the synovial fluid. These crystals then are phagocytized by synovial cells, forming calcium-phosphate-crystal microspheroids, which induce the release of activated enzymes from these cells, causing destruction of the periarticular tissues and articular surfaces.

Basic calcium-phosphate crystal is a generic term used to identify a crystal that is composed of carbonate-substituted hydroxyapatite, octacalcium phosphate, or, more rarely, tricalcium phosphate[68]. These crystals are not birefringent; thus, polarized light microscopy is not useful for identification. Furthermore, the resolution power of light microscopy is inadequate to detect the individual crystals, which are needle-shaped and less than 0.1 millimicrometer long. Both scanning and transmission electron microscopy with energy-dispersive x-ray microanalysis have been used to identify basic calcium-phosphate crystals in synovial fluid pellets. Unfortunately, there is no simple, cost-effective, readily available method to detect basic calcium-phosphate

crystals that is comparable with the use of polarized light microscopy for the detection of calcium-pyrophosphate-dihydrate and monosodium-urate-monohydrate crystals.

Aggregates of basic calcium-phosphate crystals have been found in the synovial fluid of joints undergoing acute attacks of mixed crystal deposition disease[28], calcific periarthritis, or acute arthritis. These aggregates also have been identified in the synovial fluid of patients who have erosive polyarticular disease[88], osteoarthritis of the knee[7,42,48], and rotator cuff tear arthropathy[46]. The response of synovial tissue to calcium-containing crystals, such as basic calcium-phosphate and calcium-pyrophosphate-dihydrate crystals, is low-grade inflammation with cellular proliferation. The cellular hyperplasia observed in the synovial tissue of patients who have rotator cuff tear arthropathy may be explained by the mitogenic properties of basic calcium-phosphate crystals, which have been shown to stimulate proliferation of human foreskin fibroblasts[63,64].

Synovial fibroblasts and chondrocytes, in response to certain growth factors, cytokines, and other chemical agents, synthesize the enzymes collagenase and stromelysin. Collagenase is a proteolytic enzyme that degrades interstitial collagen. Stromelysin, a metalloprotease, degrades connective-tissue components and activates procollagenase. As already noted, McCarty et al.[67], in 1981, initially identified collagenase activity in synovial fluid from patients who had rotator cuff tear arthropathy. However, this finding was not confirmed in subsequent reports[31,47,50,100]. Halverson et al.[50] suggested that this inconsistency may have been due to the presence of a low-molecular-weight inhibitor of collagenase[31], the avid binding of collagenase to collagen[63], or an artifact resulting from poor handling of specimens in preparation for the enzyme assays.

Recent investigations have focused on identifying the induction of collagenase or stromelysin gene transcription by basic calcium-phosphate crystals to elucidate the loss of collagenous structures in patients who have rotator cuff tear arthropathy. Basic calcium-phosphate crystals were found to stimulate the proliferation of cultured adult porcine articular chondrocytes and to increase collagenase messenger RNA in a dose-responsive manner[72]. Human fibroblasts have been induced by basic calcium-phosphate crystals to accumulate collagenase as well as stromelysin mRNA and to secrete collagenase, stromelysin[63,64], and ninety-two-kilodalton gelatinase[66]. It appears that basic calcium-phosphate crystals induce the synthesis of proteolytic enzymes that are responsible for the degradation of cartilage-matrix components[16].

The aggregates of hydroxyapatite crystals that have been observed throughout articular cartilage[53], but most commonly in the mid-zone[41], also may directly cause mechanical wear of cartilage. Using knee joints obtained from cadavera, Clift et al.[18] found that a higher deposition of basic calcium-phosphate crystals and an increase in the mean friction coefficient occurred in conjunction with severe fibrillation of articular cartilage. An *in vitro* investigation also suggested that crystals in synovial fluid have the potential to cause wear of articular cartilage[52]. As the presence of crystals increased, the concentration of wear debris and the size and shape of the crystals influenced the type of articular damage that was observed. The large crystal aggregates, which frequently are found in the mid-zone of articular cartilage, were studied with use of a linear elastic finite element model under short-term loading conditions[18]. The results indicated that these aggregates increase the shear stress and strain concentrations in the surrounding cartilage.

The exact origin of basic calcium-phosphate crystals remains unclear, and whether these crystals are the cause or the result of arthritis remains unanswered. It has been suggested that basic calcium-phosphate crystals are an epiphenomenon resulting from biochemical changes in the matrix of damaged cartilage and that the crystals then are shed into the synovial fluid[49]. Peri-arthropathies such as calcific rotator tendinitis or degenerative tears of the rotator tendon are conditions in which basic calcium-phosphate crystals are known to form[95]. Additional investigation is needed to fully elucidate the origin of the basic calcium-phosphate crystals and the effect that they elicit in individuals who have degenerative disease of the shoulder.

Cuff Tear Theory

In 1934, Codman[19] described a condition in which a chronic tear of the rotator cuff may result in a hygroma of the shoulder and destruction of the glenohumeral joint. He attributed the pathological changes of rotator cuff arthropathy to neglect of the ruptured rotator cuff, as retraction of the torn rotator muscles left the humeral head freely exposed under the deltoid, resulting in chronic synovitis and effusion of the bursa or joint.

In 1983, Neer et al.[75] postulated that certain chronic, massive tears would lead to a degenerated glenohumeral joint if left untreated. The mechanism of destruction of the articular cartilage was said to include mechanical and nutritional alterations in the shoulder with a rotator cuff tear. The mechanical factors that were mentioned included anteroposterior instability of the humeral head, resulting from a massive tear of the rotator cuff, and rupture or dislocation of the long head of the biceps, leading to proximal migration of the humeral head and acromial impingement. Glenohumeral articular wear was thought to occur as a result of repetitive trauma from the altered biomechanics associated with the loss of primary and secondary stabilizers of the glenohumeral joint. The nutritional status of the articular cartilage in a shoulder with a torn rotator cuff would be altered by the loss of a closed joint space and of normal glenohumeral motion. Changes in the composition of the articular cartilage then would occur because of inadequate diffusion of nutrients as the loss of a watertight joint space diminished the quantity of synovial fluid. In addition, disuse osteoporosis of the proximal part of the humerus would decrease the density of the subchondral bone in the humeral head and contribute to atrophy of the articular cartilage. Degenerative arthritis and subchondral collapse eventually would develop as a result of these changes in the articular cartilage.

This theory was based on the clinical observations and the intraoperative findings during arthroplasty in twenty-six shoulders[75]. Histological studies revealed three consistent findings: areas in the humeral head where the articular cartilage was atrophic and the subchondral bone was osteoporotic, fixed point contact between the glenoid and the humerus where the articular cartilage was denuded and the subchondral bone was sclerotic, and fragments of articular cartilage in the subsynovial layers. Normal chemical profiles of synovial fluid were obtained from twelve of the twenty-six shoulders; no other analysis of the synovial fluid, synovial tissue, or joint capsule was performed.

It is impossible to estimate accurately the number of shoulders with a rotator cuff tear that proceed to rotator cuff tear arthropathy, as several studies of cadavera have documented the age-related prevalence of rotator cuff tears[21,26,43,69]. Those studies did not show a relationship between the presence or size of the rotator cuff tear and symptoms or the prevalence of associated glenohumeral arthritis. Neer et al.[75] estimated, on the basis of Neer's observation of approximately fifty-two cases of cuff tear arthropathy in the eight-year period of the study, that cuff tear arthropathy would develop in only 4 percent of patients who have a complete tear of the rotator cuff and suggested that, because of their small size, most tears of the cuff do not lead to arthropathy.

Several authors have performed longitudinal follow-up studies of patients who had a massive rotator cuff tear, with different results[8,51,98]. Hamada et al.[51] reported the long-term radiographic results of nonoperative treatment of twenty-two patients with arthrographically proved massive rotator cuff tears. In five of the seven shoulders that were followed for more than eight years, degenerative changes had progressed radiographically. Those authors concluded that a massive tear of the cuff would progress to cuff tear arthropathy with progressive radiographic changes. In 1993, Bokor et al.[8] reported that the functional results of nonoperative treatment of arthrographically proved rotator cuff tears did not deteriorate after an average follow-up period of seven to eight years. However, objective data, such as the size of the tear and the radiographic appearance of the shoulder, were not included, and only one patient later had symptoms of rotator cuff tear arthropathy.

Arthroscopic subacromial decompression without débridement of the tendon also has been performed for the treatment of full-thickness rotator cuff tears[9,32-34,60]; however, reports on that procedure have described only short-term results and have lacked radiographic follow-up. In a retrospective study of twenty-five patients who had had arthroscopic acromioplasty and débridement of a tear of the rotator cuff with six to nine years of follow-up, seven patients had clinical and radiographic features of rotator cuff tear arthropathy[70]. The tears in that series were classified according to size, and the integrity of the subscapularis tendon was not specifically reported.

Open[4,85] and arthroscopic[9,32-34,60,71] débridement of massive tears of the rotator cuff combined with acromioplasty has been reported in patients who did not have glenohumeral arthritis. Those studies provided more objective data regarding the size of the tear and the clinical outcome. Apoil and Augereau[4] reported that rotator cuff tear arthropathy developed in more than one-fourth of fifty-six patients ten years after open débridement of a degenerative lesion of the rotator cuff. Rockwood et al.[85] reported that none of fifty-three shoulders that had a chronic, massive, irreparable tear of the supraspinatus and infraspinatus tendons had progressive deterioration of the glenohumeral joint after open acromioplasty and débridement of the rotator cuff. That series was followed for an average of six and one-half years, and shoulders followed for less than five years were compared with those followed for at least five years. Neither deterioration in the functional results nor the appearance of radiographic degenerative changes could be associated with time. Twenty shoulders had superior migration of the humeral head, defined as an acromiohumeral distance of seven millimeters or less. The subscapularis and teres minor tendons were intact in all of these patients. Preoperatively and postopera-

tively, patients were started on a specific orthopaedic-surgeon-directed rehabilitation program. After passive range of motion was restored, the patients were instructed in a program for strengthening of the remaining rotator cuff muscles, the deltoid muscle, and the scapular stabilizing muscles. Even though the supraspinatus and the infraspinatus were absent, the compressive effect of the subscapularis, teres minor, and scapular stabilizing muscles allowed active use of the shoulder. The active forward elevation of the shoulder improved from an average of 105 degrees preoperatively to an average of 140 degrees postoperatively. The result, based on relief of pain, function, range of motion, strength, and patient satisfaction, was satisfactory in forty-four (83 percent) of the fifty-three patients and unsatisfactory in the remaining nine (17 percent)[85].

The effect of a tear of the rotator cuff on the biomechanics of the shoulder has been investigated in radiographic and biomechanical studies. Inman et al.[54] used the concept of force couples to develop a theoretical model that determined the force requirements necessary for function of the shoulder joint. The force couple in the coronal plane consisted of the superiorly directed force vector of the deltoid muscle and the inferiorly directed force vector of the short external rotators of the rotator cuff. Rotation or abduction of the shoulder joint occurred as the two oppositely directed forces acted on opposite sides of the center of rotation[54]. A weak or detached supraspinatus tendon would be unable to maintain centering of the humeral head on the glenoid, and a superiorly directed force vector would result from the unbalanced force couple[62]. This concept was supported by a radiographic study comparing patients who had an arthrographically proved tear of the supraspinatus with those who had a normal shoulder[81]. The authors of that study concluded that some patients who have a rotator cuff tear have superior translation of the humeral head on the glenoid as a result of the loss of the normal depressing effect of the supraspinatus[81]. Free-body analysis of the glenohumeral joint has shown that the resultant force vector is directed superiorly during the first 60 degrees of shoulder elevation, and it also has been used to explain superior migration of the humeral head in association with a tear of the rotator cuff[82]. Although these investigators provided insight into glenohumeral biomechanics, they disregarded the contributions of the other rotator cuff muscles in maintaining joint stability.

The presence and importance of the transverse-plane force couple (Fig. 2), in which the anterior aspect of the cuff (the subscapularis) is balanced against the posterior aspect (the infraspinatus and the teres minor), was first revealed in an electromyographic study[87]. In a subsequent study, fluoroscopic examination of patients who had a massive tear of the rotator cuff revealed varying degrees of glenohumeral instability that corresponded directly to the degree of involvement of the posterior portion of the rotator cuff and the subscapularis tendon[10]. A suspension-bridge model of the shoulder, in which the leading edge of the detached rotator cuff tendon behaves biomechanically like the cable of a suspension bridge, was used to explain the nonprogressive nature of some rotator cuff tears[11]. The tension that develops on the edge of the supraspinatus tendon during the contraction of the torn rotator cuff muscle was theorized to propagate along the cable of the bridge to its point of attachment on the greater tuberosity. This allows some patients who have a large or massive tear to maintain the transverse force couple and thus to retain the ability to actively elevate the shoulder. The location of the cable (tendon) attachments on the tuberosities results in either stable or unstable glenohumeral kinematics, depending on the presence of an intact transverse force couple[10,11]. This principle has been supported clinically; Nove-Josserand et al.[78] reported that the size of the tear of the rotator cuff and the amount of degeneration of the infraspinatus muscle as seen on magnetic resonance imaging substantially affected superior migration of the humeral head.

Biomechanical studies to investigate the effect of a rotator cuff tear on the performance of the glenohumeral joint have been performed in cadavera. A dynamic shoulder-testing apparatus with preserved transverse force couples was used to investigate the effect of a torn supraspinatus tendon[70]. Full abduction was possible, and the glenohumeral kinematics were not markedly altered[70]. In another study with use of this testing apparatus, it was found that, if the transverse force couple remained functionally intact, there was sufficient compressive force to maintain concentric reduction of the humeral head and the ball-and-socket kinematics[94]. No association was found between the size of the tear and the geometry of the humeral head, disproving the concept that there is a critical ratio between the size of the rotator cuff tear and the size of the humeral head. The information from these cadaver studies is limited, however, as scapulothoracic

motion was not included and the artificial environment does not take into account the attritional, degenerative changes that occur in the rotator cuff tendons.

Rotator cuff tear arthropathy is a clinical manifestation of instability of the glenohumeral joint and loss of articular cartilage. On the basis of the existing clinical and biomechanical data, it is apparent that, if the remaining balance of the rotator cuff in the coronal and transverse planes is sufficient to maintain glenohumeral stability, then the presence of a rotator cuff tear or degenerative defect may not alter the biomechanics of the glenohumeral joint. If stability cannot be maintained and repetitive abnormal excursions of the humeral head occur on the glenoid, both in the transverse and the coronal plane, then wear and loss of the glenohumeral cartilage will result. The combination of glenohumeral instability due to loss of the primary and secondary stabilizers and loss of normal articular cartilage results in the generation of basic calcium-phosphate crystals. These crystal aggregates, which may originate from the damage to the articular cartilage or from the degenerative changes in the rotator cuff tendons, accelerate additional degenerative changes through the induction of enzymatic activity.

Diagnosis

Clinical Presentation

Rotator cuff tear arthropathy is more common in women than in men (Table I). Patients typically are elderly women with shoulder symptoms of long duration. The dominant side is most commonly affected; however, bilateral involvement is seen in approximately 60 percent of patients, in our experience. The symptoms include relatively mild or moderate joint pain, a loss of motion, and recurrent swelling of the shoulder. The pain characteristically interferes with sleep and intensifies with activity.

Although patients may report a history of having received multiple corticosteroid injections, no association has been found between the severity of the symptoms and the number of previous injections. Six of the twenty-one patients reported on by Rockwood et al.[85] had a history of multiple corticosteroid injections, and one patient had had more than twenty injections over a three-and-a-half-year period. In another report, sixteen of twenty-six patients had received previous corticosteroid injections; seven of them had not received injections until radiographic changes had developed, and only six had had more than three injections[74].

Physical examination usually reveals mild swelling of the shoulder involving the subacromial and glenohumeral joints (Fig. 3) and atrophy of the supraspinatus and infraspinatus muscles. Neer et al.[75] noted that most of the twenty-six patients specifically reported on in their series had substantial recurrent swelling of the shoulder reminiscent of hygroma of the subacromial space, as described by Codman[19], and that ecchymosis

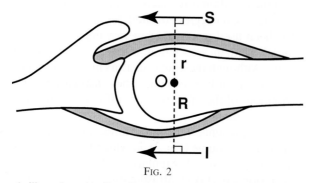

FIG. 2

Axillary view revealing the transverse force couple between the anteriorly located subscapularis muscle and the posteriorly located external rotators. These two medially directed forces are balanced and produce centering of the humeral head with compression of the head against the glenoid. S = subscapularis, I = infraspinatus, O = center of rotation, r = distance to force vector of subscapularis, and R = distance to force vector of infraspinatus.

TABLE I
SUMMARY OF THE CLINICAL FEATURES OF ROTATOR CUFF TEAR ARTHROPATHY OF THE SHOULDER JOINT

Study	No. of Patients			Age* (yrs.)	Bilateral Involvement†
	Total	Male	Female		
DeSeze[27] (1968)	3	0	3		
Lamboley et al.[56] (1977)	9	1	8	75 (67-84)	
Lequesne et al.[58] (1982)	6	0	6	75 (65-88)	1
Halverson et al.[45,47,50] (1981, 1984, 1990) and McCarty et al.[67] (1981)	30	6	24	73 (53-90)	19
Newman et al.[77] (1983)	1	0	1	75	0
Neer et al.[75] (1983)	26	6	20	69 (50-87)	5
Dieppe et al.[30] (1984)	11	1	10	77 (69-83)	9
Weiss et al.[98] (1985)	4	0	4	75 (73-86)	2
Campion et al.[14] (1988)	12	0	12	78 (64-86)	9
Klimaitis et al.[55] (1988)	2	0	2	80 (78-83)	2
Total	104	14	90	77.5	47

*The values are given as the average, with the range in parentheses.
†The values are given as the number of patients.

about the shoulder with blood-tinged effusions was present in five patients. Similarly, Williams and Rockwood[99] reported recurrent massive glenohumeral effusions in three of their twenty-one patients.

The active and passive range of motion can be severely limited because of soft-tissue contractures or fixed glenohumeral subluxation. Active glenohumeral motion may be accompanied by palpable or audible crepitus and usually is painful. Weakness of the external rotators may be profound, as specifically noted in six of the twenty-one patients who had rotator cuff tear arthropathy in the report by Williams and Rockwood[99]. Neer et al.[75] also described limitations of active glenohumeral motion in patients who had rotator cuff tear arthropathy; only two of the twenty-six patients in their

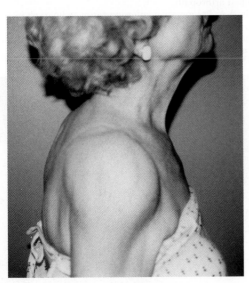

FIG. 3

Clinical photograph of a seventy-one-year-old woman who had rotator cuff tear arthropathy of the right shoulder. Swelling of the shoulder is apparent. At the time of the operation, 150 to 200 milliliters of blood-tinged fluid was evacuated.

series were able to actively elevate the shoulder above 90 degrees. In 1992, Pollock et al.[80] reported on thirty shoulders (twenty-one patients) that had a tear of the rotator cuff; the average forward elevation was 67 degrees. Glenohumeral instability secondary to a rotator cuff tear also is common in severely affected shoulders.

An association between rotator cuff tear arthropathy and arthritis of the lateral compartment of the knee was reported by Halverson et al.[50]; sixteen of their thirty patients who had rotator cuff tear arthropathy had symptomatic arthritis of the knee. The prevalence of narrowing of the lateral compartment, rather than the medial compartment, was significantly higher in this series than it was in a report of fifty-six patients who had primary osteoarthritis ($p < 0.01$)[48].

Radiographic Findings

Characteristic radiographic findings include superior migration of the humeral head with articulation with the overlying acromion, narrowing of the glenohumeral joint space, formation of osteophytes, and periarticular soft-tissue calcifications (Fig. 4-A). Occasionally, in severely affected shoulders, erosive changes are seen both in the glenohumeral joint and in adjacent structures such as the base of the coracoid process, the lateral end of the clavicle, and the anterior aspect of the acromion.

Halverson et al.[50], in a series of thirty shoulders with destructive shoulder arthropathy, identified superior subluxation of the humeral head in twenty-three shoulders and humeral head deformity in twenty. Neer et al.[75] reported an area of collapse of the proximal aspect of the humeral articular surface in all twenty-six patients in their series; they considered this finding a requirement for the diagnosis of rotator cuff tear arthropathy. Rounding-off of the greater tuberosity, as described by McCarty et al.[67], is produced by the superiorly migrated humeral head articulating chronically under the acromion. Adams[2] and Neer et al.[75], who both described thinning of the acromion and occasional acromial separation into anterior and posterior portions, thought that the acromial fragmentation was developmental in nature. An unfused acromial apophysis was noted in three of the twenty-six patients of Neer et al.[75]. Conversely, Dennis et al.[25] reported an acromial stress fracture associated with rotator cuff tear arthropathy in three patients and attributed the fracture to the mechanical forces of the superiorly directed humeral head.

Anterior or posterior instability of the glenohumeral joint may be evident on the axillary lateral radiograph. If fixed subluxation occurs, additional radiographic investigation is warranted to delineate the architecture of the glenoid. Fixed subluxation typically leads to sclerosis and formation of osteophytes, and glenoid erosion may occur at the point of contact with the humeral head (Fig. 4-B). Computed tomography is used to detect erosion, deformity, or defects of the glenoid[38,73]. Glenoid wear also may occur medially, as evidenced by destruction of the coracoid process, which is best seen on a West Point axillary radiograph[86].

Although arthrography, ultrasonography, and magnetic resonance imaging are not necessary for diagnosis, each reveals characteristic findings of a chronic rupture of the rotator cuff. Arthrography often reveals an abnormal communication (the so-called geyser sign[23]) between the glenohumeral and acromioclavicular joints that is associated with pathological distention or formation of a pseudoganglion of the acromioclavicular joint.

Treatment

Options for the treatment of rotator cuff tear arthropathy include medical management of the symptoms, arthroscopic lavage[15], arthroscopic débridement, humeral tuberoplasty[35], arthrodesis[5], constrained arthroplasty[22,59,83,84], semiconstrained arthroplasty[3,74], total shoulder arthroplasty[75], bipolar total shoulder arthroplasty[57,93,96,101], and hemiarthroplasty[5,36,80,99]. Patients who have little pain and limitation of activities of daily living should be managed with mild analgesics and gentle, function-maintaining exercises. Prostaglandins such as misoprostol have been shown *in vitro* to inhibit basic calcium-phosphate-crystal-induced mitogenesis in a dose-dependent manner; however, they remain under investigation[65]. Repeated intra-articular injections of corticosteroids are discouraged, as they have been shown to be ineffective[99] and may cause iatrogenic infection.

Arthroscopic irrigation to remove activated enzymes and crystals has been reported only recently[15] and offers only limited, short-term relief. Arthroscopic acromioplasty and tendon débridement was described in six patients who had rotator cuff tear arthropathy[33]. However, the results were not stratified according to the location of the tear, and this technique should be viewed with caution.

Elderly patients who have rotator cuff tear arthropathy may not accept glenohumeral arthrodesis or tolerate it well because of the cosmetic appearance, poor function, and the frequent bilaterality of the condition. Cofield and Briggs[20] reported the results of glenohumeral arthrodesis in a series that included twelve patients in whom the indication for the procedure was degenerative arthritis and an irreparable rotator cuff tear. Two of the patients had a pseudarthrosis, and six needed repeat operative procedures. The osteoporotic

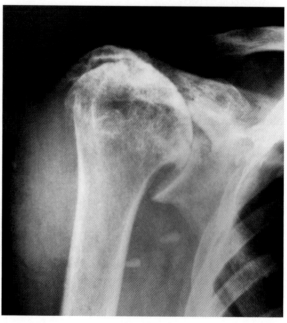

FIG. 4-A

Figs. 4-A and 4-B: Characteristic radiographic findings of rotator cuff tear arthropathy.

Fig. 4-A: Preoperative anteroposterior radiograph revealing articulation between the humerus and the acromion, rounding of the greater tuberosity, and loss of articular cartilage from the glenohumeral joint.

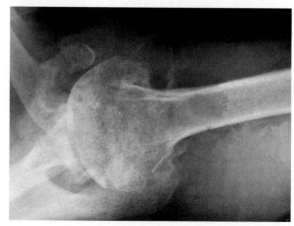

FIG. 4-B

Preoperative axillary lateral radiograph revealing loss of the articular joint space, periarticular soft-tissue calcifications, posterior fragmentation of the glenoid, and flattening of the humeral head.

bone in the scapula and the proximal part of the humerus of these elderly, usually female patients makes arthrodesis difficult. Therefore, this procedure should be reserved for patients who have a nonfunctioning deltoid muscle.

A primary indication for shoulder arthroplasty with insertion of a constrained prosthesis with cement has been a rotator cuff tear associated with arthritis of the glenohumeral joint. The fixed-fulcrum mechanics of these prostheses have resulted in high rates of mechanical failure and loosening of the glenoid component[22,59,83,84]. Loosening of the glenoid component was reported in ten of forty-nine shoulders that had been treated with a Stanmore prosthesis[59], and major complications, including dislocation of the humeral component and a bent or broken humeral neck, occurred in twenty-nine of ninety-four shoulders treated with a Michael Reese prosthesis[83,84]. One-millimeter-wide radiolucent lines were identified about the screws and the central post of the glenoid component of 30 percent of the Michael Reese prostheses that had not been revised[84]. The use of constrained shoulder arthroplasty was discouraged by Neer[76] because of the poor quality of the scapular bone, which precluded adequate fixation of the glenoid component.

Several modifications have been made to the glenoid component to provide superior mechanical coverage and to resist superior migration of the humeral component. Clayton et al.[17] reported use of a subacromial polyethylene spacer as a means of constraint against superior subluxation of the humeral component in seven patients who had an irreparable rotator cuff tear and arthritic articular surfaces. No difference was detected between the results for the seven patients who had received the spacer and those for fifteen additional patients who had had a conventional hemiarthroplasty or a total shoulder arthroplasty with use of the Neer prosthesis; according to Neer[76], the use of subacromial spacers has generally been discontinued.

Neer et al.[74-76], Amstutz et al.[3], and Gristina et al.[44] reported use of a semiconstrained prosthesis in shoulder arthroplasty. Neer et al.[74-76] used an enlarged glenoid component (one that was 200 or 600 percent larger than standard size) with a superior hood to resist superior subluxation of the humeral component in patients who had a rotator cuff tear. Use of the 600-percent-enlarged component was abandoned because of its interference with rotator cuff repair[76]. The Dana total shoulder system[3] includes a glenoid component that has a posterior hood to resist superior subluxation, as well as extended anterior and posterior lips to prevent anterior and posterior subluxation. Gristina et al. also used a hooded glenoid component to resist posterior subluxation in patients who had a rotator cuff tear.

Experience with hooded glenoid components is limited compared with that with standard, unconstrained components. In addition, few reports of total shoulder replacement have presented the results of use of semiconstrained glenoid components separately from those of use of standard components. Neer[76] noted a higher prevalence of radiolucent lines around semiconstrained glenoid components and suggested that the likelihood of loosening is greater as a result of increased stress imparted to the bone-cement interface by the added constraint. A biomechanical study performed by Orr et al.[79] with use of finite element analysis of the natural glenoid as well as various designs of glenoid components supports Neer's hypothesis. Hooded components were associated with increased compressive stresses under their superior portion and increased tensile stresses under their inferior portion. Those authors concluded that the abnormal stresses encountered with the hooded components increased the tendency for the component to tip superiorly and could lead to early loosening. Currently, there is limited information regarding the survival of these glenoid components, and they therefore should be used with caution.

Interest in semiconstrained arthroplasty was initiated in Europe with the development of the Reverse Ball-and-Socket Delta III prosthesis. De Buttet et al.[24] reported preliminary results, at an average of two years postoperatively, in seventy-one patients who had osteoarthritis and a massive rotator cuff tear. Forty-nine patients had a good or excellent result, and three had a revision because of early failure of the glenoid component. Survival analysis with prospective data collection will be necessary before this method can be recommended.

A direct association between superior migration of the humeral component due to a rotator cuff tear and loosening of the glenoid component was reported by Franklin et al.[37] in 1988. Seven of fourteen patients who had a total shoulder arthroplasty for the treatment of glenohumeral arthritis and a rotator cuff tear had loosening of the glenoid component at an average of two and one-half years postoperatively, whereas none of sixteen patients who had an intact cuff had such loosening. Those authors theorized that the eccentric superior loading of the glenoid component resulted in increased compressive stresses on its superior rim, causing it to loosen and tilt superiorly. They referred to this phenomenon as the rocking-horse glenoid and credited Gristina with first recognizing that a shift of the instant center of rotation of a glenohumeral prosthesis could result in abnormal stress on the anchorage of the glenoid component to the bone. Hemiarthroplasty was recommended, as it improved comfort and function without the risk of future loosening of the glenoid component (Figs. 5-A and 5-B).

In general, the results of hemiarthroplasty performed for rotator cuff tear arthropathy have been included in reports of hemiarthroplasty in patients who have a rotator cuff tear. Arntz et al.[5] reviewed the results of hemiarthroplasty in twelve patients who had both glenohumeral arthritis and an irreparable rotator cuff tear and diagnosed seven patients as having rotator cuff tear arthropathy. The results were not stratified according to diagnosis; however, no patient had substantial pain, and active flexion improved from an average of 71 degrees preoperatively to an average of 110 degrees postoperatively. Those authors concluded that humeral hemiarthroplasty is the procedure of choice for patients who have both glenohumeral arthritis and an irreparable rotator cuff tear.

Lohr et al.[61] compared the results of hemiarthro-

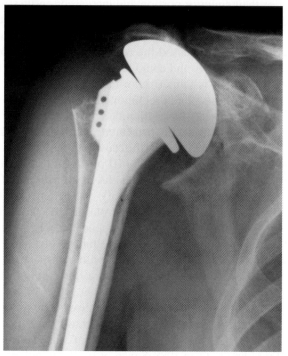

FIG. 5-A

Figs. 5-A and 5-B: Radiographs made after hemiarthroplasty.
Fig. 5-A: Anteroposterior radiograph showing superior migration of the humeral head and acromial contact.

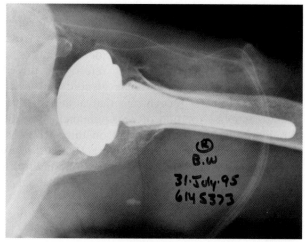

FIG. 5-B

Axillary lateral radiograph showing the humeral head replacement with contact of the head centered in the glenoid.

plasty with those of unconstrained or semiconstrained total shoulder arthroplasty in twenty-two shoulders with rotator cuff tear arthropathy. Hemiprosthetic replacement gave the poorest results with regard to relief of pain, whereas the unconstrained and semiconstrained devices had a high prevalence of radiographic and clinical loosening of the glenoid component. However, details concerning attempts at rotator cuff repair, soft-tissue balancing, and glenoid congruency were not included. Those authors concluded that rotator cuff tear arthropathy remains "one of the most difficult entities to treat."

Neer at al.[74,76] identified rotator cuff tear arthropathy as a difficult clinical syndrome to treat because of the inability to repair degenerative, nonfunctioning rotator cuff muscles. Patients with rotator cuff tear arthropathy who had a shoulder arthroplasty were placed in the limited-goals category[74], and postoperative management was aimed at achieving 20 degrees of external rotation and 90 degrees of forward elevation. A satisfactory result was obtained, with use of the limited-goals criteria, when the patient had no pain or only mild discomfort and was satisfied with the outcome.

Williams and Rockwood[99] reviewed the results of hemiarthroplasty in twenty-one shoulders with degenerative arthritis and an irreparable tear of the rotator cuff. Emphasis was placed on operative technique, which included débridement of the retracted degenerative cuff defect without an attempt to repair and balance the remaining rotator cuff tendons by altering the size of the humeral head. The correct humeral head size allows the arm to lie freely across the abdomen, the humeral head to translate 50 percent posteriorly on the glenoid surface, and the subscapularis tendon to be reattached to the cut surface of the humeral neck without bow-stringing of the tendon on the rim of the humeral head. Those authors reported a satisfactory result for eighteen of twenty-one patients with use of the limited-goals criteria of Neer et al.[74]. All patients had lower pain scores after the hemiarthroplasty, and there were no instances of postoperative instability. The average active forward elevation improved from 70 degrees preoperatively to 120 degrees postoperatively, and the average external rotation improved from 27 to 46 degrees. Williams and Rockwood concluded that humeral hemiarthroplasty provided reliable relief of pain and restored the ability to perform activities of daily living.

Pollock et al.[80] compared the results of total shoulder replacement with those of humeral hemiarthroplasty in thirty shoulders that had a rotator cuff tear. At an average of forty-one months postoperatively, relief of pain was satisfactory in eighteen of the nineteen patients who had had a hemiarthroplasty and in nine of the ten patients who had had a total shoulder arthroplasty. Twelve patients (thirteen shoulder arthroplasties) had been identified as having rotator cuff tear arthropathy, and they reported mild or no pain and had an average

TABLE II
SUMMARY OF THE REPORTED RESULTS OF HEMIARTHROPLASTY IN PATIENTS WHO HAD ROTATOR CUFF TEAR ARTHROPATHY

Study	No. of Shoulders	Pain (Preop./Postop.)*† (points)	Active Forward Elevation (Preop./Postop.)† (degrees)
Pollock et al.[80] (1992)	13	2.8/0.7	64/108
Williams and Rockwood[99] (1996)	21	2.9/0.6	70 (0-155)/120 (15-160)
Field et al.[36] (1997)	16	2.4/0.8	60 (40-80)/100 (80-130)

*0 points = no pain, 1 point = mild pain, 2 points = moderate pain, and 3 points = severe pain.
†The values are given as the average, with the range in parentheses.

increase in forward elevation of 44 degrees.

Recently, Field et al.[36] reported the results of hemiarthroplasty in sixteen patients who had rotator cuff tear arthropathy; ten of twelve patients who had normal function of the anterior portion of the deltoid and an adequate coracoacromial arch were considered to have a successful result according to the limited-goals criteria of Neer et al.[74]. All four patients who had had a previous acromioplasty and coracoacromial release had an unsuccessful outcome. The size of the humeral head was determined by its capacity to articulate with the coracoacromial arch and to maintain the ability to translate on the glenoid approximately 50 percent of its width anteriorly, posteriorly, and inferiorly. Oversizing of the head was intentionally avoided, in order to prevent an anterior shift of the head on the glenoid and tightening of the soft tissues. The reported results of hemiarthroplasty performed specifically for painful rotator cuff tear arthropathy reveal a reliable improvement in the pain-scale rating; however, gains in active forward elevation have been inconsistent (Table II)[36,80,99].

Bipolar total shoulder arthroplasty was designed in 1975 by Swanson et al.[93] for the treatment of advanced glenohumeral arthritis associated with superior migration of the humeral head and loss of function of the rotator cuff. Swanson et al. theorized that the oversized humeral head would increase the stability of the joint, increase the abductor lever arm and power, and prevent impingement of the tuberosities. The increased area of contact between the bipolar cup and the acromion and glenoid, combined with motion at two interfaces as a result of the bipolar design, was thought to decrease prosthetic contact forces and to provide relief of pain. Swanson et al.[93] reported that, at an average of five years after this procedure, thirty-five shoulders (thirty-one patients) had excellent relief of pain. Patients who had rotator cuff tear arthropathy were not specifically reported on, and the size of the humeral head, which was thirty-six to fifty millimeters in diameter, was equivalent to that used in conventional hemiarthroplasty. A 30-point shoulder-scoring system, which allotted a maximum of 10 points to three clinical categories (relief of pain, ability to perform activities of daily living, and range of motion), was devised[93].

Alterations to the original design have resulted in a lower-profile bipolar prosthesis that requires conventional resection of the humeral head, thus preserving the tuberosities. Worland et al.[101] reported the results at an average of twenty-eight months after shoulder arthroplasty with use of the modified prosthesis in twenty-two patients. Although seven patients had had a previous attempt at repair of the rotator cuff, it was not reported if an acromioplasty or a release of the acromioclavicular ligament also had been performed. Twenty-one patients had a successful result according to the limited-goals criteria[74] and an improvement in the shoulder score[93]. These results have not been duplicated by others, to our knowledge. Vrettos et al.[96] used the same type of prosthesis in seven patients who had rotator cuff tear arthropathy and reported that all but one patient had moderate-to-severe pain and were unhappy with the result. In addition, radiographs of the shoulder in varying degrees of abduction revealed no motion at the glenoid-prosthesis interface or at the bipolar polyethylene liner-humeral head articulation. Concerns that have been raised regarding the modified bipolar prosthesis include potential overstuffing of the shoulder joint, rupture of the subscapularis tendon due to the vertical orientation of the component, and the effect of polyethylene wear[13].

Overview

In summary, rotator cuff tear arthropathy of the glenohumeral joint is a clinical syndrome involving primarily the dominant extremity of elderly women and is frequently bilateral. On the basis of an extensive review of the literature, it is apparent that different authors have been describing the same clinical syndrome using different terms, which has created confusion. Rotator cuff tear arthropathy appears to be the end point in the continuum of severe degenerative changes in the glenohumeral joint. The degenerative changes that occur in the rotator cuff result in loss of the primary stabilizers of the glenohumeral joint and lead to articular wear and subsequent arthritis. As severe glenohumeral arthritis and instability develop, basic calcium-phosphate crystals are generated, inducing synovial hyperplasia and the secretion of collagenase and stromelysin enzymes. This response accounts for destruction of the collagen-containing structures[45] and may lead to ecchymotic effusions through continued tearing of the rotator cuff. This complex interplay results in glenohumeral instability and rapid destruction of articular cartilage.

If rotator cuff tear arthropathy causes relatively mild symptoms, then treatment should consist of mild anti-inflammatory medication and gentle stretching exercises to maintain or to gain a functional range of motion. A strengthening program then should be initiated to improve the active use of the arm for activities of daily living. Medical treatment with use of prostaglandins to inhibit the effects of the basic calcium-phosphate crystals appears promising yet remains experimental.

If nonoperative management fails in these patients, a humeral hemiarthroplasty is the procedure of choice as it provides reliable relief of pain and improvement in function. Both stability and the range of motion are maintained through careful soft-tissue balancing. Oversized humeral head components should be avoided. Patients who have had previous operations on the rotator cuff resulting in defects of the anterior portion of the deltoid, shortening of the acromion, and loss of the coracoacromial ligament are at risk for postoperative anterosuperior instability.

References

1. **Adams, R.:** *Illustrations of the Effects of Rheumatic Gout or Chronic Rheumatic Arthritis on All the Articulations. With Descriptive and Explanatory Statements,* pp. 1-31. London, John Churchill and Sons, 1857.
2. **Adams, R.:** *A Treatise of Rheumatic Gout or Chronic Rheumatic Arthritis of All the Joints.* Ed. 2, pp. 91-175. London, John Churchill and Sons, 1873.
3. **Amstutz, H. C.; Thomas, B. J.; Kabo, J. M.; Jinnah, R. H.;** and **Dorey, F. J.:** The Dana total shoulder arthroplasty. *J. Bone and Joint Surg.,* 70-A: 1174-1182, Sept. 1988.
4. **Apoil, A.,** and **Augereau, B.:** Antero-superior arthrolysis of the shoulder for rotator cuff degenerative lesions. In *Surgery of the Shoulder,* pp. 257-260. Edited by M. Post, B. F. Morrey, and R. J. Hawkins. St. Louis, Mosby-Year Book, 1990.
5. **Arntz, C. T.; Matsen, F. A., III;** and **Jackins, S.:** Surgical management of complex irreparable rotator cuff deficiency. *J. Arthroplasty,* 6: 363-370, 1991.
6. **Banna, A.,** and **Hume, K. P.:** Spontaneous hemarthrosis of the shoulder joint. *Ann. Phys. Med.,* 7: 180-184, 1964.
7. **Bauduin, M. P.,** and **Famaey, J. P.:** A propos d'un cas d'épaule sénile hémorragique. *Belge rhum. med. phys.,* 24: 135-140, 1969.
8. **Bokor, D. J.; Hawkins, R. J.; Huckell, G. H.; Angelo, R. L.;** and **Schickendantz, M. S.:** Results of nonoperative management of full-thickness tears of the rotator cuff. *Clin. Orthop.,* 294: 103-110, 1993.
9. **Burkhart, S. S.:** Arthroscopic treatment of massive rotator cuff tears. Clinical results and biomechanical rationale. *Clin. Orthop.,* 267: 45-56, 1991.
10. **Burkhart, S. S.:** Fluoroscopic comparison of kinematic patterns in massive rotator cuff tears. A suspension bridge model. *Clin. Orthop.,* 284: 144-152, 1992.
11. **Burkhart, S. S.:** Reconciling the paradox of rotator cuff repair versus debridement: a unified biomechanical rationale for the treatment of rotator cuff tears. *J. Arthroscopy,* 10: 4-19, 1994.
12. **Burman, M.; Sutro, C. J.;** and **Guariglia, E.:** Spontaneous hemorrhage of bursae and joints in the elderly. *Bull. Hosp. Joint Dis.,* 25: 217-239, 1964.
13. **Calton, T. F.; Fehring, T. K.; Griffin, W. L.;** and **McCoy, T. H.:** Failure of the polyethylene after bipolar hemiarthroplasty of the hip. A report of five cases. *J. Bone and Joint Surg.,* 80-A: 420-423, March 1998.
14. **Campion, G. V.; McCrae, F.; Alwan, W.; Watt, I.; Bradfield, J.;** and **Dieppe, P. A.:** Idiopathic destructive arthritis of the shoulder. *Sem. Arthrit. and Rheumat.,* 17: 232-245, 1988.
15. **Caporali, R.; Rossi, S.;** and **Montecucco, C.:** Tidal irrigation in Milwaukee shoulder syndrome. *J. Rheumatol.,* 21: 1781-1782, 1994.
16. **Cheung, H. S.,** and **Ryan, L. M.:** Role of crystal deposition in matrix degradation. In *Joint Cartilage Degradation,* pp. 209-223. Edited by J. F. Woessner, Jr., and D. S. Howell. New York, Marcel Dekker, 1993.
17. **Clayton, M. L.; Ferlic, D. C.;** and **Jeffers, P. D.:** Prosthetic arthroplasties of the shoulder. *Clin. Orthop.,* 164: 184-191, 1982.
18. **Clift, S. E.; Harris, B.; Dieppe, P. A.;** and **Hayes, A.:** Frictional response of articular cartilage containing crystals. *Biomaterials,* 10: 329-334, 1989.
19. **Codman, E. A.:** *The Shoulder. Rupture of the Supraspinatus Tendon and Other Lesions in or About the Subacromial Bursa,* pp. 478-480. Boston, privately printed, 1934.
20. **Cofield, R. H.,** and **Briggs, B. T.:** Glenohumeral arthrodesis. Operative and long-term functional results. *J. Bone and Joint Surg.,* 61-A: 668-677, July 1979.
21. **Cotton, R. E.,** and **Rideout, D. F.:** Tears of the humeral rotator cuff. A radiological and pathological necropsy study. *J. Bone and Joint Surg.,* 46-B(2): 314-328, May 1964.
22. **Coughlin, M. J.; Morris, J. M.;** and **West, W. F.:** The semiconstrained total shoulder arthroplasty. *J. Bone and Joint Surg.,* 61-A: 574-581, June 1979.
23. **Craig, E. V.:** The geyser sign and torn rotator cuff: clinical significance and pathomechanics. *Clin. Orthop.,* 191: 213-215, 1984.
24. **De Buttet, M.; Bouchon, Y.; Capon, D.;** and **Delfosse, J.:** Grammont shoulder arthroplasty for osteoarthritis with massive rotator cuff tears — report of 71 cases. *J. Shoulder and Elbow Surg.,* 6: 197, 1997.
25. **Dennis, D. A.; Ferlic, D. C.;** and **Clayton, M. L.:** Acromial stress fractures associated with cuff tear arthropathy. A report of three cases. *J. Bone and Joint Surg.,* 68-A: 937-940, July 1986.
26. **DePalma, A. F.; Gallery, G.;** and **Bennett, G. A.:** Variational anatomy and degenerative lesions of the shoulder joint. In *Instructional Course Lectures, American Academy of Orthopaedic Surgeons.* Vol. 6, pp. 255-281. Ann Arbor, J. W. Edwards, 1949.
27. **DeSeze, M.:** L'épaule sénile hémorragique. L'actualité rhumatologique. Vol. 1, pp. 107-115. Paris, Expansion Scientifique Française, 1968.
28. **Dieppe, P. A.; Doyle, D. V.; Huskisson, E. C.; Willoughby, D. A.;** and **Crocker, P. R.:** Mixed crystal deposition disease and osteoarthritis. *British. Med. J.,* 1: 150, 1978.
29. **Dieppe, P. A.; Crocker, P. R.; Corke, C. F.; Doyle, D. V.; Huskisson, E. C.;** and **Willoughby, D. A.:** Synovial fluid crystals. *Quart. J. Med.,* 48: 533-553, 1979.

30. **Dieppe, P. A.; Doherty, M.; Macfarlane, D. G.; Hutton, C. W.; Bradfield, J. W.;** and **Watt, I.:** Apatite associated destructive arthritis. *British J. Rheumatol.,* 23: 84-91, 1984.

31. **Dieppe, P. A.; Cawston, T.; Mercer, E.; Campion, G. V.; Hornby, J.; Hutton, C. W.; Doherty, M.; Watt, I.; Woolf, A. D.;** and **Hazleman, B.:** Synovial fluid collagenase in patients with destructive arthritis of the shoulder joint. *Arthrit. and Rheumat.,* 31: 882-890, 1988.

32. **Ellman, H.:** Arthroscopic subacromial decompression: analysis of one- to three-year results. *Arthroscopy,* 3: 173-181, 1987.

33. **Ellman, H.; Kay, S. P.;** and **Wirth, M.:** Arthroscopic treatment of full-thickness rotator cuff tears: 2- to 7-year follow-up study. *Arthroscopy,* 9: 195-200, 1993.

34. **Esch, J. C.; Ozerkis, L. R.; Helgager, J. A.; Kane, N.;** and **Lilliott, N.:** Arthroscopic subacromial decompression: results according to the degree of rotator cuff tear. *Arthroscopy,* 4: 241-249, 1988.

35. **Fenlin, J. M.; Rushton, S. A.;** and **Frieman, B. G.:** Tuberoplasty: creation of an acromiohumeral articulation for irreparable rotator cuff tears [abstract]. *J. Shoulder and Elbow Surg.,* 6: 225, 1997.

36. **Field, L. D.; Dines, D. M.; Zabinski, S. J.;** and **Warren, R. F.:** Hemiarthroplasty of the shoulder for rotator cuff arthropathy. *J. Shoulder and Elbow Surg.,* 6: 18-23, 1997.

37. **Franklin, J. L.; Barrett, W. P.; Jackins, S. E.;** and **Matsen, F. A., III:** Glenoid loosening in total shoulder arthroplasty. Association with rotator cuff deficiency. *J. Arthroplasty,* 31: 39-46, 1988.

38. **Friedman, R. J.; Hawthorne, K. B.;** and **Genez, B. M.:** The use of computerized tomography in the measurement of glenoid version. *J. Bone and Joint Surg.,* 74-A: 1032-1037, Aug. 1992.

39. **Galmiche, P.,** and **Deshayes, P.:** Hemarthrose essentielle récidivante. *Rev. rhumat.,* 25: 57-59, 1958.

40. **Garancis, J. C.; Cheung, H. S.; Halverson, P. B.;** and **McCarty, D. J.:** "Milwaukee shoulder" — association of microspheroids containing hydroxyapatite crystals, active collagenase, and neutral protease with rotator cuff defects. III. Morphologic and biochemical studies of an excised synovium showing chondromatosis. *Arthrit. and Rheumat.,* 24: 484-491, 1981.

41. **Genant, H. K.:** Roentgenographic aspects of calcium pyrophosphate dihydrate crystal deposition disease (pseudogout). *Arthrit. and Rheumat.,* 19 (Supplement 3): 307-328, 1976.

42. **Gibilisco, P. A.; Schumacher, H. R., Jr.; Hollander, J. L.;** and **Soper, K. A.:** Synovial fluid crystals in osteoarthritis. *Arthrit. and Rheumat.,* 28: 511-515, 1985.

43. **Grant, J. C. B.,** and **Smith, G. C.:** Age incidence of rupture of the supraspinatus tendon [abstract]. *Anat. Rec.,* 100: 666, 1948.

44. **Gristina, A. G.; Roman, R. L.; Kammire, G. C.;** and **Webb, L. X.:** Total shoulder replacement. *Orthop. Clin. North America,* 18: 445-453, 1987.

45. **Halverson, P. B.; Cheung, H. S.; McCarty, D. J.; Garancis, J.;** and **Mandel, N.:** "Milwaukee shoulder" — association of microspheroids containing hydroxyapatite crystals, active collagenase, and neutral protease with rotator cuff defects. II. Synovial fluid studies. *Arthrit. and Rheumat.,* 24: 474-483, 1981.

46. **Halverson, P. B.; Garancis, J. C.;** and **McCarty, D. J.:** Histopathological and ultrastructural studies of synovium in Milwaukee shoulder syndrome — a basic calcium phosphate crystal arthropathy. *Ann. Rheumat. Dis.,* 43: 734-741, 1984.

47. **Halverson, P. B.; McCarty, D. J.; Cheung, H. S.;** and **Ryan, L. M.:** Milwaukee shoulder syndrome: eleven additional cases with involvement of the knee in seven (basic calcium phosphate crystal deposition disease). *Sem. Arthrit. and Rheumat.,* 14: 36-44, 1984.

48. **Halverson, P. B.,** and **McCarty, D. J.:** Patterns of radiographic abnormalities associated with basic calcium phosphate and calcium pyrophosphate dihydrate crystal deposition in the knee. *Ann. Rheumat. Dis.,* 45: 603-605, 1986.

49. **Halverson, P. B.,** and **McCarty, D. J.:** Clinical aspects of basic calcium phosphate crystal deposition. *Rheumat. Dis. Clin. North America,* 14: 427-439, 1988.

50. **Halverson, P. B.; Carrera, G. F.;** and **McCarty, D. J.:** Milwaukee shoulder syndrome. Fifteen additional cases and a description of contributing factors. *Arch. Intern. Med.,* 150: 677-682, 1990.

51. **Hamada, K.; Fukuda, H.; Mikasa, M.;** and **Kobayashi, Y.:** Roentgenographic findings in massive rotator cuff tears. A long-term observation. *Clin. Orthop.,* 254: 92-96, 1990.

52. **Hayes, A.; Turner, I. G.; Powell, K. A.;** and **Dieppe, P. A.:** Crystal aggregates in articular cartilage as observed in the SEM. *J. Mater. Sci.,* 3: 75-58, 1992.

53. **Hayes, A.; Harris, B.; Dieppe, P. A.;** and **Clift, S. E.:** Wear of articular cartilage: the effect of crystals. *Proc. Inst. Mech. Eng.,* 207: 41-58, 1993.

54. **Inman, V. T.; Saunders, J. B. D. M.;** and **Abbott, L. C.:** Observations on the function of the shoulder joint. *J. Bone and Joint Surg.,* 26: 1-30, Jan. 1944.

55. **Klimaitis, A.; Carroll, G.;** and **Owen, E.:** Rapidly progressive destructive arthropathy of the shoulder — a viewpoint on pathogenesis. *J. Rheumatol.,* 15: 1859-1862, 1988.

56. **Lamboley, C.; Bataille, R.; Rosenberg, F.; Sany, J.;** and **Serre, H.:** L'épaule sénile hémorragique. A propos de 9 observations. *Rhumatologie,* 29: 323-330, 1977.

57. **Lee, D. H.,** and **Niemann, K. M. W.:** Bipolar shoulder arthroplasty. *Clin. Orthop.,* 304: 97-107, 1994.

58. **Lequesne, M.; Fallut, M.; Coulomb, R.; Magnet, J. L.;** and **Strauss, J.:** L'arthropathie destructrice rapide de l'épaule. *Rev. rhumat.,* 49: 427-437, 1982.

59. **Lettin, A. W. F.; Copeland, S. A.;** and **Scales, J. T.:** The Stanmore total shoulder replacement. *J. Bone and Joint Surg.,* 64-B(1): 47-51, 1982.

60. **Levy, H. J.; Gardner, R. D.;** and **Lemak, L. J.:** Arthroscopic subacromial decompression in the treatment of full-thickness rotator cuff tears. *Arthroscopy,* 7: 8-13, 1991.

61. **Lohr, J. F.; Cofield, R. H.;** and **Uhthoff, H. K.:** Glenoid component loosening in cuff tear arthropathy. *J. Bone and Joint Surg.,* 73-B (Supplement II): 106, 1991.

62. **Lucas, D. B.:** Biomechanics of the shoulder joint. *Arch. Surg.,* 107: 425-432, 1973.

63. **McCarthy, G. M.; Mitchell, P. G.;** and **Cheung, H. S.:** The mitogenic response to stimulation with basic calcium phosphate crystals is accompanied by induction and secretion of collagenase in human fibroblasts. *Arthrit. and Rheumat.,* 34: 1021-1030, 1991.

64. **McCarthy, G. M.; Mitchell, P. G.; Struve, J. A.;** and **Cheung, H. S.:** Basic calcium phosphate crystals cause coordinate induction and secretion of collagenase and stromelysin. *J. Cell. Physiol.,* 153: 140-146, 1992.

65. **McCarthy, G. M.; Mitchell, P. G.;** and **Cheung, H. S.:** Misoprostol, a prostaglandin E1 analogue, inhibits basic calcium phosphate crystal-induced mitogenesis and collagenase accumulation in human fibroblasts. *Calcif. Tissue Internat.,* 52: 434-437, 1993.

66. **McCarthy, G. M.; Macius, A. M.; Christopherson, P. A.; Ryan, L. M.;** and **Pourmotabbed, T.:** Basic calcium phosphate crystals induce synthesis and secretion of 92 kDa gelatinase (gelatinase B/matrix metalloprotease 9) in human fibroblasts. *Ann. Rheumat. Dis.,* 57: 56-60, 1998.

67. **McCarty, D. J.; Halverson, P. B.; Carrera, G. F.; Brewer, B. J.;** and **Kozin, F.:** "Milwaukee shoulder" — association of microspheroids containing hydroxyapatite crystals, active collagenase, and neutral protease with rotator cuff defects. I. Clinical aspects. *Arthrit. and Rheumat.,* 24: 464-473, 1981.

68. **McCarty, D. J.; Lehr, J. R.;** and **Halverson, P. B.:** Crystal populations in human synovial fluid. Identification of apatite, octacalcium phosphate, and tricalcium phosphate. *Arthrit. and Rheumat.,* 26: 1220-1224, 1983.

69. **McLaughlin, H. L.:** Rupture of the rotator cuff. *J. Bone and Joint Surg.,* 44-A: 979-983, July 1962.

70. **McMahon, P. J.; Debski, R. E.; Thompson, W. O.; Warner, J. J.; Fu, F. U.;** and **Woo, S. L.:** Shoulder muscle forces and tendon excursions during glenohumeral abduction in the scapular plane. *J. Shoulder and Elbow Surg.,* 4: 199-208, 1995.

71. **Melillo, A. S.; Savoie, F. H., III;** and **Field, L. D.:** Massive rotator cuff tears: debridement versus repair. *Orthop. Clin. North America,* 28: 117-124, 1997.

72. **Mitchell, P. G.; Struve, J. A.; McCarthy, G. M.;** and **Cheung, H. S.:** Basic calcium phosphate crystals stimulate cell proliferation and collagenase message accumulation in cultured adult articular chondrocytes. *Arthrit. and Rheumat.,* 35: 343-350, 1992.

73. **Mullaji, A. B.; Beddow, F. H.;** and **Lamb, G. H. R.:** CT measurement of glenoid erosion in arthritis. *J. Bone and Joint Surg.,* 76-B(3): 384-388, 1994.

74. **Neer, C. S., II; Watson, K. C.;** and **Stanton, F. J.:** Recent experience in total shoulder replacement. *J. Bone and Joint Surg.,* 64-A: 319-337, March 1982.

75. **Neer, C. S., II; Craig, E. V.;** and **Fukuda, H.:** Cuff-tear arthropathy. *J. Bone and Joint Surg.,* 65-A: 1232-1244, Dec. 1983.

76. **Neer, C. S., II:** *Shoulder Reconstruction,* pp. 143-272, 405-406. Philadelphia, W. B. Saunders, 1990.

77. **Newman, J. H.; Chavin, K. D.;** and **Chavin, I. F.:** Milwaukee shoulder syndrome: a new crystal-induced arthritis syndrome associated with hydroxyapatite crystals — a case report. *Delaware Med. J.,* 55: 167-169, 1983.

78. **Nove-Josserand, L.; Levigne, C.; Noel, E.;** and **Walch, G.:** Factors influencing the acromio-humeral interval in rotator cuff tears [abstract]. *J. Shoulder and Elbow Surg.,* 5: S43, 1996.

79. **Orr, T. E.; Carter, D. R.;** and **Schurman, D. J.:** Stress analyses of glenoid component designs. *Clin. Orthop.,* 232: 217-224, 1988.

80. **Pollock, R. G.; Deliz, E. D.; McIlveen, S. J.; Flatow, E. L.;** and **Bigliani, L. U.:** Prosthetic replacement in rotator cuff-deficient shoulders. *J. Shoulder and Elbow Surg.,* 1: 173-186, 1992.

81. **Poppen, N. K.,** and **Walker, P. S.:** Normal and abnormal motion of the shoulder. *J. Bone and Joint Surg.,* 58-A: 195-201, March 1976.

82. **Poppen, N. K.,** and **Walker, P. S.:** Forces at the glenohumeral joint in abduction. *Clin. Orthop.,* 135: 165-170, 1978.

83. **Post, M.; Haskell, S. S.;** and **Jablon, M.:** Total shoulder replacement with a constrained prosthesis. *J. Bone and Joint Surg.,* 62-A: 327-335, April 1980.

84. **Post, M.,** and **Jablon, M.:** Constrained total shoulder arthroplasty. Long-term follow-up observations. *Clin. Orthop.,* 173: 109-116, 1983.

85. **Rockwood, C. A., Jr.; Williams, G. R., Jr.;** and **Burkhead, W. Z., Jr.:** Debridement of degenerative, irreparable lesions of the rotator cuff. *J. Bone and Joint Surg.,* 77-A: 857-866, June 1995.

86. **Rockwood, C. A., Jr.,** and **Jensen, K. L.:** X-ray evaluation of shoulder problems. In *The Shoulder,* pp. 199-231. Edited by C. A. Rockwood, Jr., and F. A. Matsen, III. Philadelphia, W. B. Saunders, 1998.

87. **Saha, A. K.:** Dynamic stability of the glenohumeral joint. *Acta Orthop. Scandinavica,* 42: 491-505, 1971.

88. **Schumacher, H. R.; Miller, J. L.; Ludivico, C.;** and **Jessar, R. A.:** Erosive arthritis associated with apatite crystal deposition. *Arthrit. and Rheumat.,* 24: 31-37, 1981.

89. **Shephard, E.:** Swelling of the subacromial bursa: report on 16 cases. *Proc. Roy. Soc. Med.,* 56: 162-163, 1963.

90. **Smith, R. W.:** Observations upon chronic rheumatic arthritis of the shoulder [part I]. *Dublin Quart. J. Med. Sci.,* 15: 1-16, 1853.

91. **Smith, R. W.:** Observations upon chronic rheumatic arthritis of the shoulder [part II]. *Dublin Quart. J. Med. Sci.,* 15: 343-358, 1853.

92. **Snook, G. A.:** Pigmented villonodular synovitis with bony invasion. A report of two cases. *J. Am. Med. Assn.,* 184: 424-425, 1963.

93. **Swanson, A. B.; Swanson, G. G.; Sattel, A. B.; Cendo, R. D.; Hynes, D.;** and **Jar-Ning, W.:** Bipolar implant shoulder arthroplasty. Long-term results. *Clin. Orthop.,* 249: 227-247, 1989.

94. **Thompson, W. O.; Debski, R. E.; Boardman, N. D., III; Taskiran, E.; Warner, J. J.; Fu, F. H.;** and **Woo, S. L.:** A biomechanical analysis of rotator cuff deficiency in a cadaveric model. *Am. J. Sports Med.,* 24: 286-292, 1996.

95. **Uhthoff, H. K.; Sarkar, K.;** and **Maynard, J. A.:** Calcifying tendinitis. A new concept of its pathogenesis. *Clin. Orthop.,* 118: 164-168, 1976.

96. **Vrettos, B. C.; Wallace, W. A.;** and **Neumann, L.:** Bipolar hemiarthroplasty of the shoulder for the elderly patient with rotator cuff arthropathy [abstract]. In Proceedings of the British Elbow and Shoulder Society. *J. Bone and Joint Surg.,* 80-B (Supplement I): 106, 1998.

97. **Wallace, W. A.,** and **Wiley, A. M.:** The long-term results of conservative management of full-thickness tears of the rotator cuff. In Proceedings of the British Orthopaedic Association. *J. Bone and Joint Surg.,* 68-B(1): 162, 1986.

98. **Weiss, J. J.; Good, A.;** and **Schumacher, H. R.:** Four cases of "Milwaukee shoulder," with a description of clinical presentation and long-term treatment. *J. Am. Geriat. Soc.,* 33: 202-205, 1985.

99. **Williams, G. R., Jr.,** and **Rockwood, C. A., Jr.:** Hemiarthroplasty in rotator cuff-deficient shoulders. *J. Shoulder and Elbow Surg.,* 5: 362-367, 1996.

100. **Woolf, A. D.; Cawston, T. E.;** and **Dieppe, P. A.:** Idiopathic haemorrhagic rupture of the shoulder in destructive disease of the elderly. *Ann. Rheumat. Dis.,* 45: 498-501, 1986.

101. **Worland, R. L.; Jessup, D. E.; Arredondo, J.;** and **Warburton, K. J.:** Bipolar shoulder arthroplasty for rotator cuff arthropathy. *J. Shoulder and Elbow Surg.,* 6: 512-515, 1997.

The Rotator Cuff–Deficient Arthritic Shoulder: Diagnosis and Surgical Management

Craig A. Zeman, MD, Michel A. Arcand, MD, Jeffery S. Cantrell, MD,
John G. Skedros, MD, and Wayne Z. Burkhead, Jr, MD

Abstract

The symptomatic rotator cuff–deficient, arthritic glenohumeral joint poses a complex problem for the orthopaedic surgeon. Surgical management can be facilitated by classifying the disorder in one of three diagnostic categories: (1) rotator cuff–tear arthropathy, (2) rheumatoid arthritic shoulder with cuff deficiency, or (3) degenerative arthritic (osteoarthritic) shoulder with cuff deficiency. If it is not possible to repair the cuff defect, surgical management may include prosthetic arthroplasty, with the recognition that only limited goals are attainable, particularly with respect to strength and active motion. Glenohumeral arthrodesis is a salvage procedure when other surgical measures have failed. Arthrodesis is also indicated in patients with deltoid muscle deficiency. Humeral hemiarthroplasty avoids the complications of glenoid loosening and is an attractive alternative to arthrodesis, resection arthroplasty, and total shoulder arthroplasty. The functionally intact coracoacromial arch should be preserved to reduce the risk of anterosuperior subluxation. Care should be taken not to "overstuff" the glenohumeral joint with a prosthetic component. In cases of significant internal rotation contracture, subscapularis lengthening is necessary to restore anterior and posterior rotator cuff balance. If the less stringent criteria of Neer's "limited goals" rehabilitation are followed, approximately 80% to 90% of patients treated with humeral hemiarthroplasty can have satisfactory results.

J Am Acad Orthop Surg 1998;6:337-348

The patient with a symptomatic rotator cuff–deficient, arthritic glenohumeral joint poses a complex problem for the orthopaedic surgeon. Although this condition has been recognized since the early 19th century, there is no consensus on its management.[1-8] One of the difficulties is the diverse clinical presentation of patients with this disorder: some have rotator cuff–tear arthropathy (RCTA), as defined by Neer et al[1]; others have end-stage rheumatoid arthritis (RA) or degenerative arthritis with cuff tears. Different surgical solutions may be required for each presentation.[9] The surgeon must also deal with osteopenic bone, severe soft-tissue contractures, and atrophied muscles. It may be impossible to repair the cuff defect. Consequently, many of the patients who come to surgery are treated with prosthetic arthroplasty with the recognition that only limited goals are attainable, particularly with respect to strength and active motion.[1,7,9-11]

History

Between 1830 and 1860, Smith and Adams described several cases of localized shoulder arthritis associated with a large swelling about the shoulder, rotator cuff tear, biceps tendon rupture, and erosion of the superior portion of the humeral head, acromion, and distal clavicle. In his classic 1934 text, Codman described the case of a 51-year-old woman who had sustained a traumatic rotator cuff tear 6 years prior to surgery. During the operation he found, in addition to the large cuff defect, humeral head roughening, glenoid obliteration, intra-articular loose bodies, severe atrophy of the surrounding musculature, and a large fluid accumulation. He believed that these changes were the final stages of a chronically neglected large rotator cuff tear.

Dr. Zeman is in private practice in Oxnard, Calif. Dr. Arcand is in private practice in Norman, Okla. Dr. Cantrell is in private practice in Lewisville, Tex. Dr. Skedros is in private practice in Ogden, Utah. Dr. Burkhead is Clinical Associate Professor of Orthopaedic Surgery, University of Texas Southwestern Medical School, Dallas; and is in private practice with W. B. Carrell Memorial Clinic, Dallas.

Reprint requests: Dr. Zeman, W. B. Carrell Memorial Clinic, 2909 Lemmon Avenue, Dallas, TX 75204.

More than a century later, Burman and co-workers described cases of recurrent spontaneous hemorrhage into the subdeltoid bursa in elderly patients with supraspinatus tendon tears and glenohumeral arthritis. In 1968, DeSeze called this condition *l'épaule sénile hémorragique* ("hemorrhagic shoulder of the elderly"). In 1977, Neer introduced the term "cuff-tear arthropathy" to describe findings associated with a chronic full-thickness rotator cuff tear, which include restricted shoulder motion, erosions of the osseous structures of the shoulder, and an arthritic, osteopenic, and collapsed humeral head.[1] In the early 1980s, Halverson et al[12,13] described the "Milwaukee shoulder syndrome," which is in many ways similar to RCTA.

Types of Rotator Cuff Problems in Arthritic Shoulders

Surgical management of a rotator cuff–deficient arthritic shoulder can be facilitated by assigning it to one of the following diagnostic categories: (1) RCTA, (2) degenerative arthritic (osteoarthritic) shoulder with cuff deficiency, and (3) rheumatoid arthritic shoulder with cuff deficiency. Categorization is based on specific clinical, radiographic, and laboratory findings. These designations help the surgeon anticipate the quality of tissues, the natural history of the disease, and the ultimate surgical outcome.

Rotator Cuff–Tear Arthropathy

In a 1983 landmark review article, Neer et al[1] expounded on Neer's original description of RCTA. Because RCTA was found not to be associated with degenerative arthritis in other joints, they suggested that a massive rotator cuff tear is the initial event in the pathogenesis. They also described mechanical and nutritional factors that may precipitate development of RCTA (Fig. 1).

Mechanical Factors

The concept of "force couples" in the shoulder emphasizes the critical nature of mechanical factors in the dynamic stability of the glenohumeral joint.[14] For example, the glenohumeral joint is balanced anteriorly and posteriorly by the subscapularis, infraspinatus, and teres minor. Most large rotator cuff tears extend posteriorly into the infraspinatus and teres minor, leaving the subscapularis unbalanced. Due to unbalanced force couples, volitional attempts to elevate and/or rotate the arm can produce destructive forces in the glenohumeral joint. A deficient cuff may allow excessive upward migration of the humeral head, resulting in abrasion and erosion of the superior glenoid, acromioclavicular joint, and acromion. Because only about 4% of shoulders with full-thickness rotator cuff defects progress to RCTA,[1] mechanical factors do not appear to be wholly responsible for the pathologic features of RCTA described by Neer.

Nutritional Factors

As in other diarthrodial joints, the articular surfaces of the shoulder receive nutrition from synovial fluid. A full-thickness rotator cuff tear violates the closed joint space,

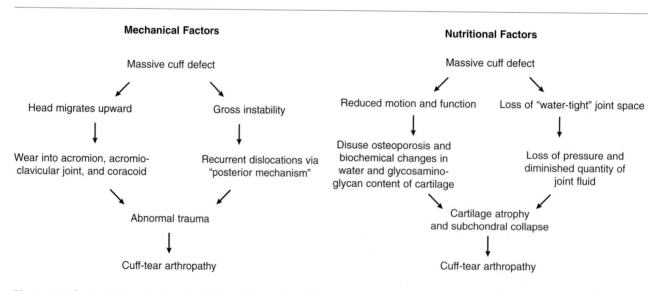

Fig. 1   Mechanical factors **(left)** and nutritional factors **(right)** that contribute to joint destruction in RCTA, according to Neer et al.[1] (Adapted with permission from Neer CS II, Craig EV, Fukuda H: Cuff-tear arthropathy. *J Bone Joint Surg Am* 1983;65:1232-1244.)

allowing synovial fluid, with its nutrients and other biochemical constituents, to leak into the subdeltoid and subacromial spaces and surrounding soft tissues. In addition, pain leads to shoulder inactivity, which reduces the delivery of synovial nutrients and produces disuse osteopenia and joint stiffness. All of these factors contribute to articular cartilage destruction.

Inflammatory Factors

The rheumatology literature contains an abundance of clinical cases that appear grossly similar to RCTA.[12-17] However, explanations of the etiology of these conditions emphasize biochemical factors, differing from Neer's emphasis on deficient cartilage nutrition and marked glenohumeral instability. In many of the cases reported by rheumatologists, crystal-induced inflammation is considered to be the cause of destruction. Halverson and coworkers identified basic calcium phosphate crystals (BCPs), such as hydroxyapatite, in the synovial tissue and fluid of shoulders with apparent inflammatory arthropathy.[12,13] They hypothesized that the crystals are formed in diseased synovium and articular cartilage and then released into the synovial fluid. Subsequent phagocytosis of these crystals by macrophages induces a phlogistic response that destroys the rotator cuff tendon and articular cartilage. As the tissue is damaged, additional crystals are released, resulting in a vicious circle. This interpretation implies that the cuff is not torn traumatically in RCTA but is severely degenerated and characterized by a 5-cm or larger defect.[2]

In 1985, Dieppe and Watt[16] reviewed the role of crystal deposition in the pathogenesis of osteoarthritis (OA). They noted that BCP crystals have been found in osteoarthritic joints, neuropathic joints, and joint tissue of healthy elderly patients and that apatite crystals in particular seem to occur in the more destructive atrophic situations. Consequently, they speculated that BCP crystals may be a product of articular surface wear, and that the crystals are produced by processes that are secondary to joint destruction and are not the inciting cause. They proposed crystal deposition as an opportunistic event in OA, with the joint damage predisposing to deposition, and the deposits in turn modifying the underlying disease. If this interpretation is correct, Milwaukee shoulder syndrome may be a localized form of erosive OA.[16,17]

Osteoarthritic Shoulder With Cuff Tear

In patients with an osteoarthritic shoulder and a cuff tear, the primary diagnosis is OA, and the associated cuff tear is traumatic or attritional.[2,18] Occasionally, hypertrophic arthritis develops after a cuff tear or repair or after a shoulder replacement.

Rheumatoid Arthritic Shoulder With Cuff Tear

Patients with RA in the shoulder and a cuff tear typically have systemic symptoms, physical signs, and radiographic and laboratory findings consistent with RA. The radiographic appearance is similar to that of RCTA, albeit commonly with more destruction.[18] Extensive rotator cuff tearing is not usual in the shoulder affected by RA.[18]

Diagnosis

History and Physical Examination

Patients with cuff-deficient, arthritic shoulders are typically elderly (seventh decade or older) and female. Most commonly, it is the dominant extremity that is involved. Patients usually present with a long history of progressively increasing pain that is worse at night and is intensified by glenohumeral motion. They also report loss of active shoulder motion. The observation by Neer et al[1] that 10 of 26 patients with RCTA had not received antecedent corticosteroid injections diminishes their importance as an etiologic factor.

Patients with OA and rotator cuff tears also relate a history of progressive pain and stiffness. It is not uncommon for these patients to relate an acute traumatic event followed by increased shoulder weakness and symptoms. Patients with rotator cuff tears and RA generally have a long history of polyarthritis and medical treatment for their systemic disease. They may have pain in other joints of the hands, wrists, elbows, hips, or knees.

In patients with RCTA, atrophy of the supraspinatus and infraspinatus muscles and weakness of external rotation and abduction are typical physical findings on clinical examination. Active and passive attempts to move the shoulder through a functional range are limited by weakness, pain, and stiffness. This is most apparent in external rotation and abduction. A rupture of the biceps tendon may be detected. A large shoulder swelling, or "fluid sign," which results from chronic, excessive fluid pressure in the subacromial bursa, may also be noted (Fig. 2). Aspiration of the fluid, which may be bloody or blood-streaked, followed by cortisone injection, is an excellent temporizing measure that can be undertaken in an attempt to avoid surgery; however, recurrence after aspiration is common.

Patients with either RA or OA can have mild swelling, but this is usually synovial-tissue thickening rather than fluid that can be aspirated. These patients may also have physical findings involving other joints, such as deformity, contractures, or instability.

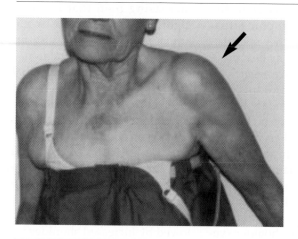

Fig. 2 The fluid sign is seen as a swelling (arrow) on the anterior aspect of this patient's shoulder. This is caused by fluid bulging from the gleno-humeral joint through a large chronic cuff tear and into the enlarged subacro-mial bursa. Less common-ly, fluid in the subdeltoid bursa can be associated with primary bursal in-volvement in RA.[18]

Imaging

There are a number of character-istic plain-radiographic findings of RCTA (Fig. 3). Erosion of the prox-imal humerus may be so extensive that the humeral head is worn beyond the surgical neck. Axillary lateral radiographs may reveal a fixed anterior or posterior gleno-humeral dislocation.

Radiographs of osteoarthritic shoulders typically show subchon-dral sclerosis, humeral head osteo-phytes, glenoid osteophytes, and posterior erosion of the glenoid.[18] In contrast to RA and RCTA, osteo-penia is not characteristic of con-ventional OA. Unlike osteoarthritic shoulders, rheumatoid shoulders are characterized by relatively sym-metrical juxta-articular erosion and relatively minimal subchondral sclerosis and osteophytosis.[18]

Patients with cuff deficiency require extra preoperative, intraop-erative, and postoperative decision making. Although magnetic reso-nance imaging is not necessary for the routine preoperative workup of patients with straightforward OA and obvious clinical and radiologic findings indicative of a full-thickness rotator cuff tear, it may be useful in patients with physical findings that are difficult to interpret (e.g., those who cannot do a lift-off or belly-press test because of pain and

motion loss). Because cuff tears may have unexpected configurations and sizes and the cuff tissue may be of poor quality, the surgeon must be prepared to use alternative methods (e.g., autografts, allografts, or tendon transfers) in reconstruction or repair. These intraoperative decisions are facilitated by preoperative knowl-edge gained with magnetic reso-nance imaging.

Differential Diagnosis

The radiographic appearance of glenohumeral joints in patients with metabolic arthritis resembles that in patients with OA; however, the rotator cuff is usually intact. In some advanced cases, the radio-graphic findings can be similar to those seen with advanced RCTA. Blood and joint-fluid chemistries and synovial biopsy can help con-firm a diagnosis of gout, pseudo-gout, hemochromatosis, and other types of metabolic arthritides.

Patients with septic arthritis are often debilitated due to a general-ized disease process such as RA.[19] In the absence of fever and an ele-vated white blood cell count, diag-nosis depends on a high level of suspicion and the findings from joint aspiration and culture. If an effusion is present, it is warm, in contrast to the cool effusion of RCTA.

Patients with Charcot (neuro-pathic) joints and osteonecrosis usually have intact rotator cuffs. Clinical workup may ultimately reveal an underlying cause, such as corticosteroid use, alcohol abuse, tabes dorsalis, or syringomyelia.

Patients with a history of hemo-philia and numerous hemarthroses may also have hemophilic arthrop-athy. Radiographs of shoulders with advanced disease may resem-ble those of shoulders with RA or, less commonly, OA. Dark pigmen-tation of the joint tissues is apparent on gross examination, and histolog-ic examination of joint cartilage reveals chondrocytes with intracel-lular iron deposits.

Indications for Surgery

The main indication for surgical management is unremitting pain that has proved resistant to a trial of nonoperative measures, including

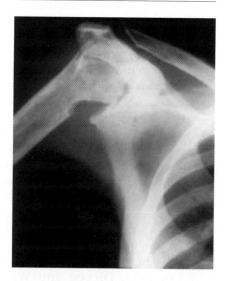

Fig. 3 Anteroposterior radiograph shows RCTA in the right shoulder of a 77-year-old man. The shoulder is in maximum active abduction. In addition to humeral head collapse, findings include periarticu-lar osteopenia, reduced acromiohumeral distance, and erosions of the glenoid, acromion, and acromioclavicular joint.

rest, oral analgesics and nonsteroidal anti-inflammatory medications, corticosteroid injections, fluid aspirations, and gentle range-of-motion exercises. Additional considerations, such as patient age, activity level, job requirements, and general health, are extremely important in individualizing a treatment plan. The integrity of the contralateral rotator cuff should also be assessed, as this may be important in planning postoperative rehabilitation. Patients who use canes or are confined to wheelchairs may, during the first few postoperative months, apply increased stresses to the contralateral shoulder; a course of preoperative stretching before a prosthetic arthroplasty may improve postoperative function.[2]

Surgical Options

Shoulder Arthrodesis

Many patients with a cuff-deficient, arthritic shoulder have poor general health and are at increased risk for major surgical complications. Shoulder arthrodesis is an extensive operation that, when combined with spica immobilization, may not be well tolerated by these individuals.[10,19,20] In addition, because of poor bone stock, these patients may have a higher failure rate than younger individuals. However, with the use of internal fixation, autogenous and allogeneic bone graft material, and aggressive medical management, glenohumeral arthrodesis is a viable option, especially in the patient with RCTA, an irreparable cuff defect, and a deficient anterior deltoid who has undergone multiple procedures.[20] However, it is infrequently the optimal surgical option in this setting.[19,20]

Resection Arthroplasty

Resection arthroplasty is not recommended for the patient with a cuff-deficient arthritic shoulder. It typically produces a flail shoulder that leaves the patient even more disabled because deltoid function is often deficient as well. Inferior instability and brachial-plexus traction neuritis are common and contribute to the severely compromised shoulder biomechanics.

Constrained Shoulder Replacement

In 1991, Laurence[21] reported on the use of polyethylene cups and large stainless-steel heads that snap-fit together to form a constrained construct. After resection of the superior two thirds of the glenoid, screws and bone cement are used to fix the cup into this region and into the coracoid and acromion. Seventy-one shoulders in 66 patients were followed up for an average of 6.8 years. All of the patients apparently had large rotator cuff defects. The remaining distal cuff tendons were surgically transected with the tuberosities and reattached more distally after placement of the prosthetic components. There was complete relief of pain in 22 patients, only minor discomfort in 35, and moderate pain in 9. Two shoulders were considered surgical failures, and 3 required revision surgery for loosening (2 after trauma). Active use of the arm was regained by 56 patients (85%), and 26 (40%) returned to gainful employment.

Once considered a solution for the patient with a cuff-deficient arthritic shoulder, constrained shoulder replacement created a whole new set of complications.[18] A theoretical advantage of this surgical option is that it provides the deltoid with a stable fulcrum on which to move the humerus when there is impairment of the normal force couple between the cuff and the deltoid due to cuff insufficiency. However, constrained shoulder replacement, which is not approved by the US Food and Drug Administration, is not considered appropriate treatment because the design produces excessive interface stresses, which can lead to rapid loosening, implant dissociation, and bone and implant fracture.[6,18,22]

Shoulder Bipolar Arthroplasty

Swanson and Swanson[8] pioneered the use of shoulder bipolar arthroplasty for treating arthritic shoulders with loss of the force-couple balance required to hold the humeral head in the glenoid during abduction. Theoretical advantages provided by the large head of this arthroplasty include the following factors: (1) smooth concentric total contact for the entire shoulder joint cavity; (2) reduction of force concentration over any one contact area and, therefore, decreased resistance to movement; (3) longer moment arm between the fulcrum and the muscle insertion, increasing the efficiency of muscle pull; and (4) prevention of impingement by the greater tuberosity against the acromion.

Lee and Niemann[23] reported on the results of shoulder bipolar arthroplasties performed on 14 patients, 13 of whom had irreparable large rotator cuff tears. Two groups were studied: 7 patients with RA who underwent a primary shoulder arthroplasty and 7 patients who underwent a secondary reconstructive procedure. No rotator cuff reconstruction was performed. The patients with RA all had good pain relief and reported satisfaction with the results of surgery. In contrast, the patients in the secondary reconstruction group had only fair pain relief, and only 4 of the 7 were satisfied with their results. The RA group had a nearly threefold greater increase in range of motion than the secondary reconstruction group. The authors concluded that bipolar arthroplasty was a good choice for treating patients with RA and massive cuff tears, but one disadvantage was the large amount of bone resection required. Fewer complications occurred when the subacromial arch was intact. If the cuff was reparable, the investigators performed a standard Neer-type hemiarthroplasty or total shoulder arthroplasty (TSA).

Nonconstrained Total Shoulder Arthroplasty

In 1982, Neer et al[9] reported on the results of nonconstrained TSA in 194 shoulders in patients treated for various diagnoses. Follow-up was from 24 to 99 months. Rotator cuff-tear arthropathy was found in 16 shoulders. Two patients (3 shoulders) had OA and a cuff defect (size not reported); both patients were paraplegic as a result of poliomyelitis. Twelve patients had large cuff tears and RA; 17 additional patients with RA had small cuff tears that were easy to repair. In the RCTA group, all but 1 patient had a successful result with "limited goals" rehabilitation. The 2 patients in the OA group were satisfied with their postsurgical results. Seven of the patients with RA and massive cuff tears had successful results on the basis of limited-goals rehabilitation criteria. The remaining 22 RA patients had satisfactory to excellent results with a full exercise rehabilitation protocol. Although lucent lines developed around the glenoid component in nearly 30% of each group, symptomatic loosening did not occur.

In 1984, Cofield[10] reported the results of 73 TSAs in 65 patients who had RA, OA, or posttraumatic arthritis and were followed up for an average of 3.8 years. Of the 31 shoulders with OA, 3 had "minor" and 3 had "major" rotator cuff tears (major tears were at least as long as the breadth of the supraspinatus tendon). Of the 29 shoulders with RA, 1 had a minor cuff tear, and 6

had major tears. Four longitudinally torn supraspinatus tendons were repaired by simple suturing. Of the 9 shoulders with major rotator cuff tears, 6 were repaired by suturing tendon directly to the cancellous bone of the proximal humerus. The major tears in the remaining 3 shoulders were repaired with fascia lata grafts. Five of the rotator cuff repairs had failed by the time of the last reported follow-up, and 1 patient had severe pain. The amount of active abduction that was achieved postoperatively was clearly related to the condition of the rotator cuff at surgery. When no complications occurred, results were predictably good. Cofield concluded that these results were superior to those obtained with shoulder fusion in patients with similar shoulder conditions.[10,19]

Hawkins et al[5] reported the results in 65 patients treated with TSA for OA and RA who were followed up for an average of 36 months. Twenty-one patients, most in the RA group, had rotator cuff tears, and all but 1 patient had satisfactory repair of the rotator cuff. The results were satisfactory in 90% of the shoulders, with no difference being noted between OA and RA patients.

Barrett et al[22] reported the results of TSA in 50 shoulders of 44 patients who were followed up for an average of 3.5 years. Nine shoulders had a tear of the rotator cuff. Three tears were less than 5 cm and were repaired; repair and/or reconstruction was attempted in the others, but all of the results were considered suboptimal. Of the 6 patients with painful shoulders at follow-up, 4 had glenoid component loosening; at the time of the original procedure, all 4 patients had had a massive tear of the rotator cuff. Two of these patients underwent revision with a hemiarthroplasty, 1 had a resection arthroplasty, and 1 elected no fur-

ther surgery. The authors theorized that in some cases the superiorly subluxated humeral head eccentrically loaded the glenoid component, ultimately producing rocking and progressive loosening of the glenoid component.

Franklin et al[6] reported an association between glenoid loosening and rotator cuff deficiency with proximal humeral migration. Of 14 patients with rotator cuff deficiency, 7 demonstrated glenoid component loosening. None of the 16 patients with an intact cuff had a loose glenoid component. The amount of superior migration of the humeral component directly correlated with the degree of glenoid loosening. The authors emphasized that an intact, functional rotator cuff can reduce eccentric glenoid loading by centering the humeral head on the glenoid during dynamic shoulder motion.

Humeral Hemiarthroplasty

Marmor[11] reported the results of humeral hemiarthroplasty in 12 shoulders of 10 patients with RA followed up for an average of 4.5 years. Five of the 12 shoulders had a rotator cuff tear (size not specified). All patients eventually had good pain relief. One patient with significant pain required an acromioplasty after the initial procedure. All but 1 patient ultimately attained increased motion.

Arntz et al used humeral hemiarthroplasty as an alternative to glenohumeral arthrodesis for the cuff-deficient arthritic shoulder. In 1993 they reported the results in 18 shoulders in 16 patients followed up for 25 to 122 months.[24] Eleven patients had RCTA. A prerequisite for surgery was a functionally intact coracoacromial arch, providing secondary stability across the anterosuperior aspect of the humeral prosthesis. A smaller prosthetic head was used to avoid pain associated with excessive tightness of the posterior capsule. Excessive shoulder tightness was also avoided by allowing 50% posterior subluxation of the humeral component on the glenoid fossa and 90 degrees of internal rotation of the abducted humerus. In all cases, the rotator cuff was not repaired because of poor tissue quality. At the final reported follow-up, 3 shoulders were pain-free, 8 shoulders were slightly painful, 4 shoulders were painful after activities that the patients described as not typical of daily use, and 3 shoulders were markedly painful and had to undergo revision procedures. Humeral component loosening was not seen.

In 1996, Williams and Rockwood[25] reported on the results of humeral hemiarthroplasty in 21 shoulders of 20 patients with irreparable rotator cuff defects and glenohumeral arthritis who were followed up for an average of 4 years. During subscapularis repair, they invariably achieved 30 degrees of external rotation. To achieve this degree of motion in 6 shoulders, the subscapularis was removed subperiosteally from the lesser tuberosity and reattached 1 to 2 cm more medially through holes drilled near the edge of the humeral osteotomy. In 2 patients with deficient subscapularis muscles, the upper 50% of the pectoralis major was transferred to the lesser tuberosity. To prevent posterior instability in patients with posterior erosion of the glenoid, the osteotomy was made in only 10 to 15 degrees of retroversion. Twelve shoulders were not painful, 6 were mildly painful, and 3 were moderately painful. Patients with moderate pain who had undergone previous operations stated that the recent surgery ameliorated their pain.[2]

When performing hemiarthroplasty on the cuff-deficient arthritic shoulder, especially in the setting of previously failed cuff surgery,

the surgeon often encounters an incompetent coracoacromial arch. Some authors have augmented the arch with bone graft. In 1991, Wiley[26] reported on four patients in whom severe superior humeral head subluxation developed after resection of the coracoacromial ligament. Three of the patients also underwent repair of a large to massive cuff tear. These four cases were selected to illustrate the potential complications of debriding the cuff without repair and the value of retaining the coracoacromial arch. Two patients had undergone humeral head replacement arthroplasty. Subsequent treatment of these patients included capsular release and bone grafting of the coracoacromial arch with a 7.5-cm-long piece of iliac-crest bone (Fig. 4). Postoperatively, both patients had significant pain relief.

In contrast to this method, Engelbrecht and Heinert[27] described the concept of augmenting the superior aspect of the glenoid with

bone from the humeral head (Fig. 5), so as to resist humeral head migration in the superior direction. Both this technique and that of Wiley seek to reestablish a stable fulcrum. The technique of Engelbrecht and Heinert seems to make better sense biomechanically, as it reestablishes the fulcrum closer to the original instant center of rotation.

In 1997, Field et al[28] reviewed the data on 16 patients who had undergone humeral hemiarthroplasty for RCTA. The surgical technique and component sizing (with use of a small humeral head) were similar to those described by Arntz et al.[24] All tears were massive and were debrided without an attempt at repair. The average age of the patients was 74 years (range, 62 to 83 years), and follow-up averaged 33 months (range, 24 to 55 months). With the use of Neer's limited-goals criteria, the results in 10 patients were rated as successful; those in 6, as unsuccessful. Of the 6 patients with unsuccessful

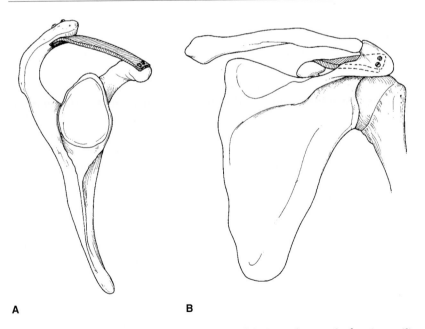

Fig. 4 Lateral-to-medial **(A)** and posteroanterior **(B)** views of a scapula showing an iliac-crest bone graft rigidly attached to the acromion and coracoid, serving to reconstitute a deficient coracoacromial arch.

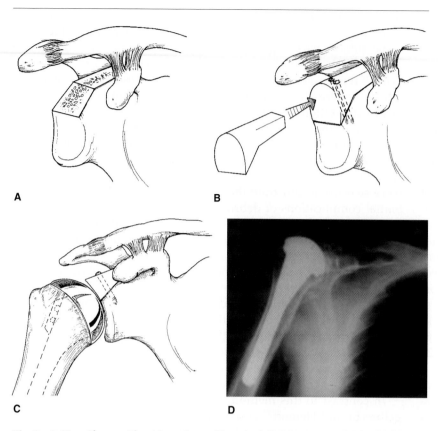

Fig. 5 **A,** Use of humeral head bone for grafting of a deficient superior pole of the glenoid serves to resist superior humeral migration. **B,** Placement of bone graft and fixation with screws. **C,** Topographic relationship of graft with prosthetic humeral head. **D,** Radiograph shows a graft in a 73-year-old man. Note the use of suture anchors for fixation into osteoporotic bone.

results, 4 had undergone at least one attempt at rotator cuff repair with acromioplasty before the index procedure, and 2 had deficient deltoid function after the rotator cuff surgery as a result of postoperative deltoid detachment. Also, 3 of these 4 patients who had previously undergone acromioplasty subsequently had anterosuperior subluxation after hemiarthroplasty. However, of the 12 patients with good deltoid function and an adequate coracoacromial arch, 10 had a successful result. This study illustrates that formal acromioplasty done in combination with repair of a torn rotator cuff may jeopardize the subsequent success of humeral hemiarthroplasty.

Humeral Hemiarthroplasty Versus Total Shoulder Arthroplasty

Lohr et al[4] briefly reported the results of RCTA in 22 shoulders in 22 patients with RCTA who were treated with either nonconstrained TSA, semiconstrained (i.e., hooded glenoid) TSA, or hemiarthroplasty. The mean follow-up period was 4 years 7 months. The hemiarthroplasty group had the poorest results for pain relief. However, the nonconstrained and semiconstrained TSA groups had a high incidence of radiologic and clinical loosening of the glenoid component. The authors concluded that although RCTA is one of the most difficult-to-treat shoulder entities, every attempt should be made to repair

the rotator cuff. In their study, nonconstrained TSA yielded the best results.

In 1992, Pollock et al[7] reviewed the results in 30 shoulders in 25 patients treated with either TSA (11 shoulders) or humeral hemiarthroplasty (19 shoulders) for glenohumeral arthritis with rotator cuff deficiency. Follow-up averaged 41 months. Seventeen arthroplasties were for RA or inflammatory arthritis, and 13 were for RCTA. Transposition of the subscapularis (Fig. 6) resulted in complete closure of superior rotator cuff defects in 15 shoulders and partial closure in 11. Four cuffs with massive defects could not be covered and were not reconstructed. Satisfactory results were achieved in all patients in the RA or inflammatory arthritis group and 11 of 13 in the RCTA group. All shoulders regained functional forward elevation and external rotation. Patient satisfaction was similar in the hemiarthroplasty and TSA groups, but the hemiarthroplasty group achieved greater postoperative range of motion. The authors concluded that hemiarthroplasty with attempted rotator cuff repair produced the best results in these patients.

A patient with OA and a small, easy-to-repair rotator cuff tear can usually be treated with a modular nonconstrained TSA. Severe bone loss in osteopenic patients generally requires fixation with polymethylmethacrylate. A deltopectoral approach is used. Many of these shoulders have osseous excrescences on the acromion and acromioclavicular joint arthritis, which can be dealt with in a standard fashion as long as the cuff is reparable. A slightly smaller humeral head or a tendency toward varus angulation during implantation will take pressure off the cuff repair. It is essential that 30 to 40 degrees of external rotation can be obtained

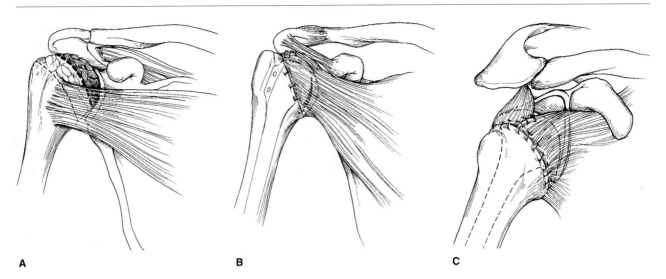

A   **B**   **C**

Fig. 6   **A,** Preoperative anteroposterior (AP) view of a right shoulder with a cuff tear and severe glenohumeral arthrosis. The broken line drawn obliquely across the proximal humeral head represents the direction of an osteotomy performed when there is an intact rotator cuff. The dotted line drawn obliquely across the more distal humeral head represents the more aggressive osteotomy used when performing an arthroplasty in shoulders with large, retracted rotator cuff tears. Postoperative AP **(B)** and oblique (superior-to-inferior) **(C)** views show use of a superiorly transposed subscapularis tendon to cover a large cuff defect; prosthetic humeral head has been recentered.

intraoperatively after repair of the subscapularis. Replacement of the glenoid is not recommended for patients with superior humeral head migration, as this finding is associated with a high incidence of glenoid loosening.

Some basic surgical principles should be emphasized before addressing specific details of this type of management. Protection of the axillary nerve is paramount, as contractures and joint deformities make it susceptible to intraoperative injury. The surgeon must have a thorough understanding of how to release joint contractures and safely mobilize the rotator cuff.[29] Mobilization may include (1) release of bursal adhesions from the subacromial and subdeltoid spaces, (2) release of the subscapularis from the capsule, (3) release of the contracted capsule from the glenoid labrum, (4) proximal mobilization of tendons,[30] (5) release or resection of the coracohumeral ligament, (6) rotator interval slide,[31] and/or (7) release of the upper 1 cm of the pectoralis major to facili-

tate exposure for mobilization of the subscapularis or the entire pectoralis major insertion if transfer is required.[2]

Neer et al[1] have stated that in rare cases a supplemental posterior incision may be needed to adequately mobilize the posterior rotators. Various methods of subscapularis lengthening may also be necessary in these stiff shoulders. If the cuff tear is small and the subscapularis tendon is of good quality, the tendon can be dissected subperiosteally off the lesser tuberosity as close as possible to the bicipital groove. This tissue can then be reattached to the anteromedial aspect of the anatomic neck with the use of suture and drill holes. For patients with massive rotator cuff tears, internal rotation contractures, and good-quality subscapularis tendon, a coronal Z-lengthening procedure is utilized. The subscapularis is not routinely separated from the joint capsule. The surgical approach is determined on the basis of whether or not the subscapularis is intact.[32]

Intact Subscapularis

Although many patients with an intact subscapularis have a negative lift-off test, they may have marked weakness with active forward flexion and external rotation. For these patients, a standard deltopectoral approach is appropriate. A more aggressive humeral osteotomy is also performed, which removes more bone than usual. The osteotomy follows a line extending laterally from approximately 1 cm above the lateral flare of the greater tuberosity to a point medially where, with firm manual downward traction on the arm, the humeral neck meets the inferior aspect of the glenoid. This satisfies three objectives: (1) it leaves an osseous margin to which the distal ends of the supraspinatus, infraspinatus, and subscapularis can be repaired; (2) it shortens the distance that the mobilized tendons must traverse; and (3) it centers the humeral head on the glenoid. Despite aggressive capsular releases inferiorly, the humeral head cannot be centered without this relatively large amount of bone resection.

When there is marked superior erosion of the glenoid, a burr is used to selectively remove bone from the inferior aspect of the glenoid until a superior shelf is created. The effective length of the subscapularis is increased by medializing the joint line, mobilizing the cuff, lowering the instant center of rotation, and using a smaller humeral head. These factors facilitate transposition of the subscapularis for covering large defects in the retracted supraspinatus tendon (Fig. 6). Preservation of the coracoacromial arch is extremely important for limiting anterosuperior migration. When the posterior glenoid is not eroded, the prosthesis should generally be retroverted more than usual (45 to 60 degrees), placing the greater part of the prosthetic head under the acromion. This maneuver ensures that, at the very least, the shoulder has captured-fulcrum mechanics[14] (Fig. 7). Although not routinely obtained, a computed tomographic scan of both shoulders can be useful for comparing glenoid version in some patients[33]; this information helps the surgeon to anticipate both the location and the amount of bone removal or augmentation that will be needed.

Deficient Subscapularis

If the patient has a positive lift-off test, the subscapularis is involved in the massive tear, and the patient has marked weakness with almost all active movements of the shoulder. In this situation, a superior approach, as described by Kessel,[34] is recommended; the acromial osteotomy facilitates increased exposure of the superior aspect of the glenohumeral joint. The acromion must be repaired accurately and securely. With an aggressive humeral osteotomy and reshaping of the glenoid with a burr, the resulting medialization of the glenoid usually allows repair of the subscapularis back to the lesser tuberosity and repair of the infraspinatus back to the greater tuberosity; however, the superior defect typically cannot be repaired. In our experience, use of humeral head bone to supplement the superior aspect of the glenoid has resulted in keeping the head centered in 3 of 5 patients followed up for more than 2 years (Fig. 5).

Deficient Deltoid

Even if the cuff defect is reparable or reconstructible, attempts at restoring motion or balancing force couples with prosthetic replacement and soft-tissue reconstruction are fruitless if the anterior deltoid is deficient due to detachment or denervation. In this case, glenohumeral fusion with the use of pelvic reconstruction plates, autogenous and/or allogeneic bone graft, scalene block anesthesia, and postoperative management of medical problems or metabolic bone disease make this an attractive alternative even for patients in their late 70s or 80s.

Postoperative Management

Postoperative management begins with preoperative education of the patient and her or his family, emphasizing that pain relief is the primary goal of surgery, and realistic expectations for range of motion and strength are typically limited.[1] On the first or second postoperative day, patients are taught passive exercises, which are continued for at least 6 weeks. These exercises may be delayed for 3 weeks if subscapularis reattachment or lengthening was performed. Between 6 and 9 weeks, depending on the size of the cuff tear and tissue quality, gentle active motion is allowed in all planes. When the rotator cuff repair is tenuous, an

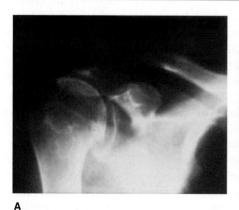
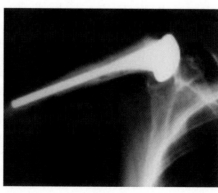
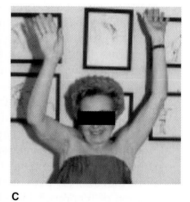

A   **B**   **C**

Fig. 7   **A,** Preoperative radiograph of a 73-year-old woman with RCTA treated with humeral hemiarthroplasty, glenoid burring, and superior transposition of the subscapularis. Radiograph **(B)** and clinical photograph **(C)** obtained 10 months after the procedure illustrate improved abduction.

abduction pillow can be used for the first 4 to 6 weeks. At approximately 3 weeks, pulley and internal-external rotation exercises on the pillow are started. When the bone graft across the superior aspect of the glenoid has united, active range of motion is initiated. Resisted strengthening is begun between 9 and 12 weeks.

In a small series compiled at our institution from 1987 to 1990, four types of surgical management were used to improve results in this group of patients: (1) bipolar prosthesis without cuff repair; (2) large-head hemiarthroplasty without cuff repair, (3) small-head hemiarthroplasty with subscapularis transposition, and (4) nonconstrained TSA with cuff repair. The results in 18 patients followed up for at least 2 years suggested that repair of large rotator cuff defects with subscapularis transposition and humeral hemiarthroplasty

with a relatively small head yielded the most reliable results.

Summary

The patient must realize that surgery will predictably provide pain relief, but that improvements in motion and strength are less predictable. The functional result will depend on the condition of the rotator cuff and deltoid muscle. The results are nearly always inferior to those that can be obtained with conventional prosthetic arthroplasty in shoulders with functionally intact cuffs.

A concerted effort must be made to repair the rotator cuff defect, resurface the arthritic humerus (hemiarthroplasty), and smooth the arthritic glenoid with a burr. Humeral hemiarthroplasty avoids the complications of glenoid loosening and is an attractive alternative to arthrodesis, resection arthroplasty,

constrained TSA, and semiconstrained TSA. The coracoacromial arch should be preserved and functionally intact to reduce the risk of anterosuperior subluxation. Care should be taken not to "overstuff" the glenohumeral joint with prosthetic components. When patients report considerably reduced internal rotation because of soft-tissue contracture, subscapularis lengthening or medialization or both are necessary to restore anterior and posterior rotator cuff balance. With the less stringent criteria of Neer's limited-goals rehabilitation, approximately 80% to 90% of patients treated with humeral hemiarthroplasty can have satisfactory results.[3,8]

Glenohumeral arthrodesis is a salvage procedure when other surgical measures have failed. It is also a viable option for patients who have undergone multiple operations and for patients with deltoid muscle deficiency.

References

1. Neer CS II, Craig EV, Fukuda H: Cuff-tear arthropathy. *J Bone Joint Surg Am* 1983;65:1232-1244.
2. Williams GR Jr, Rockwood CA Jr: Massive rotator cuff defects and glenohumeral arthritis, in Friedman RJ (ed): *Arthroplasty of the Shoulder.* New York: Thieme Medical Publishers, 1994, pp 204-214.
3. Matsen FA III, Arntz CT, Harryman DT II: Rotator cuff tear arthropathy, in Bigliani LU (ed): *Complications of Shoulder Surgery.* Baltimore: Williams & Wilkins, 1993, pp 44-58.
4. Lohr JF, Cofield RH, Uhthoff HK: Glenoid component loosening in cuff tear arthropathy [abstract]. *J Bone Joint Surg Br* 1991;73(suppl 2):106.
5. Hawkins R, Bell RH, Jallay B: Total shoulder arthroplasty. *Clin Orthop* 1989;242:188-194.
6. Franklin JL, Barrett WP, Jackins SE, Matsen FA III: Glenoid loosening in total shoulder arthroplasty: Association with rotator cuff deficiency. *J Arthroplasty* 1988;3:39-46.
7. Pollock RG, Deliz ED, McIlveen SJ,

Flatow EL, Bigliani LU: Prosthetic replacement in rotator cuff–deficient shoulders. *J Shoulder Elbow Surg* 1992;1:173-186.
8. Swanson AB, Swanson GG: Bipolar shoulder arthroplasty, in Friedman RJ (ed): *Arthroplasty of the Shoulder.* New York: Thieme Medical Publishers, 1994, pp 265-280.
9. Neer CS II, Watson KC, Stanton FJ: Recent experience in total shoulder replacement. *J Bone Joint Surg Am* 1982;64:319-337.
10. Cofield RH: Total shoulder arthroplasty with the Neer prosthesis. *J Bone Joint Surg Am* 1984;66:899-906.
11. Marmor L: Hemiarthroplasty for the rheumatoid shoulder joint. *Clin Orthop* 1977;122:201-203.
12. Halverson PB, Cheung HS, McCarty DJ, Garancis JC, Mandel N: "Milwaukee shoulder": Association of microspheroids containing hydroxyapatite crystals, active collagenase, and neutral protease with rotator cuff defects—II. Synovial fluid studies. *Arthritis Rheum* 1981;24:474-483.

13. Halverson PB, Carrera GF, McCarty DJ: Milwaukee shoulder syndrome: Fifteen additional cases and a description of contributing factors. *Arch Intern Med* 1990;150:677-682.
14. Burkhart SS: A unified biomechanical rationale for the treatment of rotator cuff tears: Debridement versus repair, in Burkhead WZ Jr (ed): *Rotator Cuff Disorders.* Baltimore: Williams & Wilkins, 1996, pp 293-312.
15. Klimaitis A, Carroll G, Owen E: Rapidly progressive destructive arthropathy of the shoulder: A viewpoint on pathogenesis. *J Rheumatol* 1988;15:1859-1862.
16. Dieppe P, Watt I: Crystal deposition in osteoarthritis: An opportunistic event? *Clin Rheum Dis* 1985;11:367-392.
17. Campion GV, McCrae F, Alwan W, Watt I, Bradfield J, Dieppe PA: Idiopathic destructive arthritis of the shoulder. *Semin Arthritis Rheum* 1988;17:232-245.
18. Cofield RH: Degenerative and arthritic problems of the glenohumeral joint, in Rockwood CA Jr, Matsen FA III

(eds): *The Shoulder*. Philadelphia: WB Saunders, 1990, vol 2, pp 678-749.

19. Cofield RH, Briggs BT: Glenohumeral arthrodesis: Operative and long-term functional results. *J Bone Joint Surg Am* 1979;61:668-677.

20. Arntz CT, Matsen FA III, Jackins S: Surgical management of complex irreparable rotator cuff deficiency. *J Arthroplasty* 1991;6:363-370.

21. Laurence M: Replacement arthroplasty of the rotator cuff deficient shoulder. *J Bone Joint Surg Br* 1991;73:916-919.

22. Barrett WP, Franklin JL, Jackins SE, Wyss CR, Matsen FA III: Total shoulder arthroplasty. *J Bone Joint Surg Am* 1987;69:865-872.

23. Lee DH, Niemann KMW: Bipolar shoulder arthroplasty. *Clin Orthop* 1994;304:97-107.

24. Arntz CT, Jackins S, Matsen FA III: Prosthetic replacement of the shoulder for the treatment of defects in the rotator cuff and the surface of the glenohumeral joint. *J Bone Joint Surg Am* 1993;75:485-491.

25. Williams GR Jr, Rockwood CA Jr: Hemiarthroplasty in rotator cuff-deficient shoulders. *J Shoulder Elbow Surg* 1996;5:362-367.

26. Wiley AM: Superior humeral dislocation: A complication following decompression and debridement for rotator cuff tears. *Clin Orthop* 1991; 263:135-141.

27. Engelbrecht E, Heinert K: More than ten years' experience with unconstrained shoulder replacement, in Kölbel R, Helbig B, Blauth W (eds); Telger TC (trans): *Shoulder Replacement*. Berlin: Springer-Verlag, 1987, pp 85-91.

28. Field LD, Dines DM, Zabinski SJ, Warren RF: Hemiarthroplasty of the shoulder for rotator cuff arthropathy. *J Shoulder Elbow Surg* 1997;6:18-23.

29. Codd TP, Flatow EL: Anterior acromioplasty, tendon mobilization, and direct repair of massive rotator cuff tears, in Burkhead WZ Jr (ed): *Rotator Cuff Disorders*. Baltimore: Williams & Wilkins, 1996, pp 323-334.

30. Warner JJP, Krushell RJ, Masquelet A, Gerber C: Anatomy and relationships of the suprascapular nerve: Anatomical constraints to mobilization of the supraspinatus and infraspinatus muscles in the management of massive rotator-cuff tears. *J Bone Joint Surg Am* 1992;74:36-45.

31. Bigliani LU, Cordasco FA, McIlveen SJ, Musso ES: Operative repair of massive rotator cuff tears: Long-term results. *J Shoulder Elbow Surg* 1992;1: 120-130.

32. Codd TP, Pollock RG, Flatow EL: Prosthetic replacement in the rotator cuff-deficient shoulder. *Techniques Orthop* 1994;8:174-183.

33. Randelli M, Gambrioli PL: Glenohumeral osteometry by computed tomography in normal and unstable shoulders. *Clin Orthop* 1986;208: 151-156.

34. Kessel L: The transacromial approach for rotator cuff rupture, in Bayley J, Kessel L (eds): *Shoulder Surgery*. New York: Springer-Verlag, 1982, pp 39-44.

JBJS

THE JOURNAL OF BONE & JOINT SURGERY

JAAOS

JOURNAL OF THE AMERICAN ACADEMY OF ORTHOPAEDIC

section five

Complications and Salvage Procedures

Clinical Outcome After Structural Failure of Rotator Cuff Repairs*

BY BERNHARD JOST, M.D.†, CHRISTIAN W. A. PFIRRMANN, M.D.†,
AND CHRISTIAN GERBER, M.D.†, ZURICH, SWITZERLAND

Investigation performed at University of Zurich, Zurich

Abstract

Background: The clinical outcome for patients with documented rerupture after open repair of one or more rotator cuff tendons is not well known. The purpose of this study was to evaluate the clinical outcomes of a consecutive series of rotator cuff reruptures after repair and to provide information concerning the advisability of rotator cuff repair in situations in which there may be a high probability of rerupture.

Methods: During prospective follow-up after rotator cuff repairs, we detected, with magnetic resonance imaging, structural failure of the repair in twenty patients, who had a mean age of fifty-nine years at the time of the rotator cuff repair. All patients were clinically examined for the purpose of this report at a mean of thirty-eight months.

Results: The reruptures invariably involved the originally torn tendon but were smaller than the original tear in sixteen of the twenty patients. Fatty degeneration of the supraspinatus and infraspinatus muscles, atrophy of the supraspinatus muscle, and glenohumeral osteoarthritis progressed significantly from the preoperative state ($p < 0.05$). At the time of the most recent follow-up, the subjective shoulder value averaged 75 percent of the value for a normal shoulder. Eleven patients were very satisfied with the result, six were satisfied, two were disappointed, and one was dissatisfied. The mean relative score according to the system of Constant and Murley had increased from 49 percent of the score for a normal shoulder preoperatively to 83 percent postoperatively ($p = 0.0001$). Pain had decreased significantly, and the ranges of active, pain-free forward elevation and abduction as well as the abduction strength had improved significantly ($p < 0.05$). The clinical outcome was significantly correlated with the size of the postoperative tear, the stage of postoperative fatty muscle degeneration of the infraspinatus and subscapularis, the postoperative acromiohumeral distance, and the degree of postoperative glenohumeral osteoarthritis ($p < 0.05$).

Conclusions: This study documents that an attempt at rotator cuff repair significantly decreases pain ($p = 0.0026$) and significantly improves function ($p = 0.0005$) and strength ($p = 0.0137$) even if magnetic resonance imaging documents that the repair has failed. This finding suggests that the potential for rerupture should not be considered a formal contraindication to an attempt at repair if optimal functional recovery is the goal of treatment.

*No benefits in any form have been received or will be received from a commercial party related directly or indirectly to the subject of this article. No funds were received in support of this study.
†Department of Orthopedics (B. J. and C. G.) and Division of Diagnostic Radiology (C. W. A. P.), University of Zurich, Balgrist, Forchstrasse 340, 8008 Zurich, Switzerland. E-mail address for Christian Gerber: cgerber@balgrist.unizh.ch.

Rates of rerupture after open rotator cuff repair have been reported to range from 13 percent[1] (fourteen of 108) to 68 percent[16] (fifteen of twenty-two)[1,10,14,16,21,25,32], depending on the size of the original tear. The functional outcome for patients with a rerupture is not well known. With the success of arthroscopic débridement[7,8,26,37], the question arises regarding whether an attempt at rotator cuff repair necessitating more postoperative rehabilitation is justified if débridement yields satisfactory results and the chance of failure of the repair is high. The purpose of this study was to identify and analyze a consecutive series of patients with structural failure defined by magnetic resonance imaging criteria after open rotator cuff repair; to assess their preoperative state in terms of pain, function, and strength; and to determine whether progression of degenerative changes in terms of muscle atrophy, fatty muscle degeneration, and glenohumeral osteoarthritis could be identified. Finally, we sought to determine the relevance of the preoperative history, intraoperative findings, and sizes of the original and repeat tears relative to the end result.

Materials and Methods

Twenty rotator cuff reruptures were identified with postoperative magnetic resonance imaging in a series of sixty-five consecutive patients who had had a repair of a full-thickness tear of the rotator cuff. Of the twenty patients who had a rerupture, thirteen were men and seven were women; the mean age at the time of the index operation was fifty-nine years (range, forty-seven to seventy-one years). The reruptures were diagnosed with the use of established magnetic resonance imaging criteria[15,24,27]. Initially, eight patients had had a tear of one tendon (the supraspinatus), ten had had a tear of two tendons (the supraspinatus and the subscapularis in five and the supraspinatus and the infraspinatus in five), and two patients had had a tear of three tendons.

TABLE I
DATA ON THE PATIENTS

Case	Age at Index Op. (yrs.)	Gender	Duration of Follow-up (mos.)	No. of Previous Ops.	Torn Tendons at Index Op.	Duration of Symptoms (mos.)	History of Trauma
1	59	M	40	0	Supraspinatus	10	No
2	66	F	45	0	Supraspinatus	12	No
3	56	M	34	0	Supraspinatus	48	Yes
4	61	M	42	0	Supraspinatus	10	No
5	64	M	33	0	Supraspinatus	14	Yes
6	71	F	27	0	Supraspinatus	24	No
7	67	M	34	0	Supraspinatus	10	No
8	56	F	39	0	Supraspinatus	8	Yes
9	47	M	40	1	Supraspinatus, subscapularis	11	Yes
10	51	M	33	0	Supraspinatus, subscapularis	18	Yes
11	51	M	39	0	Supraspinatus, subscapularis	6	Yes
12	67	M	47	0	Supraspinatus, subscapularis	8	No
13	55	M	33	0	Supraspinatus, subscapularis	5	Yes
14	56	F	49	0	Supraspinatus, infraspinatus	3	Yes
15	55	F	27	0	Supraspinatus, infraspinatus	36	No
16	68	F	30	0	Supraspinatus, infraspinatus	8	Yes
17	49	F	29	1	Supraspinatus, infraspinatus	3	Yes
18	64	M	38	0	Supraspinatus, infraspinatus	7	No
19	56	M	47	0	Supraspinatus, infraspinatus, subscapularis	36	No
20	58	M	48	0	Supraspinatus, infraspinatus, subscapularis	11	Yes
Mean	59		38			14	

Seventeen patients had involvement of the dominant side (Table I).

Findings at the Index Operation

In eleven of the twenty patients, the quality of the tendon of the supraspinatus muscle had been judged to be fair or poor on the basis of unusually poor holding power for sutures or brittle, myxomatous macrostructure. After mobilization of the torn musculotendinous units, the tendons were grasped with nonresorbable sutures according to the modified Mason-Allen technique[11,12]. Both strands of one stitch were brought through the tuberosity and knotted over two holes of a thin titanium plate with seven rounded holes (Stratec Synthes SA, Oberdorf, Switzerland), which served as a cortical bone augmentation device[11,12]. The titanium plate does not cut the sutures and does not interfere with assessment of the operatively treated shoulder with magnetic resonance imaging. In one patient (Case 14), the supraspinatus tendon was unexpectedly found to be too far retracted and too degenerated to allow complete reinsertion on the greater tuberosity, so only a partial repair could be performed. An anterior acromioplasty was performed in sixteen of the twenty patients. An acromioplasty was avoided if postoperative anterosuperior subluxation seemed likely due to difficulties in obtaining an optimal closure of the rotator interval; this was the case for massive tears involving the supraspinatus and the subscapularis (four patients). Furthermore, five patients had a tenotomy or tenodesis of the tendon of the long head of the biceps muscle because it was either degenerated or partially ruptured. The decision to perform a tenotomy rather than a tenodesis was based on cosmetic considerations for the individual patient (there may be bulging of the biceps muscle after tenotomy). In four patients,

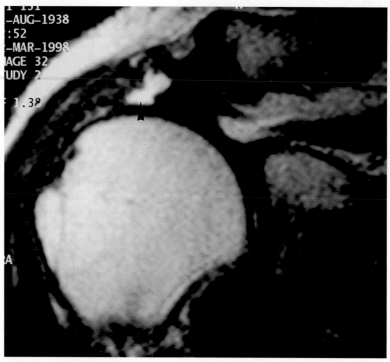

FIG. 1

Case 3. Postoperative T2-weighted coronal magnetic resonance image of a right shoulder, showing a small rerupture in the anterior part of the supraspinatus tendon (arrowhead), which was seen thirty-four months after a supraspinatus repair.

the long head of the biceps tendon was already torn at the index operation.

Postoperative Rehabilitation

Ten patients wore an abduction splint on the arm for six weeks postoperatively because the intraoperative quality of the supraspinatus had been thought to be poor (five patients), the reinserted supraspinatus tendon had been under tension (three patients), or the index operation was a reoperation for a failed repair of a rotator cuff tendon (two patients). The remaining ten patients, most of whom had had a large subscapularis lesion, wore only a sling for six weeks. Immediately postoperatively, passive range-of-motion exercises were begun within the range that had been found to be safe intraoperatively. Active range-of-motion exercises were started after six weeks. Strengthening of the rotator cuff muscles was begun after twelve weeks.

Complications

No patient had hematoma, wound dehiscence, infection, stiffness necessitating manipulation, deltoid dehiscence, or neural injury. At the time of the most recent follow-up, only one patient (Case 8) had had a reoperation; this patient had had an arthroscopic débridement because of persistent pain.

Clinical Assessment

At the most recent follow-up evaluation, clinical assessment was performed, in a standardized fashion, for the purpose of this study by a single examiner (B. J.) who was not the operating surgeon (C. G.). The clinical assessment consisted of a structured interview and a detailed physical examination including all elements needed for assessment of shoulder function according to the system of Constant and Murley[5,6]. This score is based on a scale of 100 points. A maximum of 35 points is assigned for subjective variables (pain, activities of daily living, and functional use of the arm); 40 points, for range of motion; and 25 points, for quantitative measurement of abduction strength.

Active shoulder motion was measured with the patient sitting. The range of flexion was assessed in the sagittal plane as the angle between the humeral shaft and the midthoracic line (not the vertical). Abduction was always measured with simultaneous maximal abduction of both arms as the angle of the humeral shaft with the midthoracic line. Active external rotation was assessed, according to the method of Constant and Murley[5,6], while the patient performed five functional external rotation movements without touching the head with the hand. Internal rotation was determined by the spinous process that the patient could reach with the thumb. Abduction strength was measured with the patient standing and the arm abducted to 90 degrees in the scapular plane with the elbow extended and the forearm pronated. The resistance of an Isobex dynamometer (Cursor SA, Bern, Switzerland) was applied to the wrist, and three consecutive measurements of a duration of five seconds each (the B mode of the device) were averaged to measure the strength. One point was attributed per 0.48 kilogram of strength measured[6]. If 90 degrees of abduction was not achieved, abduction strength was automatically considered to be zero. The total score obtained was also related to the age and gender-matched normal values that had been identified by Constant[5], and the respective value was called the relative Constant score. In addition, the patients estimated the value of the operatively treated shoulder as a percentage of the value for an entirely normal shoulder (that is, 100 percent). This value was called the subjective shoulder value.

Although clinical data on both shoulders were collected for comparison of the treated and contralateral limbs, the high prevalence of symptomatic disease of the contralateral shoulder precluded the use of the contralateral side for meaningful comparison.

Radiographic Assessment

For all twenty patients, postoperative radiographic assessment included standardized radiographs (anteroposterior radiographs with the arm in neutral rotation and axillary lateral radiographs) and magnetic resonance imaging. Magnetic resonance imaging was performed with a 1.0-tesla scanner (Siemens, Erlangen, Germany). Continuity or rerupture of the tendon was assessed on coronal oblique T2-weighted and proton-density-weighted images as well as short inversion recovery sequences according to established magnetic resonance imaging criteria[15,24,27]. When a fluid-equivalent signal or nonvisualization of the supraspinatus, infraspinatus, or subscapularis tendon was found on at least one T2-weighted or fat-suppressed section, the diagnosis of a full-thickness rerupture was made[27]. Additionally acquired parasagittal T1-weighted turbo spin-echo magnetic resonance images parallel to the glenohumeral joint were obtained for qualitative and quantitative assessment of the rotator cuff muscles[36]. The slices covered the rotator cuff from the humeral tuberosities to the medial third of the scapula. Cross-sectional areas of the supraspinatus were measured on the most lateral image on which the scapular spine was in contact with the scapular body (Y-shaped view)[36]. Intramuscular fatty degeneration and atrophy of the muscle bellies were assessed as described by Goutallier et al.[14] for computed tomography scanning and validated by Fuchs et al.[9] for magnetic resonance imaging.

The preoperative radiographic assessment included magnetic resonance imaging (nineteen patients) or computed tomography scanning (one patient) and standard radiographs. In order to compare the preoperative and postoperative extents of the rotator cuff defect, the sizes of the tears were assessed on the basis of the maximal mediolateral and anteroposterior diameters. Preoperative and postoperative glenohumeral osteoarthritic changes were assessed on standard radiographs according to the classification of Samilson and Prieto[31].

Statistical Methods

The Mann-Whitney U test was used for unpaired groups, and the Wilcoxon test was used for paired

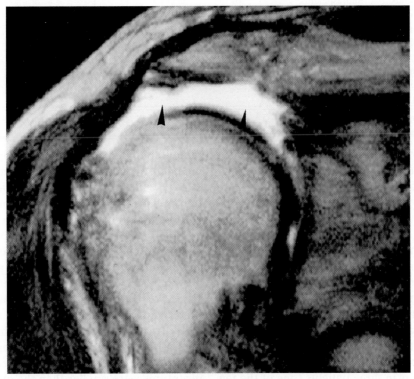

FIG. 2

Case 12. Postoperative T2-weighted coronal magnetic resonance image of a right shoulder with a large rerupture of the entire supraspinatus tendon with marked retraction (arrowheads) as well as extension into the infraspinatus, which was seen forty-seven months after a supraspinatus and subscapularis repair.

TABLE II

COMPARISON OF PREOPERATIVE AND POSTOPERATIVE STRUCTURAL PARAMETERS AS SEEN ON MAGNETIC RESONANCE IMAGING

| | Torn Tendons | | Size of Tear (mm^2) | | Fatty Degeneration $(stage^{9,14})$ | | | |
| | | | | | Supraspinatus | | Infraspinatus | |
Case	Preop.	Postop.	Preop.	Postop.	Preop.	Postop.	Preop.	Postop.
1	Supraspinatus	Supraspinatus	236	25	1	1	0	1
2	Supraspinatus	Supraspinatus	603	38	1	1	1	1
3	Supraspinatus	Supraspinatus	393	38	0	0	0	0
4	Supraspinatus*	Supraspinatus	550*	80	2*	2	2*	2
5	Supraspinatus	Supraspinatus	589	94	1	1	1	1
6	Supraspinatus	Supraspinatus	294	251	1	1	1	1
7	Supraspinatus	Supraspinatus	1374	353	2	4	1	1
8	Supraspinatus	Supraspinatus	314	785	1	3	1	2
9	Supraspinatus, subscapularis	Supraspinatus, infraspinatus	1413	50	1	1	1	2
10	Supraspinatus, subscapularis	Supraspinatus, subscapularis	2159	565	4	4	1	2
11	Supraspinatus, subscapularis	Supraspinatus	2159	589	2	2	1	2
12	Supraspinatus, subscapularis	Supraspinatus, infraspinatus	471	1295	1	2	2	2
13	Supraspinatus, subscapularis	Supraspinatus, subscapularis	2355	1963	1	2	1	2
14	Supraspinatus, infraspinatus	Supraspinatus	2159	392	3	4	2	3
15	Supraspinatus, infraspinatus	Supraspinatus, infraspinatus	687	471	1	2	2	3
16	Supraspinatus, infraspinatus	Supraspinatus	1766	1099	1	4	2	2
17	Supraspinatus, infraspinatus	Supraspinatus, infraspinatus	1570	2159	2	4	1	4
18	Supraspinatus, infraspinatus	Supraspinatus, infraspinatus	707	2355	1	2	1	4
19	Supraspinatus, infraspinatus, subscapularis	Supraspinatus, infraspinatus	1178	942	2	3	2	4
20	Supraspinatus, infraspinatus, subscapularis	Supraspinatus	2159	1256	2	2	2	3

*Finding was on a computed tomography scan.

groups. The level of significance was set at p < 0.05. Spearman's correlation coefficient was used to test relationships between variables.

Results

Imaging

The mean acromiohumeral distance measured on a true anteroposterior radiograph with the forearm in neutral rotation decreased significantly (p = 0.01), from ten millimeters (range, seven to thirteen millimeters) before the operation to 8.4 millimeters (range, four to twelve millimeters) at the time of follow-up at a mean of thirty-eight months (range, twenty-seven to forty-nine months) postoperatively. The distance was less than seven millimeters in three patients (one of the ten who initially had had a two-tendon tear and both of the patients who initially had had a three-tendon tear), reflecting a large rotator cuff tear[34]. On the axillary lateral

radiograph, the humeral head appeared centered in nineteen of the twenty patients. In one patient (Case 17), who had sustained a traumatic posterior dislocation of the shoulder with the rotator cuff tear, the head was slightly subluxated posteriorly.

Osteoarthritic changes, as assessed according to the classification of Samilson and Prieto[31], had increased significantly (p = 0.002) from the preoperative to the postoperative evaluation, but never by more than one stage. At the time of follow-up, stage-II osteoarthritis was found in four patients (three who had originally had a two-tendon tear and one who had had a three-tendon tear). Three of these four patients had a retear that was larger than the original tear. Overall, sixteen reruptures were smaller than the original tear and four (one in the one-tendon-tear group and three in the two-tendon-tear group) were larger than the initial tear. The mean decrease in the tear size from the pre-

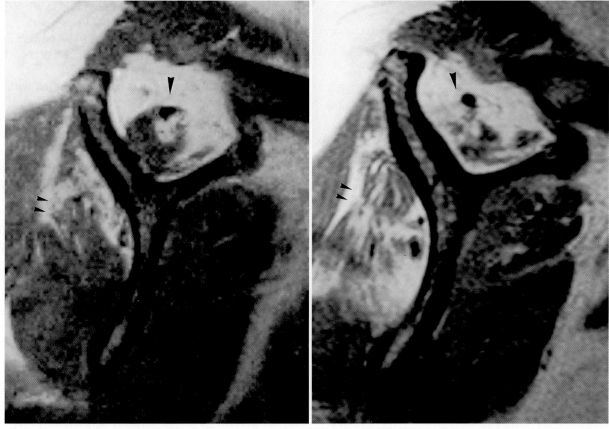

FIG. 3-A   FIG. 3-B

Case 14. T1-weighted parasagittal magnetic resonance images of a right shoulder, made before (Fig. 3-A) and forty-nine months after (Fig. 3-B) operative repair of a large supraspinatus and infraspinatus tear. The repair structurally failed in the supraspinatus tendon. A comparison of the preoperative and postoperative radiographs shows progressive atrophy and fatty degeneration of the supraspinatus muscle (single arrowhead) and the infraspinatus muscle (double arrowheads).

operative to the postoperative evaluation was significant for the entire series of twenty patients (p = 0.045) and for the ten patients who originally had had a two-tendon tear (p = 0.032), but it was not found to be significant for the eight patients who had had a one-tendon tear (p = 0.078), probably because of the small number of patients.

Structural failure always involved the repaired tendon and always involved the supraspinatus (Fig. 1). It extended into an infraspinatus that had been intact at the time of the index operation in only two patients (Fig. 2).

Fatty muscle degeneration of the supraspinatus progressed in ten patients (two of the eight who had originally had a one-tendon tear, seven of the ten who had had a two-tendon tear, and one of the two who had had a three-tendon tear). Progression of fatty muscle degeneration was significant in the entire series (p = 0.002) and in the patients who had had a two-tendon tear (p = 0.016), but it was not found to be significant, with the numbers available, in the patients who had had a one-tendon tear (p = 0.5). Fatty muscle degeneration of the infraspinatus progressed in twelve patients (two who had originally had a one-tendon tear, eight who had had a two-tendon tear, and two who had had a

three-tendon tear). The progression was significant in the entire series (p = 0.0005) and in the patients who had had a two-tendon tear (p = 0.007), but it was not found to be significant in the patients who had had a one-tendon tear (p = 0.5). In the two-tendon-tear group, fatty muscle degeneration of the infraspinatus progressed in four of the five patients in whom the tendon of the infraspinatus had been intact at the index operation and in the four patients in whom the infraspinatus had not been successfully repaired (Figs. 3-A and 3-B) (Table II). Fatty muscle degeneration of the subscapularis was not found to have progressed significantly (p = 0.147), with the numbers available.

Muscle atrophy of the supraspinatus could be assessed in a standardized fashion on eleven preoperative magnetic resonance images and on all postoperative images. The postoperative cross-sectional area as seen on the Y-shaped image decreased significantly in ten of the eleven patients (p = 0.007); nine of the ten had originally had a two-tendon tear.

Clinical Evaluation

Eleven patients were very satisfied with the result, six were satisfied, two were disappointed, and one was dissatisfied. No patient thought that the shoulder was

TABLE III
POSTOPERATIVE CLINICAL RESULTS

Case	Relative Constant[5,6] Score* (percent)	Subjective Shoulder Value† (percent)	Patient Satisfaction
1	100	100	Very satisfied
2	100	90	Very satisfied
3	79	50	Satisfied
4	80	60	Very satisfied
5	100	100	Very satisfied
6	100	90	Satisfied
7	100	100	Very satisfied
8	74	80	Disappointed
9	94	100	Very satisfied
10	88	90	Very satisfied
11	54	50	Satisfied
12	61	50	Satisfied
13	88	80	Very satisfied
14	96	80	Very satisfied
15	100	90	Satisfied
16	100	70	Very satisfied
17	49	50	Not satisfied
18	73	50	Satisfied
19	78	70	Very satisfied
20	54	50	Disappointed

*The relative Constant score is given as a percentage of an age and gender-related normal value[5,6].

†The subjective shoulder value represents the patient's estimation of the value of the operatively treated shoulder as a percentage of the value of an entirely normal shoulder.

worse than it had been preoperatively. At the time of follow-up, the mean subjective shoulder value was 75 percent of the value for a normal shoulder. The mean relative Constant score increased from 49 percent preoperatively to 83 percent at the most recent follow-up evaluation (p = 0.0001). Nine patients had a relative Constant score of at least 90 percent (Table III). Patients with a one-tendon tear at the index operation were not found to have a significantly higher mean relative postoperative Constant score than those with a two-tendon tear (92 compared with 80 percent, p = 0.1457). The Constant score correlated well with the subjective shoulder value (r = 0.82, p < 0.0001). Pain decreased significantly (p = 0.0026), with eight patients being pain-free (a Constant score of 15 points) and only one patient having severe pain (a Constant score of 0 points). The ability to carry out activities of daily living was significantly improved (p = 0.0002), with ten patients having no limitations (a Constant score of 10 points), as was functional use of the arm (p = 0.0005), with thirteen patients having no limitations (a Constant score of 10 points). Except for external rotation (p = 0.1805), the ranges of active motion increased significantly (p ≤ 0.0006). The mean abduction strength improved significantly (p = 0.0137), from 1.7 to 3.2 kilograms (Table IV). Except for postoperative abduction

strength (4.8 compared with 2.2 kilograms, p = 0.0021), the results for the patients who had been operated on for a one-tendon tear were not found to be significantly better than the results for those who had had a two or three-tendon tear (Table V).

The sixteen patients who had been treated with an acromioplasty were not found to have better clinical results (p = 0.143), with the numbers available, than the four who had not. We also found no difference in the clinical outcome for the nine patients who had had a rupture of the long head of the biceps tendon, a biceps tenotomy, or a biceps tenodesis (p = 0.38). Three patients (Cases 17, 18, and 19) with rupture of the infraspinatus at the index operation were not able to actively externally rotate the treated shoulder at the time of follow-up and had a positive lag sign[17] for the supraspinatus and infraspinatus.

The small number of reruptures (four) that were larger than the initial tear did not allow for statistical comparison of preoperative and postoperative parameters in this group. The mean postoperative subjective shoulder value in this group (58 percent) was not found to be significantly different (p = 0.058) from the value for the sixteen patients in whom the rerupture was smaller than the initial tear (79 percent). The four patients with the larger reruptures had a mean relative Constant score of 64 percent postoperatively (45 percent preoperatively) compared with 88 percent postoperatively for the sixteen patients with the smaller reruptures (p = 0.016). All four patients with the larger reruptures had an improvement in the absolute Constant score, although one (Case 17) had only 2 points of improvement. The mean postoperative score for pain in this group (6.3 points) did not improve compared with the mean preoperative score (6.8 points), and the patients with the larger reruptures had more pain postoperatively (6.3 points) than did the patients with the smaller reruptures (12.6 points) (p = 0.03). Except for external rotation, which decreased from 31 degrees preoperatively to 16 degrees postoperatively, the active ranges of motion in the group with the larger reruptures improved compared with the preoperative ranges. Flexion improved from 90 to 124 degrees; abduction, from 91 to 113 degrees; and internal rotation, from 6 to 8.5 points. With the numbers available, no significant difference could be detected between the active ranges of motion of the patients with the larger reruptures and those of the patients with the smaller reruptures (124 compared with 151 degrees for flexion [p = 0.108], 113 compared with 158 degrees for abduction [p = 0.118], 16 compared with 40 degrees for external rotation [p = 0.088], and 8.5 compared with 8.8 points for internal rotation [p = 0.773]). Abduction strength in the four patients who had the larger reruptures was 1.7 kilograms compared with 3.6 kilograms in the patients with the smaller reruptures (p = 0.13). No preoperative or intraoperative risk factors for the development of a rerupture that was larger than the initial tear could be identified.

TABLE IV

COMPARISON OF PREOPERATIVE AND POSTOPERATIVE CLINICAL PARAMETERS IN THE ENTIRE SERIES OF TWENTY PATIENTS

Component	Preop.	Postop.	P Value*
Subjective shoulder value† (percent)		75	
Constant score[5,6]			
Total			
Absolute (points)	40	69	0.0001
Relative‡ (percent)	49	83	0.0001
Pain (points)	5	11.4	0.0026
Activities of daily living (points)	3.7	8.3	0.0002
Functional use of arm (points)	4.5	8.7	0.0005
Active mobility			
Flexion (degrees)	104	146	0.0002
Abduction (degrees)	105	149	0.0006
External rotation (degrees)	39	35	0.1805
Internal rotation (Constant score) (points)	6.4	8.7	0.0001
Abduction strength§ (kg)	1.7	3.2	0.0137

*The p values were determined with use of the Wilcoxon signed-rank test (level of significance, $p < 0.05$).

†The subjective shoulder value represents the patient's estimation of the value of the operatively treated shoulder as a percentage of the value of an entirely normal shoulder.

‡The relative Constant score is given as a percentage of an age and gender-related normal value[5,6].

§The abduction strength was measured with an Isobex dynamometer.

Correlation Between Preoperative and Postoperative Functional and Imaging Parameters

The postoperative Constant score as well as the postoperative abduction strength ($r = -0.75$, $p = 0.0001$, and $r = -0.61$, $p = 0.004$, respectively) correlated significantly with the size of the rerupture but not with the size of the preoperative tear ($r = -0.24$, $p = 0.303$, and $r = -0.08$, $p = 0.73$).

There was no correlation between the postoperative Constant score and fatty muscle degeneration of the supraspinatus ($r = -0.27$, $p = 0.246$ preoperatively and $r = -0.21$, $p = 0.378$ postoperatively). The Constant score correlated significantly with postoperative fatty muscle degeneration of the infraspinatus ($r = -0.55$, $p = 0.012$) and the subscapularis ($r = -0.51$, $p = 0.023$) but not with preoperative fatty degeneration of either the infraspinatus ($r = -0.11$, $p = 0.653$) or the subscapularis ($r = -0.3$, $p = 0.204$).

The degree of osteoarthritis seen on the postoperative radiographs was also significantly correlated with the postoperative Constant score ($r = -0.63$, $p = 0.003$) and the size of the rerupture ($r = 0.8$, $p < 0.0001$) but not with the size of the preoperative tear ($r = 0.38$, $p = 0.094$) or postoperative pain ($r = 0.29$, $p = 0.214$).

The postoperative acromiohumeral distance correlated significantly with the postoperative Constant score ($r = 0.52$, $p = 0.02$), the size of the rerupture ($r = -0.59$, $p = 0.006$), and postoperative fatty degeneration of the infraspinatus ($r = -0.61$, $p = 0.004$) but not with postoperative fatty degeneration of the supraspinatus ($r = -0.281$, $p = 0.23$).

Return to Work

Preoperatively, nineteen patients were working in their original occupation and one was retired. Eight of the nineteen patients had a strenuous job. Postopera-

tively, fifteen patients returned to their original occupation, after an average of 3.5 months (range, 0.5 to ten months); two patients who had been performing manual work changed to a less strenuous job; and two patients were receiving a disability pension.

Discussion

Rerupture or structural failure after rotator cuff repair is a well known and frequently encountered complication[1,10,14,16,21,25,32]. In studies reported in the literature, reruptures have usually been diagnosed with sonography[1,10,16], arthrography[4], or arthrography together with computed tomography[14]. Thomazeau et al.[32] and Knudsen et al.[21] recently used magnetic resonance imaging for evaluation after rotator cuff repairs. Magnetic resonance imaging is considered to be the primary investigative tool for evaluation after rotator cuff repairs[15] and the noninvasive imaging modality of choice for patients with suspected rotator cuff disease[24]. It is especially helpful for differentiating full and partial-thickness tears of the supraspinatus tendon from intact tendons, a differential diagnosis that may be impossible to accomplish with a physical examination[18,24]. The sensitivity and specificity of magnetic resonance imaging are higher than those of sonography or arthrography[2], especially for full-thickness tears[18,24].

In the current study, the postoperative structural integrity of the rotator cuff was assessed with magnetic resonance imaging. All of the twenty reruptures involved the supraspinatus (either alone or with one of the other tendons), as did all of the original ruptures that were treated at the index operation. Lesions of the most superior part of the subscapularis were difficult to identify with use of the magnetic resonance imaging sequences (without arthrography) employed for this study, which may explain why a postoperative lesion of this

TABLE V
COMPARISON OF POSTOPERATIVE CLINICAL PARAMETERS
BETWEEN PATIENTS WITH A ONE-TENDON TEAR AND THOSE WITH A TWO-TENDON TEAR

Component	One-Tendon Tear (N = 8)	Two-Tendon Tear (N = 10)	P Value*
Subjective shoulder value† (percent)	84	71	0.1728
Constant score[5,6]			
Total			
Absolute (points)	76	66	0.1457
Relative‡ (percent)	92	80	0.1457
Pain (points)	11	11.5	0.9654
Activities of daily living (points)	7.4	9	0.4598
Functional use of arm (points)	9.5	8.5	0.7618
Active mobility			
Flexion (degrees)	154	139	0.2370
Abduction (degrees)	160	143	0.9654
External rotation (degrees)	48	31	0.0831
Internal rotation (Constant score) (points)	9.8	8	0.0676
Abduction strength§ (kg)	4.8	2.2	0.0021

*The p values were determined with use of the Mann-Whitney U test (level of significance, $p < 0.05$).

†The subjective shoulder value represents the patient's estimation of the value of the operatively treated shoulder as a percentage of the value of an entirely normal shoulder.

‡The relative Constant score is given as a percentage of an age and gender-related normal value[5,6].

§The abduction strength was measured with an Isobex dynamometer.

tendon was detected in only two patients.

The rerupture was smaller than the initial tear in sixteen of the twenty patients. When it was larger, the clinical result was inferior and the patient was less satisfied, although there was still improvement compared with the preoperative state. Three of the larger reruptures had extended posteriorly into the infraspinatus tendon with concomitant functional weakness of this muscle, as documented by the inability to actively externally rotate the arm with the elbow at the side. These observations are in agreement with the concept that a single-tendon lesion of the supraspinatus does not influence the motion pattern of the glenohumeral joint[23,33], but the integrity of the infraspinatus is essential for a good clinical result[1,34] because it maintains an intact centering mechanism[1,3,23,33]. The functional importance of the infraspinatus is also demonstrated by the significant correlation of postoperative fatty degeneration of this muscle with the postoperative acromiohumeral distance and the clinical outcome; this correlation was not seen for the supraspinatus.

Glenohumeral osteoarthritis progressed significantly ($p = 0.002$), especially in patients with a two or three-tendon tear, and was associated with larger reruptures and less favorable clinical outcomes. This was also observed by Petersson[28], but Bellumore et al.[1] did not find that progression of osteoarthritis influenced the end result. In our series, osteoarthritis did not correlate with postoperative pain.

A key question for patients and surgeons is whether structural failure is identical to clinical failure. Our study documents that failed rotator cuff repairs provide significant improvement compared with the preoperative state. The overall excellent clinical outcome is related not only to successful treatment of pain but also to a gain in overhead motion and strength. Nineteen of the twenty patients felt that they had improvement compared with the preoperative state, and seventeen of the twenty patients were satisfied with the result. On the average, the patients rated the value of the operatively treated shoulder as being 75 percent of the value of a completely normal shoulder. Although the rate of patient satisfaction in our study was lower than that reported in studies of patients with successfully repaired rotator cuffs[16], it was at least in the range of the satisfaction rate of 63 to 90 percent reported for patients treated with arthroscopic débridement[7,8]. Subjectively unsatisfactory results were caused either by postoperative pain (one patient) or by inappropriately high expectations of patients who originally had had a very large tear (two patients).

Four of the twenty patients were completely asymptomatic, and the rerupture would have been impossible to detect on physical examination alone. In fact, in sixteen of the patients, despite the structural failure of the repair, pain relief and restoration of active mobility were comparable with those associated with a postoperatively intact cuff[1,10,16]. Interestingly, we documented not only a significant decrease in pain and an improvement in overall function but also a significant improvement in measured abduction strength. Whereas quantitative measurements of strength after successful repairs of the rotator cuff have been either reported postoperatively[13,16,19,22,35] or compared with preoperative measurements[10,20,21,30,32], we know of only a few studies that have documented strength before and after failed repairs[21,32], and we do not know of any study of an entire series of such patients. The improvement of measured strength that was found in our series of reruptures was hitherto considered to be consistent with only so-called intact repairs[32]. The postoperative strength did correlate with the size of the rerupture, as was observed by Rokito et al.[30], but our data show that a watertight cuff is not mandatory for recovery of abduction strength of greater than four kilograms, as was previously believed[32]. Whereas pain relief and functional improvement have also been reported after open[29] and arthroscopic[7,8,26,37] débridement, we are not aware of any documentation of improvement of measured abduction strength in patients who had a rerupture after open repair of the rotator cuff, and we consider our observation that strength was improved by partial healing to be of importance.

In conclusion, patients with a rerupture after rotator cuff repair still had significant improvement compared with the preoperative state. The rerupture usually was smaller than the original tear, and the structural failures were tolerated well, with good pain relief and functional improvement, including abduction strength. This finding suggests that the potential for structural failure should not be considered to be a formal contraindication to an attempt at rotator cuff repair if optimal functional recovery is the goal of treatment.

References

1. **Bellumore, Y.; Mansat, M.;** and **Assoun, J.:** Résultats de la chirurgie réparatrice de la coiffe des rotateurs. Corrélation radio-clinique. *Rev. chir. orthop.,* 80: 582-594, 1994.
2. **Burk, D. L., Jr.; Karasick, D.; Kurtz, A. B.; Mitchell, D. G.; Rifkin, M. D.; Miller, C. L.; Levy, D. W.; Fenlin, J. M.;** and **Bartolozzi, A. R.:** Rotator cuff tears: prospective comparison of MR imaging with arthrography, sonography, and surgery. *AJR: Am. J. Roentgenol.,* 153: 87-92, 1989.
3. **Burkhart, S. S.:** Arthroscopic treatment of massive rotator cuff tears. Clinical results and biomechanical rationale. *Clin. Orthop.,* 267: 45-56, 1991.
4. **Calvert, P. T.; Packer, N. P.; Stoker, D. J.; Bayley, J. I. L.;** and **Kessel, L.:** Arthrography of the shoulder after operative repair of the torn rotator cuff. *J. Bone and Joint Surg.,* 68-B(1): 147-150, 1986.
5. **Constant, C. R.:** Age related recovery of shoulder function after injury. Thesis, University College, Cork, Ireland, 1986.
6. **Constant, C. R.,** and **Murley, A. H.:** A clinical method of functional assessment of the shoulder. *Clin. Orthop.,* 214: 160-164, 1987.
7. **Ellman, H.; Kay, S. P.;** and **Wirth, M.:** Arthroscopic treatment of full-thickness rotator cuff tears: 2- to 7-year follow-up study. *Arthroscopy,* 9: 195-200, 1993.
8. **Esch, J. C.; Ozerkis, L. R.; Halgager, J. A.; Kane, N.;** and **Lilliott, N.:** Arthroscopic subacromial decompression: results according to the degree of rotator cuff tear. *Arthroscopy,* 4: 241-249, 1988.
9. **Fuchs, B.; Weishaupt, D.; Zanetti, M.; Hodler, J.;** and **Gerber, C.:** Fatty degeneration of the muscles of the rotator cuff: assessment by computed tomography versus magnetic resonance imaging. *J. Shoulder and Elbow Surg.,* 8: 599-605, 1999.
10. **Gazielly, D. F.; Gleyze, P.;** and **Montagnon, C.:** Functional and anatomical results after rotator cuff repair. *Clin. Orthop.,* 304: 43-53, 1994.
11. **Gerber, C.; Schneeberger, A. G.; Beck, M.;** and **Schlegel, U.:** Mechanical strength of repairs of the rotator cuff. *J. Bone and Joint Surg.,* 76-B(3): 371-380, 1994.
12. **Gerber, C.; Schneeberger, A. G.; Perren, S. M.;** and **Nyffeler, R. W.:** Experimental rotator cuff repair. A preliminary study. *J. Bone and Joint Surg.,* 81-A: 1281-1290, Sept. 1999.
13. **Gore, D. R.; Murray, M. P.; Sepic, S. B.;** and **Gardner, G. M.:** Shoulder-muscle strength and range of motion following surgical repair of full-thickness rotator-cuff tears. *J. Bone and Joint Surg.,* 68-A: 266-272, Feb. 1986.
14. **Goutallier, D.; Postel, J.-M.; Bernageau, J.; Lavau, L.;** and **Voisin, M.-C.:** Fatty muscle degeneration in cuff ruptures. Pre- and postoperative evaluation by CT scan. *Clin. Orthop.,* 304: 78-83, 1994.
15. **Gusmer, P. B.; Potter, H. G.; Donovan, W. D.;** and **O'Brien, S. J.:** MR imaging of the shoulder after rotator cuff repair. *AJR: Am. J. Roentgenol.,* 168: 559-563, 1997.
16. **Harryman, D. T., II; Mack, L. A.; Wang, K. Y.; Jackins, S. E.; Richardson, M. L.;** and **Matsen, F. A., III:** Repairs of the rotator cuff. Correlation of functional results with integrity of the cuff. *J. Bone and Joint Surg.,* 73-A: 982-989, Aug. 1991.
17. **Hertel, R.; Ballmer, F. T.; Lambert, S. M.;** and **Gerber, C.:** Lag signs in the diagnosis of rotator cuff rupture. *J. Shoulder and Elbow Surg.,* 5: 307-313, 1996.
18. **Hodler, J.; Kursunoglu-Brahme, S.; Snyder, S. J.; Cervilla, V.; Karzel, R. P.; Schweitzer, M. E.; Flannigan, B. D.;** and **Resnick, D.:** Rotator cuff disease: assessment with MR arthrography versus standard MR imaging in 36 patients with arthroscopic confirmation. *Radiology,* 182: 431-436, 1992.
19. **Iannotti, J. P.; Bernot, M. P.; Kuhlman, J. R.; Kelley, M. J.;** and **Williams, G. R.:** Postoperative assessment of shoulder function: a prospective study of full-thickness rotator cuff tears. *J. Shoulder and Elbow Surg.,* 5: 449-457, 1996.
20. **Kirschenbaum, D.; Coyle, M. P., Jr.; Leddy, J. P.; Katsaros, P.; Tan, F., Jr.;** and **Cody, R. P.:** Shoulder strength with rotator cuff tears. Pre- and postoperative analysis. *Clin. Orthop.,* 288: 174-178, 1993.
21. **Knudsen, H. B.; Gelineck, J.; Sojbjerg, J. O.; Olsen, B. S.; Johannsen, H. V.;** and **Sneppen, O.:** Functional and magnetic resonance imaging evaluation after single-tendon rotator cuff reconstruction. *J. Shoulder and Elbow Surg.,* 8: 242-246, 1999.
22. **Leroux, J.-L.; Hebert, P.; Mouilleron, P.; Thomas, E.; Bonnel, F.;** and **Blotman, F.:** Postoperative shoulder rotators strength in stages II and III impingement syndrome. *Clin. Orthop.,* 320: 46-54, 1995.
23. **Loehr, J. F.; Helmig, P.; Søjbjerg, J.-O.;** and **Jung, A.:** Shoulder instability caused by rotator cuff lesions. An in vitro study. *Clin. Orthop.,* 304: 84-90, 1994.
24. **Magee, T. H.; Gaenslen, E. S.; Seitz, R.; Hinson, G. A.;** and **Wetzel, L. H.:** MR imaging of the shoulder after surgery. *AJR: Am. J. Roentgenol.,* 168: 925-928, 1997.
25. **Mansat, P.; Cofield, R. H.; Kersten, T. E.;** and **Rowland, C. M.:** Complications of rotator cuff repair. *Orthop. Clin. North America,* 28: 205-213, 1997.
26. **Ogilvie-Harris, D. J.,** and **Demazière, A.:** Arthroscopic debridement versus open repair for rotator cuff tears. A prospective cohort study. *J. Bone and Joint Surg.,* 75-B(3): 416-420, 1993.
27. **Owen, R. S.; Iannotti, J. P.; Kneeland, J. B.; Dalinka, M. K.; Deren, J. A.;** and **Oleaga, L.:** Shoulder after surgery: MR imaging with surgical validation. *Radiology,* 186: 443-447, 1993.

28. **Petersson, C. J.:** Degeneration of the gleno-humeral joint. An anatomical study. *Acta Orthop. Scandinavica*, 54: 277-283, 1983.
29. **Rockwood, C. A., Jr.; Williams, G. R., Jr.;** and **Burkhead, W. Z., Jr.:** Débridement of degenerative, irreparable lesions of the rotator cuff. *J. Bone and Joint Surg.*, 77-A: 857-866, June 1995.
30. **Rokito, A. S.; Zuckerman, J. D.; Gallagher, M. A.;** and **Cuomo, F.:** Strength after surgical repair of the rotator cuff. *J. Shoulder and Elbow Surg.*, 5: 12-17, 1996.
31. **Samilson, R. L.,** and **Prieto, V.:** Dislocation arthropathy of the shoulder. *J. Bone and Joint Surg.*, 65-A: 456-460, April 1983.
32. **Thomazeau, H.; Boukobza, E.; Morcet, N.; Chaperon, J.;** and **Langlais, F.:** Prediction of rotator cuff repair results by magnetic resonance imaging. *Clin. Orthop.*, 344: 275-283, 1997.
33. **Thompson, W. O.; Debski, R. E.; Boardman, N. D.; Taskiran, E.; Warner, J. J.; Fu, F. H.;** and **Woo, S. L.:** A biomechanical analysis of rotator cuff deficiency in a cadaveric model. *Am. J. Sports Med.*, 24: 286-292, 1996.
34. **Walch, G.; Maréchal, E.; Maupas, J.;** and **Liotard, J. P.:** Traitement chirurgical des ruptures de la coiffe des rotateurs. Facteurs de pronostic. *Rev. chir. orthop.*, 78: 379-388, 1992.
35. **Walker, S. W.; Couch, W. H.; Boester, G. A.;** and **Sprowl, D. W.:** Isokinetic strength of the shoulder after repair of a torn rotator cuff. *J. Bone and Joint Surg.*, 69-A: 1041-1044, Sept. 1987.
36. **Zanetti, M.; Gerber, C.;** and **Hodler, J.:** Quantitative assessment of the muscles of the rotator cuff with magnetic resonance imaging. *Invest. Radiol.*, 33: 163-170, 1998.
37. **Zvijac, J. E.; Levy, H. J.;** and **Lemak, L. K.:** Arthroscopic subacromial decompression in the treatment of full thickness rotator cuff tears: a 3- to 6-year follow-up. *Arthroscopy*, 10: 518-523, 1994.

Failed Repair of the Rotator Cuff: Evaluation and Treatment of Complications

Evan H. Karas, MD

Joseph P. Iannotti, MD

Surgical repair of a tear of the rotator cuff usually provides relief of pain.[1-7] Restoration of strength is somewhat less predictable, but the rate of overall patient satisfaction after primary repair of the rotator cuff has been reported to be as high as 91% in a series of 340 shoulders.[2,4] Improved surgical techniques that have been developed over the last several decades have been largely responsible for this success. However, surgical repairs can fail. These failures present diagnostic and therapeutic challenges, because they may have multiple causes. Identification of the cause in a given patient requires a thorough evaluation that includes a complete history, physical examination, and review of the radiographs and the ancillary studies. Only then can an effective treatment plan be established. Although the results of repair of recurrent tears of the rotator cuff have not been as satisfactory as those of primary repair,[7,8-11] proper diagnosis and treatment can greatly increase the chance for success.

The major reasons for failure of repair of the rotator cuff are an incomplete or incorrect diagnosis; postoperative complications; errors in surgical technique; and errors in or poor performance of postoperative rehabilitation, or both. A combination of these factors may be responsible for a poor result in a given patient. The clinical evaluation of these parameters must be extremely thorough in order to avoid failure of treatment.

A careful history, including a review of the medical record, surgical notes, and preoperative and postoperative imaging studies, must be obtained. This information should allow the preoperative diagnosis to be established on the basis of both the clinical data and the anatomic abnormalities. An inaccurate or incomplete diagnosis or an error in the execution of the surgical procedure or the postoperative rehabilitation program may then be revealed. Accurate definition of all of the factors resulting in failure of the initial procedure is the first step in deciding on future treatment and improving the likelihood of a successful revision when surgery is indicated.

Errors in Diagnosis

Physical examination and injection tests help to define the patient's current problems. Care must be taken to specifically identify referred pain due to thoracic outlet syndrome and lesions of the cervical spine. Pain secondary to cervical lesions often presents in a dermatomal pattern over the posterior and lateral aspects of the shoulder; the pain may radiate to the occiput and the thoracic spine. Tenderness to palpation and a decreased range of motion of the neck are indicative of cervical disk disease. Provocative maneuvers, such as the Spurling test for diskogenic disease and the Wright[12] and Adson[13] tests for thoracic-outlet syndrome,[14,15] may be helpful if the results are positive. The Spurling test is performed by passive lateral bending and ipsilateral rotation of the neck. A positive test reproduces radicular symptoms. With the Adson test, the arm is positioned in extension with ipsilateral rotation of the neck. With the Wright test, the arm is placed in extension and abduction. The Adson and Wright tests are positive when they reproduce the symptoms of the upper extremity and the hand. If selective injection of lidocaine into the subacromial space or the acromioclavicular joint, or both, relieves pain, the cervical spine may be eliminated from consideration.

Neuropathies of the suprascapular and axillary nerves also may mimic disease of the rotator cuff and cause misdiagnoses. The suprascapular nerve, a branch of the superior trunk of the brachial plexus, may be compressed beneath the suprascapular ligament in the suprascapular notch[16] or by a ganglion in the spinoglenoid notch.[17] In addition, if a superior capsular release was performed during the original procedure, it is possible that dissection more than 2 cm medial to the superior aspect of the glenoid rim had resulted in iatrogenic suprascapular nerve injury.

Clinical presentation of these neuropathies usually consists of pain in the posterior aspect of the shoulder with accompanying muscle weakness specific to the site of nerve compression.

Proximal compression at the suprascapular notch or iatrogenic injury at this level denervates both the supraspinatus and the infraspinatus, while more distal compression at the spinoglenoid notch causes selective weakness of the infraspinatus. Similarly, weakness of the deltoid and the teres minor secondary to postoperative neuropathy of the axillary nerve may have a presentation very similar to that of a tear of the rotator cuff. Electromyographic analysis can help to confirm these diagnoses.[16,18,19] Magnetic resonance imaging (MRI) is the only useful imaging modality for defining neuropathy of the suprascapular nerve as a cause of failed rotator cuff surgery. It may reveal space-occupying lesions such as a ganglion cyst, or it may show severe muscle atrophy without a defect of the cuff.

Acromioclavicular joint arthropathy also can complicate the clinical presentation of disorders of the rotator cuff and can lead to failures in diagnosis and treatment. Careful clinical examination of the acromioclavicular joint, including direct palpation for tenderness and cross-arm adduction maneuvers, should be performed routinely for patients who have a possible lesion of the cuff. Imaging studies may be useful for diagnosing residual abnormalities of the acromioclavicular joint, a common cause of persistent pain following rotator cuff surgery. A Zanca radiograph (an anteroposterior radiograph made with the x-ray beam centered on the acromioclavicular joint with 15° of cephalic angulation) shows the full extent of the joint and may reveal lesions that were missed on routine anteroposterior radiographs. If radiographs are inconclusive and a lesion of the acromioclavicular joint is strongly suspected, a bone scan may confirm the diagnosis and lead to appropriate treatment.

An unrecognized os acromiale can cause persistent pain after subacromial decompression and repair of the rotator cuff. This lesion is most readily identified on routine axillary radiographs of the shoulder or on axial MRIs of the acromion. If small fragments are mobile and painful, they can be excised with reattachment of the deltoid to the remaining edge of the acromion. Larger lesions may require excision of the intervening synchondrosis and fixation with a tension-band wire with use of local bone graft obtained from a simultaneous acromioplasty.

Lesions of the biceps tendon and the superior glenoid labrum often are found in patients who have impingement syndrome and rotator cuff tears.[20] Failure to recognize and treat these problems appropriately can lead to a poor surgical result. An arthroscopic mini-open repair offers the advantage of improved visualization of the biceps tendon and its attachment to the superior aspect of the labrum. A finding of tenderness of the biceps tendon to palpation on physical examination, and a positive result on the Speed or the Yergason test, are suggestive of but nonspecific for biceps tendinitis.[21] The Yergason test is performed by resisting supination and flexion of the forearm. The Speed test is performed by resisting flexion of the elbow and the shoulder with the elbow in 90° of flexion and the shoulder in approximately 30° of flexion. Both tests are performed to evaluate referred pain to the long head of the biceps tendon. Standard radiographs are not particularly helpful for assessing the status of the biceps tendon. An axial radiograph of the intertubercular sulcus may provide indirect evidence of a lesion of the biceps tendon.[22] Arthroscopy is the most useful tool for delineating severe lesions of the biceps tendon. Tendon fraying and labral detachments can be both assessed accurately and treated arthroscopically. These intra-articular structures may be difficult to visualize and treat during routine open repair of defects of the cuff that are less than 2 cm long. Additionally, arthroscopy can be helpful for distinguishing internal posterosuperior glenoid impingement or secondary subtle glenohumeral instability,[23,24] especially in athletes who have pain during the late cocking phase (marked external rotation and abduction) of throwing.

Errors in Surgical Technique

Errors in the surgical technique of acromioplasty and rotator cuff repair can undermine the results of treatment of even the most accurately diagnosed lesions of the cuff. These errors include inadequate surgery and intraoperative complications. Inadequate surgeries include those in which a lesion of the biceps tendon or the labrum, or both, is missed; those in which arthropathy of the acromioclavicular joint is missed, as discussed previously; and inadequate acromioplasty. Intraoperative complications include fracture of the acromion, detachment or denervation of the deltoid, and failure to preserve the coracoacromial arch in patients who have an irreparable tear of the cuff.

The principles of acromioplasty include removal of sufficient bursa for adequate evaluation of the underlying rotator cuff and adequate removal of anteroinferior acromial bone without excessively shortening or narrowing the acromion. Inadequate anterior acromioplasty has been reported by many investigators as a common source of failures requiring revision surgery.[8,9,25-29]

In a study by Flugstad and associates,[26] 15 of 19 patients who had failure of surgical treatment for impingement syndrome were found to have residual acromial spurs. Of 117 patients who had a failed acromioplasty in a study by Rockwood and Williams,[29] all 90 who had recurrent symptoms of impingement had a residual anterior acromion at the time of surgery. DeOrio and Cofield[9] also demonstrated the importance of adequate subacromial decompression in their study of failed rotator cuff repairs; more than 50% of their 27 patients had not had an acromioplasty during the first, unsuccessful, operation.

Removal of an excessive amount of the anterior or lateral portion of the acromion may be associated with a fracture of the acromion or with detachment of the deltoid and a poor surgical result.[30] In the early development of techniques for repair of the rotator cuff, radical acromionectomy or subtotal lateral acromionectomy was advocated for subacromial decompression.[31-34] More recently, however, it has become clear that the acromion serves a necessary function in providing a strong attachment point and fulcrum for the powerful deltoid muscle. In 1981, Neer and Marberry[35] reported on 30 patients who had had removal of 80% of the acromion with resultant adhesions of the deltoid to the rotator cuff, deltoid retraction, and loss of the acromial fulcrum. Attempted surgical correction in 20 of these patients was unsuccessful. It is now accepted that acromionectomy is fraught with complications and should be abandoned.[17,25,33]

Frank acromial fractures can occur either intraoperatively or postoperatively.[30] Careful visualization and palpation of the thickness of the acromion is necessary to avoid this complication. Meticulous surgical technique, with emphasis on the correct angle of progression of the osteotome and with great care taken not to lever on the acromion with a subacromial retractor, is mandatory. An intraoperative fracture should be identified readily at the time of surgery and corrected with open reduction and internal fixation to prevent a painful nonunion and consequent deltoid weakness. Acromial fractures also have been reported after arthroscopic subacromial decompression[29] (Fig. 1), emphasizing the need for excellent visualization of the undersurface of the acromion and careful control of bone removal. Excessive use or trauma, or both, during the postoperative period also can cause an excessively thinned acromion to fracture.

The manner in which the deltoid is handled during an acromioplasty and rotator cuff repair is critical to a successful result. Avoidance of lateral acromionectomy to prevent deltoid retraction and scarring of the rotator cuff has been discussed previously. However, deltoid detachment from an intact acromion can still occur. The technique for removing and repairing the origin of the deltoid from the acromion can help to minimize the occurrence of this complication. In 1972, Neer[36] reported a method of acromioplasty in which a limited portion of the deltoid origin is removed subperiosteally from the anterior acromion and the acromioclavicular joint. Blunt dissection between the anterior and lateral heads of the deltoid muscle then allows exposure of the rotator cuff without excessive acromial destruction or deltoid detachment.[36] The deltoid-splitting technique was modified by Bigliani and Rodosky[37] to provide better access to the posterior cuff tendons without necessitating additional deltoid origin detachment.

Arthroscopic acromioplasty and mini-open repair of the rotator cuff theoretically should decrease the prevalence of detachment of the deltoid. To our knowledge, there have been no reported cases of detachment of the deltoid after mini-open or arthroscopic techniques. However, the senior one of us (JPI) has seen such detachment after both arthroscopic mini-open repair of the cuff and arthroscopic acromioplasty alone. Therefore, it is possible for this complication to occur with both arthroscopic techniques.

Reattachment of the deltoid to the acromion after repair of a tear of the rotator cuff is crucial. If an inadequate soft-tissue cuff of fascia remains on the acromion, or if excessive deltoid detachment is necessary for repair of a massive tear, then the deltoid should be reattached to the osseous edge of the acromion and the clavicle (if necessary) through drill holes. If the lateral portion of the clavicle has been resected, the deltoid must be repaired to the leading edge

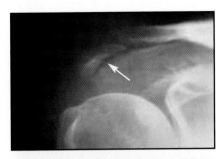
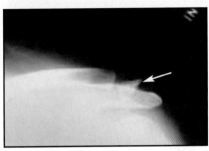

Fig. 1 Postoperative fractures of the acromion (arrows). (Top, Reproduced with permission from Naranja RJ, Iannotti JP, Gartsman GM: Complications of rotator cuff surgery, in Norris TR (ed): *Orthopaedic Knowledge Update: Shoulder and Elbow*. Rosemont, IL, American Academy of Orthopedic Surgeons, 1997, pp 157-166.)

of the trapezius fascia. Improper reattachment may result in retraction of the deltoid and may substantially compromise the functional result. When poor-quality deltoid tissue is encountered, an extended period of protected mobilization of the shoulder may be necessary.

Examination of the shoulder of a patient who has deltoid detachment reveals a defect at the deltoid origin from the acromion and a prominence of the deltoid distal to the defect that is accentuated by active elevation of the arm (Fig. 2, *left*). An MRI may be helpful for confirming this diagnosis (Fig. 2, *right*). Surgical repair of a retracted deltoid should proceed as soon as possible. Prolonged retraction leads to scarring and subsequent stiffness, pain, and loss of shoulder function.

Sher and associates (personal communication, Sher JS, Warner JJ, Gross Y, et al, 1996.) reported on 24 patients who

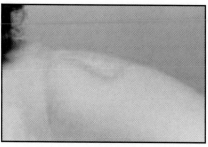 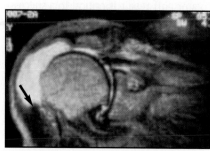

Fig. 2 Postoperative detachment of the deltoid. **Left,** Clinical evaluation reveals a defect that is accentuated by attempted active elevation of the arm. **Right,** T2-weighted magnetic resonance image demonstrates detachment and retraction of the origin of the deltoid (arrow). (Reproduced with permission from Naranja RJ, Iannotti JP, Gartsman GM: Complications of rotator cuff surgery, in Norris TR (ed): *Orthopaedic Knowledge Update: Shoulder and Elbow.* Rosemont, IL, American Academy of Orthopadic Surgeons, 1997, pp 157-166.)

had had either deltoid repair (for an acute tear) or rotational deltoidplasty of the middle deltoid anteriorly (for a chronic tear) to reconstruct a postsurgical deltoid disruption. At an average of 39 months, 16 patients (67%) had an unsatisfactory clinical result. The poor results were associated with a previous lateral acromionectomy; involvement of the middle deltoid; duration of symptoms of more than 12 months; and a concomitant, poorly compensated for, massive rotator cuff tear. Conversely, a satisfactory result was associated with an acute disruption isolated to the anterior deltoid, an intact acromion, and preserved function of the rotator cuff.

Iatrogenic deltoid denervation is a serious complication of rotator cuff surgery. Knowledge of the anatomy of the terminal branches of the axillary nerve as they relate to the splitting of the deltoid muscle is critical. The axillary nerve arises from the posterior cord of the brachial plexus near the coracoid process and then courses through the quadrilateral space to reach the posterior aspect of the shoulder. While in the quadrilateral space, it divides into posterior and anterior terminal branches, which supply the posterior one-third and the anterior two-thirds of the deltoid muscle, respectively. The anterior branch travels approximately 5

cm inferior to the lateral and anterior margin of the acromion, and is perpendicular to the direction of the muscle fibers. The deltoid split, therefore, should not extend beyond this distance. A stay suture can be placed at the apex of this split to prevent its propagation from excessive deltoid retraction. Furthermore, Burkhead and associates[38] showed that, in some smaller patients, the nerve may be located slightly closer than 5 cm from the acromial margin.

Axillary nerve neuropathy initially presents as weakness in abduction and forward elevation of the shoulder. Chronic disorders are accompanied by deltoid atrophy. Loss of sensation in the dermatome overlying the lateral deltoid is variable, as the cutaneous nerves supplying this area often arise from the posterior terminal branches of the axillary nerve.

Electromyography should be used when denervation of the deltoid is suspected postoperatively, both to confirm the diagnosis and to establish the nature of the injury as either a neurapraxia or a neurotmesis. Neurapraxias can be managed expectantly, with institution of passive range-of-motion exercises to prevent stiffness of the shoulder. Nerve transections should be evaluated for recovery on a monthly basis; nerve repair can be considered if no improvement is evident by 3

to 4 months and if it is warranted by the degree of the functional impairment. However, these recommendations are based on results obtained after repair of axillary nerve injuries secondary to dislocation of the shoulder or surgery for anterior stabilization in which the nerve was injured at its larger, main-branch region.[39] There is little information in the literature with regard to the treatment of terminal branch lesions after cuff repair. Leffert[40] described rotational deltoidplasty with excision of the denervated portion of the muscle as a valuable alternative to nerve repair for this problem.

The importance of the coracoacromial arch in providing anterosuperior stability for the humeral head has been the subject of several recent investigations.[41,42] Lazarus and associates[41] demonstrated anterosuperior escape of the humeral head from beneath the coracoacromial arch in five of six cadaver shoulders after coracoacromial ligament release and anterior acromioplasty. In a more elaborate cadaver model, Flatow and associates (personal communication, Flatow EL, Raimondo Ra, Kelkar R, et al, 1996.) demonstrated that this superior migration is most severe in the presence of large rotator cuff tears, especially when the edges of the tear approach the equator of the humeral head. Repair of the rotator cuff tears restored nearly normal glenohumeral kinematics in their patients. Failure to recognize the role of the coracoacromial arch in shoulders with a torn rotator cuff may lead to clinically evident anterosuperior instability (Fig. 3). In an attempt to circumvent this problem, Flatow and associates[43] recently described a technique of limited subacromial decompression and reattachment of the coracoacromial ligament in patients with a massive irreparable rotator cuff tear.

Postoperative Complications

Complications of repair of the rotator cuff include infection, heterotopic ossification, frozen shoulder, and recurrent tearing. Because these complications can be related both to the surgical technique and to the postoperative rehabilitation, they will be discussed separately.

Postoperative infections may be difficult to diagnose, as they often present in a delayed and unimpressive fashion. Superficial wound infections are characterized by erythema with or without drainage, induration, warmth, and fever. These findings may be subtle initially and may be overlooked as normal postoperative inflammation. Laboratory and imaging studies are often unrevealing at this stage. If left to worsen, these infections eventually will manifest themselves as wound dehiscence, drainage, cellulitis, and lymphadenopathy. Treatment is most successful if begun early and based on positive cultures. A heightened awareness of this potential problem is critical, and aspiration of the joint or the wound should not be delayed in suspicious cases. Intravenous administration of anti-staphylococcal and antistreptococcal antibiotics (first-generation cephalosporin) should be initiated after surgical debridement and exploration of the extent of the infection. If the infection does not pass deep to an intact repair of the cuff, then the repair can be left intact if this allows for adequate debridement of necrotic tissue. If the infection extends into the shoulder joint, then it should be debrided arthroscopically. The subacromial space and the biceps tendon sheath should be debrided in an open fashion. Nonabsorbable suture and any metallic suture anchors should be removed. Closed suction drains should be left in place, and antibiotics should be given intravenously as dictated by the results of gram stains and specimens of intraoperative cultures.

Heterotopic ossification is rare after acromioplasty and repair of the rotator cuff. It occurs in approximately 3% to 5% of patients, in our experience, but not all of these patients are symptomatic. Copious irrigation to remove all bone fragments after acromioplasty reduces the chance of heterotopic bone formation. When ossification occurs in the subacromial space or in the space created by resection of the lateral portion of the clavicle, it can be a source of pain (Fig. 4). The diagnosis is best made with use of routine radiographs. Lesions that cause severe pain or that limit motion can be treated with excision. Preoperative bone scans help to delineate mature lesions when they do not display markedly increased uptake of radioisotope. In our center, low-dose irradiation (7 Gy in a single dose) given within the first 48 hours after resection, or indomethacin given orally for 6 weeks, has been successful in preventing recurrence. This regimen is based on its effectiveness in patients who have had a total hip arthroplasty; we are unaware of any scientific data that support its use specifically for heterotopic ossification of the shoulder.

Postoperative stiffness after rotator cuff repair can lead to severe functional limitations. Bigliani and associates[8,25] reported on five patients who had frozen shoulder after the procedure. Those authors attributed the failures to inadequate postoperative rehabilitation and they recommended gentle pendulum exercises and passive elevation in the scapular plane, beginning on the first or second postoperative day, as preventive measures. One must be careful to identify patients who have a severe loss of motion of the shoulder preoperatively, as they are at higher risk for frozen-shoulder syndrome during the postoperative period. Passive shoulder-stretching exercises should be initiated, and a nearly full range of motion should be achieved before the cuff is repaired. If rehabilitation fails to restore motion, then manipulation with the patient under anesthesia followed by arthroscopic capsular release for shoulders that are resistant to manipulation should be performed. The patient can be brought back to the operating room at a later date, after motion of the shoulder

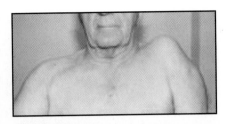

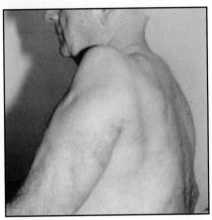

Fig. 3 Top, Coracoacromial arch insufficiency. (Reproduced with permission from Naranja RJ, Iannotti JP, Gartsman GM: Complications of rotator cuff surgery, in Norris TR (ed): *Orthopaedic Knowledge Update: Shoulder and Elbow.* Rosemont, IL, American Academy of Orthopadic Surgeons, 1997, pp 157-166.) **Bottom,** Attempted shoulder evaluation results in superior migration of the humeral head.

has been restored, for definitive surgical treatment of the lesion of the cuff.

More recently, Mormino and associates[44] reported on 13 patients who had subdeltoid adhesions after rotator cuff repair. These patients had arthroscopic release of the adhesions, which was universally successful in alleviating pain. The average score according to the system of the University of California at Los Angeles increased from 14.8 to 30.1 points. These authors postulated that the adhesions acted as a functional tenodesis, thus altering the normal biomechanics of the shoulder by preventing rolling of the humeral head on the glenoid. This restriction of motion is distinct from that secondary to capsular contracture or to scarring in the classic frozen shoulder

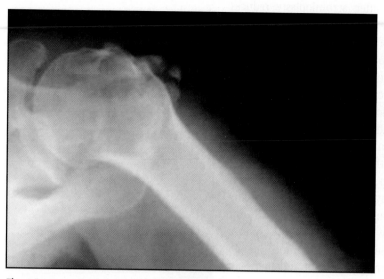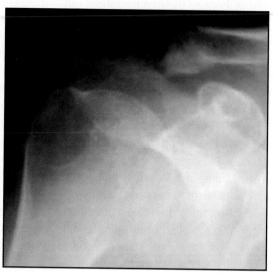

Fig. 4 Postoperative heterotopic ossification. **Left,** Axillary radiograph demonstrating heterotopic bone in the vicinity of an anterior acromioplasty. **Right,** Zanca (acromioclavicular joint) radiograph demonstrating heterotopic bone formation in the space created by resection of the lateral portion of the clavicle. ((Reproduced with permission from Naranja RJ, Iannotti JP, Gartsman GM: Complications of rotator cuff surgery, in Norris TR (ed): *Orthopaedic Knowledge Update: Shoulder and Elbow*. Rosemont, IL, American Academy of Orthopadic Surgeons, 1997, pp 157-166.)

and has been termed the captured shoulder. Early mobilization of the shoulder postoperatively may reduce the prevalence of this complication. However, all of the patients in this series began therapy on the first postoperative day. These authors did not explore factors that may have been associated with the development of the adhesions.

Persistent Rotator Cuff Defects

Persistent defects of previously repaired rotator cuff tendons may be related to an inadequate initial repair of the cuff, poor-quality tendon or bone, persistent impingement, or improper physical therapy. The results of clinical evaluation and radiographs must be evaluated concomitantly in order to determine the presence of a persistent defect as well as its relative clinical importance.

Persistent impingement usually is related to inadequate acromioplasty. Inadequate repair of the original tear may be secondary to improper identification of thickened, hypertrophic subacromial bursal tissue as rotator cuff tendon or to

inadequate mobilization of the torn tendons with consequent tension on the site of the repair. Bigliani and associates[25] identified the cause of 11 of 31 failed repairs as secondary to inadequate mobilization. Observation of the ease with which the bursal tissue pulls away from the underlying rotator cuff, as well as the differential motion of the bursa as compared with that of the rotator cuff with rotation of the humeral head, should serve as guides with which to determine the proper tissue to repair.

Overly intensive physical therapy during the early postoperative period may lead to avulsion of the tendon before healing. This mechanism was associated with five of the 31 failures in the series of Bigliani and associates.[25] In addition, Neviaser and Neviaser[10] found that early use of weights was a factor leading to failure of repair of rotator cuff tears. Rehabilitation must be tailored individually to intraoperative observations of the repair in each patient. A small tear that is repaired without detachment of the deltoid will withstand more intensive thera-

py than will a large or massive tear necessitating takedown and repair of the deltoid origin. Intraoperative assessment of the quality of the tissue and the amount of tension on the site of the repair also will help to guide therapy.

The identification of persistent defects of the cuff with use of imaging modalities can be difficult. The most useful study in the postoperative setting is arthrography. Communication of contrast medium between the subacromial and glenohumeral joint spaces was reported to be 100% sensitive and 96% specific for the diagnosis of full-thickness rotator cuff tears in series ranging from 20 to 805 shoulders.[45-47] Ultrasonography also has been used successfully to delineate full-thickness defects in the shoulder postoperatively. Accurate interpretation of sonographic images requires an extremely experienced sonographer who has the frequent opportunity to correlate the readings with the intraoperative findings. The sensitivity for the diagnosis of postoperative tears of the cuff approached 95% overall, and failure to visualize a supraspinatus musculotendinous unit was virtually 100% predictive of a complete tear, in series of 50[48] and 72[49] patients. Unlike preoperative MRI scans, postoperative scans do not delineate partial rotator cuff tears accurately. Persistent full-thickness tears can be assessed accurately when there is a well-defined defect in the tendon that displays high signal intensity on T2-weighted images (Fig. 5).

The clinical importance of a persistent full-thickness tear must be integrated within the context of the growing body of literature defining the presence of asymptomatic or minimally symptomatic tears. These data come from cadaver studies, imaging studies of shoulders after repair, clinical series of shoulders that have had subacromial decompression without repair of a massive tear, and imaging studies of asymptomatic individuals.

DePalma and associates,[50] in their classic study of 108 cadavera, determined the prevalence of defects of the rotator cuff relative to aging. Although no specimens from individuals who had died before the fifth decade of life had a tear of the rotator cuff, 33% from those who had died in the fifth decade and 100% from those who had died in the seventh decade had a complete tear. Of these specimens, 44 were obtained during autopsies on patients for whom the history and the findings on physical examination had been negative for a lesion of the rotator cuff.

Calvert and associates[45] used arthrography to study 20 shoulders after repair of the rotator cuff. They found that 18 of the shoulders had a persistent defect and that 17 of the 18 had satisfactory relief of the preoperative pain. Harryman and associates,[51] in a larger, more detailed study, performed bilateral ultrasonography on 122 patients after repair of the cuff. Of 105 patients who had a postoperative defect of the cuff, 94 were satisfied with the decrease in pain. Persistent defects were related to a decreased range of motion of the shoulder and to an

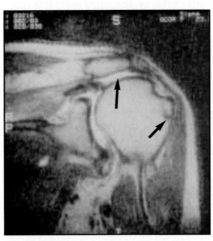

Fig. 5 T2-weighted magnetic resonance image, made in the coronal plane, of a recurrent defect of the rotator cuff. There is a full-thickness, high-signal-intensity defect in the supraspinatus tendon (large arrow). Note the bone trough and the suture through the bone tunnel (small arrow).

inability to perform activities of daily living. Additionally, the subjective results associated with intact repairs of recurrent tears were as successful as those associated with intact repairs of primary tears. The size of the tear was not related to the subjective assessment of function or pain relief at the latest follow-up evaluation if the repair had remained intact. However, a repair of a large defect is less likely to heal than is a small tear.

These results are not surprising, given the recent reports in the literature concerning the results of imaging of asymptomatic shoulders. With use of ultrasonography of the contralateral, asymptomatic shoulder of 73 patients who had a unilateral tear, Harryman and associates[51] noted rotator cuff defects in 40 (55%). Sher and associates[52] performed MRI on 96 asymptomatic shoulders and found an over-all prevalence of full-thickness and partial-thickness tears of 15% and 20%. All but one full-thickness defect was in a patient who was more than 60 years old.

Finally, the clinical importance of postoperative defects of the cuff must be

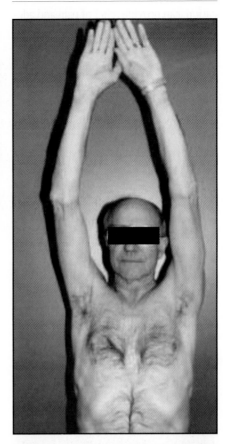

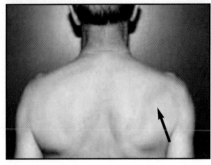

Fig. 6 This patient had an excellent result 2 years after debridement of a massive rotator cuff tear. **Top,** The range of motion is excellent. **Bottom,** There is marked atrophy of the infraspinatus (arrow).

interpreted in light of the evidence that acromioplasty and partial debridement or partial repair of a portion of the cuff is successful for the treatment of some large degenerative tears. Rockwood and associates[53,54] showed that this technique, coupled with intensive postoperative rehabilitation, can provide relief of pain and adequate function. Selection of the patients is critical, as the best results have been in patients who have had preoperative forward elevation of the shoulder above the horizontal plane, an intact long head of the biceps, and excellent function of the deltoid[53,54] (Fig. 6). Less favorable results have been noted in patients who have had a previous operation, anterior deltoid dysfunction, or a biceps tendon tear.[53,54] Although detachment of the cuff can provide favorable results in selected patients, we recommend repair of the cuff whenever possible.

To establish a treatment plan for patients in whom recurrent defects of the cuff are suspected, the results of imaging studies must be interpreted within the context of each patient's clinical presentation. Symptomatic patients who have subacromial crepitus, weakness of abduction and external rotation, and positive lag signs on external rotation as noted on physical examination are potential candidates for repeat repair. Findings at the time of the reoperation, including the size and location of the recurrent defect and the quality of the tendon and its degree of retraction and ability to be mobilized, will help to determine whether repeat repair of the torn edges of the tendon to bone is justified. A discussion of the patient's goals and expectations preoperatively is also important for guiding intraoperative decisions.

In conclusion, there are many potential causes of failure of rotator cuff repair. The categories of incomplete and incorrect diagnosis, errors of surgical technique or postoperative rehabilitation, and postoperative complications are convenient for classification, but it must be remembered that there may be several causes of failure in any given patient. Clinical evaluation is most dependent on a careful history, a review of the medical record and the preoperative imaging studies, and a physical examination with use of injection tests as indicated. On the basis of this evaluation, a definitive diagnosis or a limited differential diagnosis often can be established. The selective use of additional imaging studies and diagnostic arthroscopy will define the anatomic abnormalities. These lesions must be correlated carefully with the clinical findings in order to determine their relative importance and to choose the appropriate treatment.

References

1. Cofield RH: Rotator cuff disease of the shoulder. *J Bone Joint Surg* 1985;67A:974–979.

2. Hawkins RJ, Misamore GW, Hobeika PE: Surgery for full-thickness rotator-cuff tears. *J Bone Joint Surg* 1985;67A:1349–1355.

3. Iannotti JP: Full-thickness rotator cuff tears: Factors affecting surgical outcome. *J Am Acad Orthop Surg* 1994;2:87–95.

4. Neer CS II, Flatow EL, Lech O: Tears of the rotator cuff: Long term results of anterior acromioplasty and repair. *Orthop Trans* 1988;12:735.

5. Petersson C: Long-term results of rotator cuff repair, in Bayley I, Kessel L (eds): *Shoulder Surgery*. Berlin, Germany, Springer-Verlag, 1982, pp 64–69.

6. Samilson RL, Binder WF: Symptomatic full thickness tears of the rotator cuff: An analysis of 292 shoulders in 276 patients. *Orthop Clin North Am* 1975;6:449–466.

7. Wolfgang GL: Surgical repair of tears of the rotator cuff of the shoulder: Factors influencing the result. *J Bone Joint Surg* 1974;56A:14–26.

8. Bigliani LU, McIlveen SJ, Cordasco FA, et al: Operative management of failed rotator cuff repairs. *Orthop Trans* 1988;12:674.

9. DeOrio JK, Cofield RH: Results of a second attempt at surgical repair of a failed initial rotator-cuff repair. *J Bone Joint Surg* 1984;66A:563–567.

10. Neviaser RJ, Neviaser TJ: Reoperation for failed rotator cuff repair: Analysis of 46 cases. *Orthop Trans* 1989;13:509.

11. Sahlstrand T: Operations for impingement of the shoulder: Early results in 52 patients. *Acta Orthop Scand* 1989;60:45–48.

12. Wright IS: The neurovascular syndrome produced by hyperabduction of the arms: The immediate changes produced in 150 normal controls, and the effects on some persons of prolonged hyperabduction of the arms, as in sleeping, and in certain occupations. *Am Heart J* 1945;29:1–19.

13. Adson AW: Surgical treatment for symptoms produced by cervical ribs and the scalenus anticus muscle. *Surg Gynecol Obstet* 1947;85:687–700.

14. Leffert RD: Thoracic outlet syndrome: Orthopaedic perspective on diagnosis and treatment. *Orthop Trans* 1988;12:190.

15. Leffert RD: Thoracic outlet syndrome, in Gelberman RH (ed): *Operative Nerve Repair and Reconstruction*. Philadelphia, PA, JB Lippincott, 1991, vol 2, pp 1177–1195.

16. Rengachary SS, Burr D, Lucas S, et al: Suprascapular entrapment neuropathy: A clinical, anatomical, and comparative study. Anatomical study and comparative study. *Neurosurgery* 1979;5:447–455.

17. Neviaser TJ, Ain BR, Neviaser RJ: Suprascapular nerve denervation secondary to attenuation by a ganglionic cyst. *J Bone Joint Surg* 1986;68A:627–628.

18. Donovan WH, Kraft GH: Rotator cuff tear versus suprascapular nerve injury: A problem in differential diagnosis. *Arch Phys Med Rehabil* 1974;55:424–428.

19. Drez D Jr: Suprascapular neuropathy in the differential diagnosis of rotator cuff injuries. *Am J Sports Med* 1976;4:43–45.

20. Neer CS II, Bigliani LU, Hawkins RJ: Rupture of the long head of the biceps related to subacromial impingement. *Orthop Trans* 1977;1:111.

21. Yergason RM: Supination sign. *J Bone Joint Surg* 1931;13:160.

22. Cone RO, Danzig L, Resnick D, et al: The bicipital groove: Radiographic, anatomic, and pathologic study. *Am J Roentgenol* 1983;141:781–788.

23. Lombardo SJ, Jobe FW, Kerlan RK, et al: Posterior shoulder lesions in throwing athletes. *Am J Sports Med* 1977;5:106–110.

24. Snyder SJ, Karzel RP, Del Pizzo W, et al: SLAP lesions of the shoulder. *Arthroscopy* 1990;6:274–279.

25. Bigliani LU, Cordasco FA, McIlveen SJ, et al: Operative treatment of failed repairs of the rotator cuff. *J Bone Joint Surg* 1992;74A:1505–1515.

26. Flugstad D, Matsen FA, Larry I, et al: Failed acromioplasty: Etiology and prevention. *Orthop Trans* 1986;10:229.

27. Hawkins RJ, Chris AD, Kiefer GN: Failed anterior acromioplasties. *Orthop Trans* 1987;11:233.

28. Packer NP, Calvert PT, Bayley JI, et al: Operative treatment of chronic ruptures of the rotator cuff of the shoulder. *J Bone Joint Surg* 1983;65B:171–175.

29. Rockwood CA Jr, Williams GR: The shoulder impingement syndrome: Management of surgical treatment failures. *Orthop Trans* 1992;16:739–740.

30. Matthews LS, Burkhead WZ, Gordon S, et al: Acromial fracture complicating arthroscopic subacromial decompression. *J Shoulder Elbow Surg* 1994;3:256–261.

31. Armstrong JR: Excision of the acromion in treatment of the supraspinatus syndrome: Report of ninety-five excisions. *J Bone Joint Surg* 1949;31B:436–442.

32. Hammond G: Complete acromionectomy in the treatment of chronic tendinitis of the shoulder: A follow-up of ninety operations on

eighty-seven patients. *J Bone Joint Surg* 1971;53A:173–180.

33. McLaughlin HL: Lesions of the musculotendinous cuff of the shoulder: I. The exposure and treatment of tears with retraction. *J Bone Joint Surg* 1944;26:31–51.

34. Smith-Petersen MN, Aufranc OE, Larson CB: Useful surgical procedures for rheumatoid arthritis involving joints of the upper extremity. *Arch Surg* 1943;46:764–770.

35. Neer CS II, Marberry TA: On the disadvantages of radical acromionectomy. *J Bone Joint Surg* 1981;63A:416–419.

36. Neer CS II: Anterior acromioplasty for the chronic impingement syndrome in the shoulder: A preliminary report. *J Bone Joint Surg* 1972;54A:41–50.

37. Bigliani LU, Rodosky MW: Techniques of repair of large rotator cuff tears. *Tech Orthop* 1994;9:133–140.

38. Burkhead WZ Jr, Scheinberg RR, Box G: Surgical anatomy of the axillary nerve. *J Shoulder Elbow Surg* 1992;1:31–36.

39. Petrucci FS, Morelli A, Raimondi PL: Axillary nerve injuries: 21 cases treated by nerve graft and neurolysis. *J Hand Surg* 1982;7A:271–278.

40. Leffert RD: Neurological problems, in Rockwood CA Jr, Matsen FA III (eds): *The Shoulder*. Philadelphia, PA, WB Saunders, 1990, vol 2, pp 750–773.

41. Lazarus MD, Yung SW, Sidles JA, et al: Abstract: Anterosuperior humeral displacement: Limitation by the coracoacromial arch. *J Shoulder Elbow Surg* 1996;5:S7.

42. Moorman CT III, Deng XH, Warren RF, et al: Abstract: The coracoacromial ligament: Is it the appendix of the shoulder? *J Shoulder Elbow Surg* 1996;5(suppl):S9.

43. Flatow EL, Pollock RG, Bigliani LU: Coracoacromial ligament preservation in rotator cuff surgery. *Tech Orthop* 1994;9:97–98.

44. Mormino MA, Gross RM, McCarthy JA: Captured shoulder: A complication of rotator cuff surgery. *Arthroscopy* 1996;12:457–461.

45. Calvert PT, Packer NP, Stoker DJ, et al: Arthrography of the shoulder after operative repair of the torn rotator cuff. *J Bone Joint Surg* 1986;68B:147–150.

46. Mink JH, Harris E, Rappaport M: Rotator cuff tears: Evaluation using double-contrast shoulder arthrography. *Radiology* 1985;157:621–623.

47. Stiles RG, Otte MT: Imaging of the shoulder. *Radiology* 1993;188:603–613.

48. Drakeford MK, Quinn MJ, Simpson SL, et al: A comparative study of ultrasonography and arthrography in evaluation of the rotator cuff. *Clin Orthop* 1990;253:118–122.

49. Olive RJ Jr, Marsh HO: Ultrasonography of rotator cuff tears. *Clin Orthop* 1992;282:110–113.

50. DePalma AF, Callery G, Bennett GA: Part I: Variational anatomy and degenerative lesions of the shoulder joint, in Blount WP, Banks SW (eds): American Academy of Orthopaedic Surgeons *Instructional Course Lectures VI*. Ann Arbor, MI, JW Edwards, 1949, pp 255–281.

51. Harryman DT II, Mack LA, Wang KY, et al: Repairs of the rotator cuff: Correlation of functional results with integrity of the cuff. *J Bone Joint Surg* 1991;73A:982–989.

52. Sher JS, Uribe JW, Posada A, et al: Abnormal findings on magnetic resonance images of asymptomatic shoulders. *J Bone Joint Surg* 1995;77A:10–15.

53. Rockwood CA Jr: The management of patients with massive rotator cuff defects by acromioplasty and rotator cuff debridement. *Orthop Trans* 1986;10:622.

54. Rockwood CA, Williams GR, Burkhead WZ: Debridement of degenerative, irreparable lesions of the rotator cuff. *J Bone Joint Surg* 1995;77A:857–866.

Transfer of the Latissimus Dorsi Muscle After Failed Repair of a Massive Tear of the Rotator Cuff

A TWO TO FIVE-YEAR REVIEW*

BY ANTHONY MINIACI, M.D., F.R.C.S.(C)†, TORONTO, AND MARK MACLEOD, M.D., F.R.C.S.(C)‡, LONDON, ONTARIO, CANADA

Investigation performed at The Toronto Hospital, Western Division, University of Toronto, Toronto, and the London Health Sciences Centre, University of Western Ontario, London

Abstract

Introduction: Seventeen patients with an average age of fifty-five years (range, thirty-two to seventy-seven years) who had ongoing pain and impaired function following failed operative treatment of a massive tear of the rotator cuff were managed with a transfer of the latissimus dorsi muscle as a salvage operation.

Methods: The patients were examined at an average of fifty-one months (range, twenty-four to seventy-two months) after the operation. Pain, function, and satisfaction were assessed with use of a questionnaire, visual analog and ordinal scales, physical examination, and the University of California at Los Angeles shoulder score.

Results: Fourteen of the seventeen patients were found to have significant relief of pain (p < 0.0001) and a significant improvement in function (p < 0.001 for all activities except lifting more than fifteen pounds [6.8 kilograms], for which the p value was <0.0036) and were satisfied with the result of the operative procedure. Fifteen patients stated that they would have the operative procedure again under similar circumstances. Seven of eight patients with a detached or nonfunctional anterior portion of the deltoid had substantial improvement. Three operations were classified as failures because the patients were not satisfied with the result and had ongoing pain and impaired function. All three failures were in patients who had a work-related injury. Overall, six patients had a work-related injury, and only three of them had a satisfactory result. There were three complications, all related to contracture of a hypertrophic axillary scar.

Conclusions: The results in this series indicate that transfer of the latissimus dorsi muscle is a reasonable approach for salvage after failed operative treatment of a massive tear of the rotator cuff.

Tears of the rotator cuff are common orthopaedic problems that may cause pain and impaired function. Massive tears increase the complexity of the problem,

and management of these lesions remains a somewhat controversial area. Many operative solutions have been proposed[2,3,5-8,10-15,17-21,23-26]. When these approaches fail, the situation is difficult, with few available options for treatment. Reasons for failure include inadequate decompression[4,9,22], failure of repair[4,9,16,22], and detachment of the deltoid with impaired function[4,16,22]. A reoperation after these failures does not necessarily relieve pain[4,9,16,22] or improve function, especially if the deltoid is one of the causes of failure. For these reasons, we have searched for operative techniques that could potentially salvage those situations. One such repair is the transfer of the latissimus dorsi muscle, as described by Gerber et al.[12]. The objective of the present retrospective study was to analyze one surgeon's experience with transfer of the latissimus dorsi muscle to manage patients in whom operative treatment of a massive defect of the rotator cuff had failed. We evaluated the results at a minimum of two years after the operative procedure.

Materials and Methods

The retrospective study included seventeen patients who had been managed between January 1990 and October 1995 by one of us (A. M.). The patient's history; the results of clinical examination; preoperative radiographs; and subjective questionnaires documenting preoperative and postoperative pain, function, and satisfaction were analyzed.

Twelve patients were male and five were female. Ten patients had involvement of the dominant extremity. Eleven patients had had one previous operative procedure, four had had two, and two had had at least three. The anterior portion of the deltoid was thought to be detached or nonfunctional in eight of the seventeen patients, and there was clinical evidence of disruption of the subscapularis in four of the seventeen patients. All patients had preoperative pain and an objective lack of active motion in forward elevation, abduction, and external rotation. All described an inability to use the upper extremity to perform activities of daily living and work. Clinical examination revealed positive impingement signs and weakness of external rotation and on supraspinatus testing in all patients. Six of the patients had a work-related injury and were collecting Workers' Compensation benefits.

Preoperative radiographic examination demonstrated proximal humeral migration in all patients, mild

*No benefits in any form have been received or will be received from a commercial party related directly or indirectly to the subject of this article. No funds were received in support of this study.

†The Toronto Hospital, Western Division, University of Toronto, 399 Bathurst Street, ECW 1-036, Toronto, Ontario M5T 2S8, Canada.

‡London Health Sciences Centre, University of Western Ontario, London, Ontario N6A 5A5, Canada.

degenerative glenohumeral arthritis with sclerosis of the glenoid and the greater tuberosity in seven, and joint-space narrowing with an osteophytic spur in one. Nine patients had no obvious evidence of radiographic osteo-arthritis at the glenohumeral joint.

Every patient had an initial exploration of the deltoid, the acromion, and the subacromial space. If the failure of the operation was believed to be due solely to inadequate decompression or failure of repair, or both, a repeat decompression or a repeat repair and decompression was performed and the patient did not have a latissimus dorsi transfer. The present series includes only patients who had previously had an adequate operation and did not have tissue available for a repeat repair of the cuff.

The four patients with absence, attenuation, or a tear of the subscapularis all had a positive lift-off test. At the time of the index operation, two of these four patients had complete absence of the subscapularis with no identifiable tissue present. These patients had the transfer of the latissimus dorsi muscle at that time despite previous literature suggesting that the absence of the subscapularis is a relative contraindication to the procedure[12]. In these patients, the latissimus dorsi was anchored to bone troughs both laterally and anteriorly along the neck of the humerus and medially to any remnant of the rotator cuff that was available. The other two patients with a positive lift-off test did have some soft tissue remaining anteriorly in the position of the subscapularis. One patient had what we considered to be a partial tear of the superior portion of the subscapularis tendon. The tendon was thickened and frayed. The remaining tissue was adequate, and the latissimus dorsi could be transferred to it. The fourth patient had what appeared to be a thin atrophic subscapularis. We were not sure about its function, but it was adequate to hold the sutures for the muscle transfer.

In eight of the seventeen patients, anterior deltoid weakness was evident on physical examination and was believed to be related to detachment or impaired function, or both. These patients also demonstrated severe anterior and superior migration of the humeral head, which was easily seen and palpated in the subacromial region. In each patient, the tissue attached to the acromion was found to be thin and atrophic at the time of the operation and attempts were made to advance healthier tissue.

Function, pain, and satisfaction were evaluated clinically with use of both ordinal and visual analog scales. The overall status of each shoulder was assessed with use of the University of California at Los Angeles shoulder score[1], which is also used to evaluate pain, function, range of motion, and strength. Function was evaluated by determining the degree of difficulty that the patient had with the performance of ten different activities (hair-combing, dressing, perineal care, sleeping on the shoulder, washing under the contralateral arm, pulling ten pounds [4.5 kilograms] or more, using the hand overhead or at shoulder level, working or performing daily activities, and lifting fifteen pounds [6.8 kilograms] or more). The degree of difficulty with these activities was rated on a 4-point scale, with 0 points indicating that the activity was not difficult; 1 point, that it was slightly difficult; 2 points, that it was moderately difficult; 3 points, that it was very difficult but not impossible; and 4 points, that it was impossible. Pain at work, at rest, and at night were also evaluated with use of a 4-point scale, with 0 points indicating no pain; 1 point, occasional mild pain; 2 points, frequent mild-to-moderate pain; 3 points, moderate-to-severe pain; and 4 points, severe pain. In addition, the patient indicated the degree of pain and function on a visual analog scale, which was an open-ended, unmarked 100-millimeter line.

Finally, overall satisfaction with the shoulder and with the procedure was assessed with use of a questionnaire as well as a visual analog scale.

Data were analyzed statistically with the Student t test for paired data and multiple analysis of variance as indicated. Analysis of variance was used to determine whether there was a significant difference between the group of patients who had weakness of the deltoid and the group who had a normal deltoid. The means and standard deviations for all of the measured parameters were analyzed.

Operative Procedure

All of the operative procedures were performed with the patient in lateral decubitus and rolled anteriorly about 10 to 15 degrees, with the bed in a slight reverse Trendelenburg position and the patient stabilized with a sandbag. The arm and shoulder were prepared and draped free to the anterior and posterior midlines to allow for dissection of the latissimus dorsi. The rotator cuff was first exposed through an antero-superior approach. Various incisions had been previously used, and these incisions were utilized in all patients. The anterior portion of the deltoid, the acromion, the acromioclavicular joint, and the subacromial space were assessed. An attempt was made in all patients to free up enough healthy tissue to perform a primary repair. Once the surgeon was convinced that a repeat repair could not be performed (Fig. 1), attention was turned to the latissimus dorsi transfer. The procedure was performed as described by Gerber et al.[12], with an incision paralleling the latissimus dorsi through the axilla and then turning at right angles to the humerus near the attachment of the latissimus dorsi tendon (Fig. 2). This incision was used in the first six patients, but because of complications with hypertrophic axillary scarring the incision was changed to a modified z-plasty in the axilla to prevent contracture in the subsequent eleven patients. The incision for the first limb of the z-plasty was made parallel to the anterior border of the latissimus dorsi tendon, beginning distally and directed

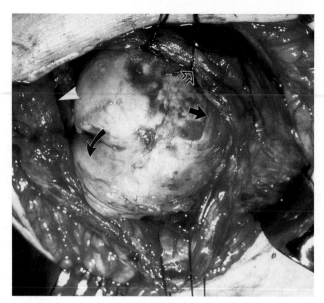

FIG. 1

Operative photograph showing a massive tear of the rotator cuff that was not reparable with any local closure technique. Previous attempts at débridement and repair had failed. The detached deltoid (open arrow) was thin and attenuated. The previous acromioplasty (white arrowhead) was adequate. The subscapularis (straight black arrow) is seen attached to the lesser tuberosity. The substance of the subscapularis is very thin and atrophic. Some posterior rotator cuff tissue, probably the teres minor (curved black arrow), is present. There is early arthropathy of the glenohumeral joint.

toward the posterior axillary fold. The incision stopped approximately two to three centimeters before reaching the posterior axillary fold, and then a second limb was made at approximately 135 degrees to the first limb and was directed toward the head of the patient in a supero-medial direction. The second limb was approximately three to four centimeters in length. A third limb was then made at approximately an 80-degree angle to the second limb and was extended parallel to the arm in the direction of the hand. This limb was also approximately three to four centimeters in length, so a triangular incision was made in the area of the posterior axillary fold. Finally, a fourth limb was cut perpendicular to the third limb and approximately perpendicular to the line of the

arm to allow for adequate exposure of the latissimus dorsi and its attachment onto the humeral shaft.

The latissimus dorsi was dissected free, with the surgeon taking care not to injure the neurovascular structures on its undersurface, which come from proximal to distal and can be damaged. Division of these structures will devitalize the tendon transfer. The tendon was followed to its osseous attachment on the humerus. It is imperative that the tendon attachment to the humerus be visualized to reduce the risk of neurovascular injury and to improve the probability of obtaining tendon tissue of adequate width and length. Maximum internal rotation helps the surgeon to visualize the attachment of the tendon to the humerus. The surgeon must be careful when detaching the tendon. The radial nerve lies just distal to the tendon and should at least be palpated or visualized. If the surgeon is not satisfied with the latissimus dorsi tendon, the teres major can also be obtained at this point (Fig. 3). Both tendons and muscles were obtained in one patient in this series because we thought that the size of the defect and the latissimus tendon were mismatched.

Once the tendon had been detached it was retracted, the undersurface of the latissimus dorsi was visualized, and the neurovascular pedicle was identified and dissected free. The muscle was mobilized by operative dissection as close to the muscle origin as necessary to ensure adequate proximal migration. The tendon was prepared by using two number-1 nonabsorbable sutures of different colors, with one color running down each edge of the tendon. The use of different colors helped to ensure that the tendon was not twisted during passage.

The interval between the posterior portion of the deltoid and the long head of the triceps was then identified and dissected. With the two muscles retracted, the posterior aspect of the acromion was palpated and a long curved clamp was passed from anterior to posterior under the acromion, exiting between the posterior portion of the deltoid and the long head of the triceps. Spreading the jaws of the clamp fashioned the passageway that allowed excursion of the tendon so that the

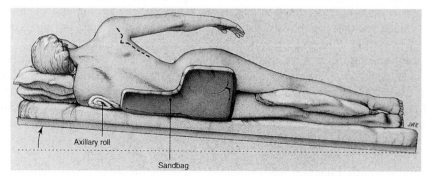

FIG. 2

Drawing showing the patient in lateral decubitus, stabilized with a sandbag and with an axillary roll in place. An incision is made along the anterolateral border of the latissimus dorsi muscle. At the posterior axillary fold, a v incision is made to avoid crossing the axillary fold directly and thus to avoid contracture. (Reprinted, with permission, from: Miniaci, A.: Latissimus dorsi transfer for irreparable rotator cuff insufficiency. Op. Tech. Orthop., 8: 247, 1998.)

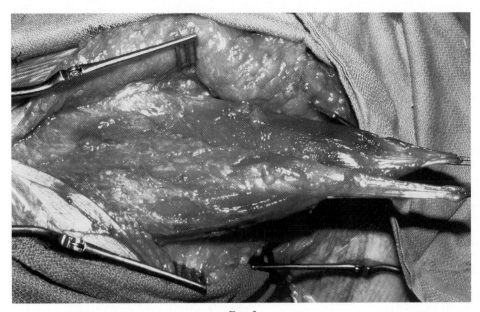

FIG. 3

Operative photograph showing a free and mobile latissimus dorsi muscle-and-tendon unit (inferior) ready for transfer. In this patient, the teres major (superior) was also used to complete the repair. The tendon of the teres major is usually shorter, and the muscle is bulkier. Additional transfer of the teres major is possible but is not often necessary. Only one of the seventeen patients in the present series needed transfer of the teres major in addition to the latissimus dorsi.

tendon could be passed anteriorly. After passage of the tendon, its lateral edge was sutured through drill-holes into a bone trough in the greater tuberosity, in a manner similar to that described for standard repair of the rotator cuff. Medially, the tendon was attached to any remaining mobile cuff tissue. Anteriorly, the leading edge of the latissimus dorsi was sutured to the free edge of the subscapularis muscle (Fig. 4). Alternatively, when the subscapularis was totally absent, an anterior bone trough was used to anchor the leading edge of the tendon. The shoulder was moved through a full range of motion to ensure that there was not excessive tension on the repair. A suction drain was placed posteriorly to eliminate the dead space for twenty-four to forty-eight hours. The wound was closed, and bulky compressive dressings were applied.

Postoperative Protocol

Postoperatively, a shoulder immobilizer was used for comfort. We made sure that there was not excessive tension on the repair with the arm at the side and that the patient felt comfortable using only a sling without abduction. Physical therapy consisted of passive forward elevation as well as internal and external rotation for six weeks, after which a program of progressive stretching and strengthening was begun. Although recovery was variable, it typically took about six to twelve months.

Results

The seventeen patients were evaluated at a minimum of two years (average, fifty-one months; range, twenty-four to seventy-two months) after the latissimus dorsi transfer was done following failure of treat-

ment of a massive tear of the rotator cuff. The average age at the time of follow-up was fifty-five years (range, thirty-two to seventy-seven years).

Three of the six patients who had a work-related injury had a failure, and these were the only failures in the series. Two of those patients stated that they would not have the procedure again under similar circumstances, but the third stated that he would still choose to have the operation. This patient noted some subjective

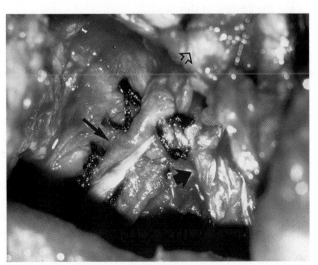

FIG. 4

Operative photograph showing a completed repair of a rotator cuff defect with a transferred latissimus dorsi tendon. Anteriorly the tendon is attached to the subscapularis (thick black arrow), and laterally a bone trough in the greater tuberosity is used to anchor the lateral edge of the latissimus dorsi tendon into the greater tuberosity (thin black arrow). The detached deltoid (open arrow) is retracted with sutures.

TABLE I

RESULTS OF TRANSFER OF THE LATISSIMUS DORSI

	Mean and Standard Deviation		P Value
	Preop.	Postop.	
Pain			
Ordinal scale* (points)			
At work	3.9 ± 0.24	1.2 ± 1.16	<0.0001
At rest	3.7 ± 0.47	1.1 ± 1.36	<0.0001
At night	3.8 ± 0.39	1.2 ± 1.33	<0.0001
Visual analog scale† (mm)	86.1 ± 12.90	26.0 ± 32.00	<0.0001
Function			
Ordinal scale‡ (points)			
Hair-combing	3.4 ± 0.71	1.8 ± 1.13	<0.0001
Dressing	3.1 ± 0.67	1.5 ± 1.12	<0.0001
Perineal care	3.2 ± 0.91	1.6 ± 0.96	<0.0001
Sleeping on shoulder	3.8 ± 0.39	1.7 ± 1.49	<0.0001
Washing under contralat. arm	2.9 ± 0.97	1.4 ± 1.00	<0.0001
Pulling ≥10 lbs. (≥ 4.5 kg)	3.5 ± 0.62	2.2 ± 1.15	<0.0001
Working overhead	3.9 ± 0.33	2.8 ± 1.19	<0.001
Working at shoulder level	3.8 ± 0.44	2.8 ± 0.86	<0.0001
Activities of daily living or work	3.7 ± 0.59	2.1 ± 0.86	<0.0001
Lifting ≥15 lbs. (≥ 6.8 kg)	3.9 ± 0.33	3.3 ± 0.77	<0.0036
Visual analog scale† (mm)	13.8 ± 9.90	56.1 ± 29.70	<0.0001
UCLA shoulder score[1]§ (points)	6.8 ± 1.50	16.4 ± 6.10	<0.0001
Overall satisfaction with shoulder on visual analog scale† (mm)	10.9 ± 7.10	68.5 ± 29.40	<0.0001
Overall satisfaction with procedure on visual analog scale† (mm)		75.3 ± 28.00	0.0018
Active range of motion (degrees)			
Forward elevation	41.8 ± 27.60	100.6 ± 43.40	<0.0001
External rotation	18.2 ± 10.30	30.9 ± 14.40	<0.0001

*0 points = none; 1 point = mild, occasional; 2 points = mild to moderate, frequent; 3 points = moderate to severe; and 4 points = severe.
†The visual analog scale consisted of an open-ended, unmarked 100-millimeter line.
‡0 points = not difficult, 1 point = slightly difficult, 2 points = moderately difficult, 3 points = very difficult but not impossible, and 4 points = impossible.
§UCLA = University of California at Los Angeles.

improvement, but this did not translate into an improvement in the outcome measures that were used to evaluate the results in this study.

Pain: As demonstrated on the ordinal scale, all but three patients had significant relief of pain at work, at rest, and at night (p < 0.0001 for all three) (Table I). The score according to the visual analog scale also improved significantly (p < 0.0001), from an average of 86.1 millimeters preoperatively to an average of 26.0 millimeters postoperatively. The operation was considered to have failed in the three patients who had little pain relief, as the primary purpose of the operation was to alleviate pain.

Function: Interestingly, function improved for all of the activities rated with the ordinal scale (p < 0.001 for all except lifting fifteen pounds [6.8 kilograms] or more, for which the p value was <0.0036) (Table I). The patients' subjective assessment of function on the visual analog scale also improved significantly (p < 0.0001), from an average of 13.8 millimeters preoperatively to an average of 56.1 millimeters after the operation (Table I). In addition, both the active and the passive range of motion improved in forward elevation and in internal and external rotation (p < 0.0001) (Table I).

Overall shoulder score: The University of California

at Los Angeles shoulder score[1], which was used to provide a general overall assessment of the shoulder, also improved significantly (p < 0.0001), from an average of 6.8 points preoperatively to an average of 16.4 points postoperatively (Table I).

Patient satisfaction: Overall, fourteen of the seventeen patients were satisfied with the improvement following the operative procedure, and this was reflected by the improvement (from an average of 10.9 millimeters preoperatively to an average of 68.5 millimeters postoperatively; p < 0.0001) in the overall satisfaction with the shoulder as indicated on the visual analog scale. All fourteen of the patients who were satisfied with the improvement of the shoulder stated unequivocally that they would have the procedure again under similar circumstances, although a few expressed concern over the duration of recovery and the time needed for rehabilitation.

Success of the procedure: On the basis of these assessments, fourteen of the seventeen patients were deemed to have had a successful operative procedure, whereas the procedure was considered to have failed in three.

Comparison of results for patients who had an intact deltoid with those for patients in whom the deltoid was not intact: The patients were divided into two groups according to whether or not the deltoid was intact. Eight patients were believed to have either a detached or an attenuated deltoid, and nine had an intact deltoid. With the numbers available, we could not detect any significant differences, either preoperatively or post-operatively, between the groups with regard to pain, function, range of motion, University of California at Los Angeles shoulder score, or the overall satisfaction with the shoulder. This finding suggested to us that the patients had similar amounts of disability before the operation and had similar levels of success after the procedure.

Complications: No operative infections or neurovascular injuries were encountered in this series. Three patients had contracture of the incision in the axilla with hypertrophic scarring. All three were treated with injections of corticosteroids, and one patient had limitation of abduction and forward elevation related to the contracture. The scar for this patient was subsequently revised with a z-plasty in the axilla, which allowed the patient more motion. The three patients who had hypertrophic scarring were among the first six to be managed, and because of this complication the remaining eleven patients had a modified z-plasty-type incision through the axilla. Hypertrophic axillary scarring has not been a problem since.

Discussion

The literature dealing with revision after failed attempts at rotator cuff repair is sparse. Various authors[4,9,22] have suggested that the cause of failure must be determined before revision is attempted. The usual causes of failure include inadequate decompression, failure of repair, and detachment of the deltoid with impaired function. Nevertheless, reoperations to treat these problems do not necessarily guarantee success. Both Bigliani et al.[4] and Neviaser and Neviaser[22] noted some relief of pain, not necessarily associated with improved function, following repeat attempts at repair. DeOrio and Cofield[9] reported that, of twenty-four patients who were available for follow-up after management with a second attempt at repair of a failed repair, fourteen (58 percent) had a poor result. Patients who have a detached deltoid and an irreparable defect probably have an even poorer prognosis. The present series represents a subset of patients in whom no local tissue remained and previous attempts at operative treatment had failed to provide pain relief or improved function. The transfer of the latissimus dorsi muscle in these patients was effective. Pain relief, the primary goal of this operative procedure, was achieved in fourteen of the seventeen patients. The range of motion and function also improved, a finding that had not been totally expected. Despite the significant improvement in function, none of these patients would be considered as having normal or nearly normal function. The patients' subjective rating of function on

TABLE II
RESULTS ACCORDING TO WHETHER
OR NOT THE DELTOID WAS INTACT*

	Deltoid Detached (N = 8)	Deltoid Intact (N = 9)
Mean age *(yrs.)*	57.8	52.0
Pain on visual analog scale† *(mm)*		
Preop.	89.1 ± 7.90	83.6 ± 16.00
Postop.	24.0 ± 24.00	27.7 ± 40.00
Function on visual analog scale† *(mm)*		
Preop.	16.7 ± 11.00	11.3 ± 8.20
Postop.	55.0 ± 26.00	57.0 ± 34.00
UCLA shoulder score[1]‡ *(points)*		
Preop.	7.4 ± 1.77	6.3 ± 1.10
Postop.	15.5 ± 4.78	17.1 ± 3.98
Overall satisfaction with shoulder on visual analog scale† *(mm)*		
Preop.	13.3 ± 10.90	8.9 ± 6.90
Postop.	72.9 ± 22.20	64.6 ± 35.50
Active range of motion *(degrees)*		
Forward elevation		
Preop.	35.0 ± 28.00	47.8 ± 28.00
Postop.	101.3 ± 45.40	100 ± 44.40
External rotation		
Preop.	13.8 ± 6.90	22.2 ± 12.00
Postop.	30.0 ± 13.60	31.7 ± 15.80

*The values are given as the mean and standard deviation.
†The visual analog scale consisted of an open-ended, unmarked 100-millimeter line.
‡UCLA = University of California at Los Angeles.

the visual analog scale, although significantly improved from the preoperative rating, was only 56.1 millimeters after the operation. The University of California at Los Angeles shoulder score[1], which was used in this series to provide an overall impression of the status of the shoulder, improved to an average of only 16.4 points, which would, at best, be considered fair. This reflects the fact that the patients were still moderately disabled. The most important finding, however, was that there was a significant overall improvement between the preoperative and postoperative University of California at Los Angeles shoulder scores.

The subset of eight patients in whom the anterior portion of the deltoid was detached or nonfunctional had substantial improvement. Seven of the eight patients had relief of pain, had improvement with regard to function and the range of motion, and were quite satisfied with the result of the procedure. Our subjective examination revealed that the patients eventually were able to raise the arm, and, although superior subluxation was not totally eliminated, the patients seemed to be able to control the humerus from subluxating superiorly when the arm was in forward elevation. Preoperatively, our subjective impression was that the patients with detachment of the deltoid had more difficulty with activities of daily living and had a smaller active range of motion than the patients in whom the deltoid was intact. However, this impression could not be demonstrated statistically. Detachment of the deltoid as well as a massive irreparable defect in the rotator cuff did not seem to preclude the use of the latissimus dorsi transfer, as both groups (those with and those without detachment of the deltoid) seemed to have marked improvement after the operation (Table II). As previous reports[4,9] have failed to show improvement following a repeat operative attempt at repair of the rotator cuff in patients with an abnormal deltoid, we were encouraged by our results.

It is difficult to determine the true effect of the transferred latissimus dorsi tendon. Some might argue that soft-tissue interposition may have played a role in the reduction of the pain. Although this may be true, the tendon itself is quite thin, and it is difficult to imagine that soft-tissue interposition was the only reason for the improvement. It may be that some of the positive effect of the transfer was either due to active muscle contraction or simply due to a tethering or tenodesis effect of the transferred tendon. Clinically, it appeared that the latissimus dorsi was contracting when it was palpated during elevation of the shoulder. Whether the tendon acts as a passive restraint or an active muscle transfer, the humeral head is centered better in the glenoid and is maintained there, allowing the deltoid better mechanical advantage for elevation of the arm.

Four of the patients in the present series had absence, attenuation, or a tear of the subscapularis. It is not possible to draw significant conclusions on the basis of four patients; however, we can report that, although technically the repair was difficult, the latissimus dorsi transfer was possible as the tendon was anchored anteriorly onto the humerus or into local surrounding tissue, which provided good fixation of the tendon. Our impression is that even patients in whom the subscapularis is absent can benefit from this procedure and, therefore, we do not consider absence of the subscapularis to be a contraindication.

One of the intriguing findings in this study was the trend of poor results for patients receiving Workers' Compensation benefits. All three of the failures were in this subgroup: three of the six patients who were receiving such compensation had an unsatisfactory outcome. This finding, as always, is difficult to explain as there was documentable evidence of a serious lesion and it was made very clear before the procedure that we did not expect the patients to obtain enough improvement to be able to return to work. Whatever the reason, this group posed the greatest challenge, and there were no apparent distinguishing features to explain the failures.

Fortunately, complications were not common, although infection or neurovascular injury could be a problem with this procedure because of the extent of the operative dissection and the proximity of vital structures to the latissimus dorsi tendon. The one problem that was noted was related to the skin incision, which we initially made across the posterior axillary fold. This resulted in three hypertrophic scar contractures at the axilla in the first six patients managed with this type of incision. One patient needed a revision of the operative scar to correct the problem as it caused discomfort and limited motion. Subsequently, the incision was modified to a z-type axillary incision, and to date this has eliminated the problem.

There were weaknesses in this study. The group was not totally homogeneous, we performed a retrospective review, and some minor variations in the operative procedure were made; however, the group consisted of patients for whom, it was believed, there were no other treatment options and who represented what we thought to be the worst-case scenario. All patients were operated on and followed by one surgeon. We believe that the outcomes, although only fair, were quite favorable when compared with the preoperative status. We did not include in the present study any primary repairs of massive defects of the rotator cuff, a procedure that was suggested by Gerber et al.[12] As a result of the favorable outcomes in this series, we now also consider using the latissimus dorsi transfer as the primary procedure for the treatment of an irreparable massive defect. Of course, that situation is rare, and decompression and repair of the rotator cuff with local tissue remains our first choice for the treatment of massive defects.

In conclusion, transfer of the latissimus dorsi muscle for salvage after a failed attempt at operative repair of a massive defect of the rotator cuff is an effective procedure. Our patients reported marked relief of pain and improvement of function, although the shoulders were by no means normal or nearly normal. The procedure seems possible even when the subscapularis is weak or can no longer be identified. In addition, patients with the combined problem of a massive defect of the rotator cuff with anterosuperior subluxation and a detached anterior portion of the deltoid have a favorable outcome after this procedure. We suggest that transfer of the latissimus dorsi be used as an alternative operation in difficult situations in which a patient with a massive defect of the rotator cuff has had a failure of a previous procedure.

References

1. **Amstutz, H. C.; Sew Hoy, A. L.;** and **Clarke, I. C.:** UCLA anatomic total shoulder arthroplasty. *Clin. Orthop.,* 155: 7-20, 1981.
2. **Apoil, A.,** and **Augereau, B.:** Antero-superior arthrolysis of the shoulder for rotator cuff degenerative lesions. In *Surgery of the Shoulder,* pp. 257-260. Edited by M. Post, B. F. Morrey, and R. J. Hawkins. St. Louis, Mosby-Year Book, 1990.
3. **Augereau, B.:** Rekonstruktion massiver Rotatorenmanschettenrupturen mit einem Deltoidlappen. *Orthopäde,* 20: 315-319, 1991.

4. **Bigliani, L. U.; Cordasco, F. A.; McIlveen, S. J.;** and **Musso, E. S.:** Operative treatment of failed repairs of the rotator cuff. *J. Bone and Joint Surg.,* 74-A: 1505-1515, Dec. 1992.

5. **Burkhart, S. S.:** Arthroscopic treatment of massive rotator cuff tears: clinical results and biomechanical rationale. *Orthop. Trans.,* 14: 173, 1990.

6. **Burkhart, S. S.; Nottage, W. M.; Ogilvie-Harris, D. J.; Kohn, H. S.;** and **Pachelli, A.:** Partial repair of irreparable rotator cuff tears. *Arthroscopy,* 10: 363-370, 1994.

7. **Cofield, R. H.:** Subscapularis muscle transposition for repair of chronic rotator cuff tears. *Surg., Gynec. and Obstet.,* 154: 667-669, 1982.

8. **Debeyre, J.; Patte, D.;** and **Elmelik, E.:** Repair of ruptures of the rotator cuff of the shoulder. With a note on advancement of the supraspinatus muscle. *J. Bone and Joint Surg.,* 47-B(1): 36-42, 1965.

9. **DeOrio, J. K.,** and **Cofield, R. H.:** Results of a second attempt at surgical repair of a failed initial rotator-cuff repair. *J. Bone and Joint Surg.,* 66-A: 563-567, April 1984.

10. **Dierickx, C.,** and **Vanhoof, H.:** Massive rotator cuff tears treated by a deltoid muscular inlay flap. *Acta Orthop. Belgica,* 60: 94-100, 1994.

11. **Franklin, J. L.; Barrett, W. P.; Jackins, S. E.;** and **Matsen, F. A., III:** Glenoid loosening in total shoulder arthroplasty. Association with rotator cuff deficiency. *J. Arthroplasty,* 3: 39-46, 1988.

12. **Gerber, C.; Vinh, T. S.; Hertel, R.;** and **Hess, C. W.:** Latissimus dorsi transfer for the treatment of massive tears of the rotator cuff. A preliminary report. *Clin. Orthop.,* 232: 51-61, 1988.

13. **Ha'eri, G. B.,** and **Wiley, A. M.:** Advancement of the supraspinatus muscle in the repair of ruptures of the rotator cuff. *J. Bone and Joint Surg.,* 63-A: 232-238, Feb. 1981.

14. **Hawkins, R. J.; Misamore, G. W.;** and **Hobeika, P. E.:** Surgery for full-thickness rotator-cuff tears. *J. Bone and Joint Surg.,* 67-A: 1349-1355, Dec. 1985.

15. **Mikasa, M.:** Trapezius transfer for global tear of the rotator cuff. In *Surgery of the Shoulder,* pp. 196-199. Edited by J. E. Bateman and R. P. Welsh. Philadelphia, B. C. Decker, 1984.

16. **Miniaci, A.,** and **MacLeod, M.:** Latissimus dorsi muscle transfer as a salvage procedure for failed surgical treatment of massive rotator cuff tears [abstract]. *J. Shoulder and elbow Surg.,* 6: 179, 1997.

17. **Nasca, R. J.:** Rotator cuff grafts. *Orthop. Trans.,* 9: 50, 1985.

18. **Neer, C. S., II; Watson, K. C.;** and **Stanton, F. J.:** Recent experience in total shoulder replacement. *J. Bone and Joint Surg.,* 64-A: 319-337, March 1982.

19. **Neer, C. S., II; Craig, E. V.;** and **Fukuda, H.:** Cuff-tear arthropathy. *J. Bone and Joint Surg.,* 65-A: 1232-1244, Dec. 1983.

20. **Neviaser, J. S.:** Ruptures of the rotator cuff of the shoulder. New concepts in the diagnosis and operative treatment of chronic ruptures. *Arch. Surg.,* 102: 483-485, 1971.

21. **Neviaser, R. J.,** and **Neviaser, T. J.:** Transfer of subscapularis and teres minor for massive defects of the rotator cuff. In *Shoulder Surgery,* pp. 60-63. Edited by I. Bayley and L. Kessel. New York, Springer, 1982.

22. **Neviaser, R. J.,** and **Neviaser, T. J.:** Reoperation for failed rotator cuff repair: analysis of fifty cases. *J. Shoulder and Elbow Surg.,* 1: 283-286, 1992.

23. **Ozaki, J.; Fujimoto, S.;** and **Masuhara, K.:** Repair of chronic massive rotator cuff tears with synthetic fabrics. In *Surgery of the Shoulder,* pp. 185-191. Edited by J. E. Bateman and R. P. Welsh. Philadelphia, B. C. Decker, 1984.

24. **Paavolainen, P.; Slatis, P.;** and **Bjorkenheim, J. M.:** Transfer of the tuberculum majus for massive ruptures of the rotator cuff. In *Surgery of the Shoulder,* pp. 252-256. Edited by M. Post, B. F. Morrey, and R. J. Hawkins. St. Louis, Mosby-Year Book, 1990.

25. **Patte, D.; Goutallier, D.;** and **Scheffer, J. C.:** Large cuff ruptures: repair results by muscle advancement. In *Surgery of the Shoulder,* pp. 248-251. Edited by M. Post, B. F. Morrey, and R. J. Hawkins. St. Louis, Mosby-Year Book, 1990.

26. **Rockwood, C. A., Jr.; Williams, G. R., Jr.;** and **Burkhead, W. Z., Jr.:** Débridement of degenerative, irreparable lesions of the rotator cuff. *J. Bone and Joint Surg.,* 77-A: 857-866, June 1995.

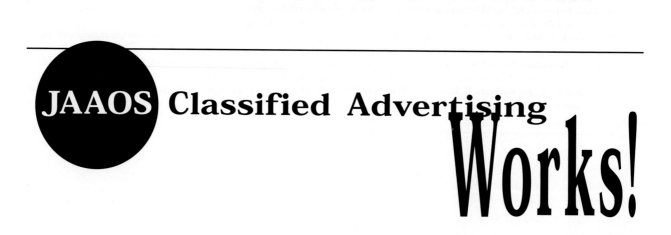

Painful Shoulder After Surgery for Rotator Cuff Disease

Gerald R. Williams, Jr, MD

Abstract

Persistent shoulder pain after surgery for rotator cuff disease may be caused by conditions that are either extrinsic or intrinsic to the shoulder. Extrinsic causes of persistent shoulder pain include cervical radiculopathy, suprascapular neuropathy, abnormalities of scapular rotation (due to long-thoracic or spinal-accessory neuropathy), and adjacent or metastatic neoplasms. Causes of persistent pain that are intrinsic to the shoulder include both intra-articular conditions (e.g., glenohumeral osteoarthritis, adhesive capsulitis, recurrent anterior subluxation, and labral and bicipital tendon abnormalities) and extra-articular conditions (e.g., persistent subacromial impingement, persistent or recurrent rotator cuff defects, acromioclavicular arthropathy, and deltoid muscle deficiency). Successful management requires an accurate diagnosis, maximal rehabilitation, judicious use of surgical intervention, and a well-motivated patient. The results of revision surgery in patients with persistent subacromial impingement, with or without an intact cuff, are inferior to reported results after primary acromioplasty or rotator cuff repair.

J Am Acad Orthop Surg 1997;5:97-108

Rotator cuff disease is a common cause of shoulder disability, particularly in patients beyond the fourth decade of life. Anterior acromioplasty, combined with rotator cuff repair when indicated, generally provides predictable pain relief and improved function.[1] However, when pain continues in spite of surgery for rotator cuff disease, patient management becomes more complicated and less predictable. It is important to recognize that persistent rotator cuff disease is only one of the many potential causes for such pain (Table 1). Possible extrinsic causes include cervical radiculopathy; suprascapular, long-thoracic, or spinal-accessory neuropathy; and adjacent or metastatic neoplastic disease. Potentially causative intrinsic shoulder disorders may be intra-articular, such as osteoarthritis, adhesive capsulitis, recurrent anterior subluxation, and labral or bicipital tendon abnormalities, or extra-articular, such as subacromial impingement, persistent or recurrent rotator cuff defect, acromioclavicular joint arthropathy, and deltoid insufficiency. Successful management begins with an accurate identification of the underlying pathologic process responsible for the pain.

Evaluation

In most cases, an initial diagnostic impression can be formulated on the basis of the history, physical examination, and routine radiography. Additional studies that may be useful include arthrography, ultrasonography, magnetic resonance (MR) imaging, electromyography, and scintigraphy. Selective injections into the subacromial space and the acromioclavicular joint can help localize the pain or quantitate how much pain is attributable to each area when both are involved. Diagnostic arthroscopy may be useful, especially when extrinsic disorders have been excluded, the previously performed acromioplasty has been judged adequate by radiographic criteria, and the rotator cuff is intact.

Extrinsic Shoulder Disorders

It is important to recognize that persistent pain after rotator cuff surgery may be the result of pathologic processes extrinsic to the

Dr. Williams is Assistant Professor, University of Pennsylvania School of Medicine, and Attending Surgeon, Shoulder and Elbow Service, Hospital of the University of Pennsylvania, Philadelphia.

Reprint requests: Dr. Williams, Department of Orthopaedic Surgery, University of Pennsylvania, Shoulder and Elbow Service, Penn Musculoskeletal Institute, 1 Cupp Pavilion, Presbyterian Medical Center, 39th and Market Streets, Philadelphia, PA 19104.

Table 1
Causes of Persistent Shoulder Pain After Rotator Cuff Surgery

Extrinsic shoulder pathology
    Brachial plexopathy
    Cervical radiculopathy
    Long-thoracic neuropathy
    Neoplasm
    Reflex sympathetic dystrophy
    Spinal-accessory neuropathy
    Suprascapular neuropathy
    Thoracic outlet syndrome
Intrinsic shoulder pathology
    Intra-articular
        Adhesive capsulitis
        Articular cartilage defect
        Bicipital tendinitis
        Instability
        Labral tears
        Osteoarthritis
    Extra-articular
        Acromioclavicular arthropathy
        Deltoid insufficiency
        Rotator cuff defect
        Subacromial impingement

shoulder. In addition, an extrinsic cause of persistent pain (e.g., cervical radiculopathy) may coexist with an intrinsic cause (e.g., recurrent rotator cuff defect), in which case diagnostic injection into the subacromial space may help distinguish between the intrinsic and extrinsic components of the pain.

When an extrinsic cause for the persistent pain has been identified, treatment should be directed accordingly.

Of the extrinsic causes of persistent shoulder pain, cervical radiculopathy involving the fifth or sixth cervical root is perhaps the most common. The symptoms of neck pain accompanied by radiation into the upper extremity, numbness, or paresthesias suggest this diagnosis. Routine radiography may reveal cervical spondylosis or neural foraminal encroachment. If indicated, MR imaging of the cervical spine and electromyography may confirm the diagnosis.

Long-thoracic and spinal-accessory neuropathies result in scapular winging and poor scapular rotation during overhead elevation. Secondary impingement symptoms may develop as scapular rotation lags behind glenohumeral elevation. Although true scapular winging is an uncommon cause of persistent pain after rotator cuff surgery, many patients will exhibit varying degrees of scapulothoracic dysfunction. Scapulothoracic and scapulohumeral rhythm should be observed in all patients with persistent symptoms after acromioplasty or cuff repair. In patients with severe scapular dysfunction associated with winging, electromyography may confirm the neurologic lesion.

Suprascapular neuropathy may also result in impingement-like symptoms because of the posterior cuff weakness that results from chronic nerve compression. Patients present with severe atrophy of either the supraspinatus and infraspinatus or the infraspinatus alone. This is associated with weakness of external rotation with the arm at the side. Electromyography is helpful in confirming the diagnosis and localizing the site of compression to the infraspinatus alone or to both the supraspinatus and the infraspinatus. Magnetic resonance imaging may reveal a ganglion cyst compressing the suprascapular nerve (Fig. 1).

Neoplastic processes are a very rare but devastating cause of persistent shoulder pain after rotator cuff surgery. The apical lung fields should always be inspected on shoulder radiographs, because apical lung tumors (i.e., Pancoast tumors) cause referred shoulder pain through extension to the brachial plexus or cervical roots. If a lung mass is suspected, appropriate chest radiographs and medical consultation are indicated. Persistent pain may also be caused by direct involvement of the shoulder by a neoplastic process. Magnetic resonance imaging may be used to further characterize masses or unusual prominences discovered on physical examination (Fig. 2).

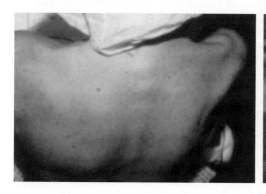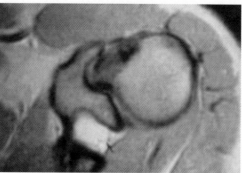

Fig. 1 Left, Severe atrophy of the supraspinatus and infraspinatus muscles in a patient with continued pain after arthroscopic acromioplasty. **Right,** MR image depicts a ganglion cyst compressing the suprascapular nerve.

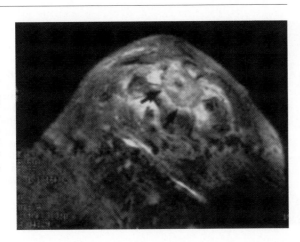

Fig. 2 Patient had persistent pain associated with a tender mass in the region of the trapezius after arthroscopic acromioplasty. MR imaging revealed a soft-tissue mass that proved to be metastatic carcinoma from the lung.

Intrinsic Shoulder Disorders

Causes of persistent pain that are intrinsic to the shoulder include both intra-articular conditions (e.g., glenohumeral osteoarthritis, adhesive capsulitis, recurrent anterior subluxation, and labral and bicipital tendon abnormalities) and extra-articular conditions (e.g., persistent subacromial impingement, persistent or recurrent rotator cuff defects, acromioclavicular arthropathy, and deltoid muscle deficiency).

Intra-articular Causes of Persistent Pain

Unrecognized glenohumeral disorders may be responsible for persistent postsurgical shoulder pain. Intra-articular causation should be suspected when postoperative radiographs reveal adequate decompression of the supraspinatus outlet, and the acromioclavicular joint is asymptomatic.

Articular Cartilage Abnormalities

Glenohumeral osteoarticular disease may be a cause of persistent pain in at least two circum-

stances: (1) unrecognized or underappreciated preoperative osteoarthritis and (2) cuff tear arthropathy, or Milwaukee shoulder syndrome. Primary glenohumeral osteoarthritis is characterized by subchondral sclerosis and cyst formation, glenohumeral joint-space narrowing and osteophyte formation, asymmetric posterior glenoid wear, and an intact or repairable rotator cuff.[2] The management of primary osteoarthritis does not differ substantially whether or not there has been prior impingement or rotator cuff surgery.

Cuff tear arthropathy is characterized by destruction of the glenohumeral articular surfaces, accompanied by chronic, massive rotator cuff insufficiency and proximal humeral migration, that persists or recurs in spite of one or more previous attempts at cuff repair.[3] Persistent pain may be improved by humeral hemiarthroplasty.[4,5] Functional improvement is less predictable than pain relief, especially if the coracoacromial ligament was sacrificed during previous cuff repair.

Traumatic articular cartilage defects of the humerus and glenoid may cause persistent shoulder pain in the absence of generalized artic-

ular degeneration. A history of a single traumatic event is often elicited. Examination may reveal painful glenohumeral crepitus during glenohumeral rotation. Radiographs and MR images are often normal. In this circumstance, diagnostic arthroscopy may be necessary to confirm a humeral or glenoid articular defect (Fig. 3).

Adhesive Capsulitis

The hallmark of capsular contracture or adhesive capsulitis is a symmetric decrease in both active and passive range of motion, which can be localized or can involve all planes of motion. Localized posterior capsular contracture is common with subacromial impingement syndrome and is characterized not only by limited elevation but also by decreased cross-body adduction and internal rotation, both of which are more pronounced with the arm at 90 degrees of elevation in or anterior to the scapular plane. The presence of localized posterior capsular contracture postoperatively is a sign of an incompletely rehabilitated shoulder and can be a factor contributing to continued pain and disability. Generalized capsular contracture is less common with primary rotator cuff disease or subacromial impingement syndrome than localized posterior contracture. It is characterized by loss of motion in all planes (especially passive external rotation with the arm at the side) and is an important source of persistent pain and disability after surgery for rotator cuff disease.

The initial management of adhesive capsulitis consists of physiotherapy for joint mobilization and capsular stretching. If motion cannot be restored through the use of nonoperative joint-mobilization techniques, then closed manipulation or surgical capsular release is indicated. Postoperative frozen

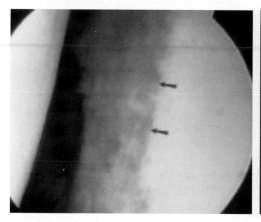
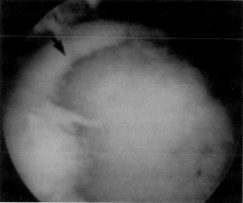

Fig. 3 Arthroscopic images of patients with continued pain after open acromioplasty and rotator cuff repair. **Left,** One patient had an articular defect of the anterior glenoid. **Right,** Other patient had an articular defect of the humeral head.

shoulder is often unresponsive to closed manipulation. Traditionally, surgical capsular release was performed through an anterior deltopectoral approach in combination with subscapularis lengthening.[6] Arthroscopic capsular release has recently been reported as an alternative,[7,8] but this procedure requires advanced arthroscopic surgical skills and may be contraindicated in the presence of extra-articular adhesions.

Recurrent Anterior Subluxation

In patients less than 40 years of age, particularly those who engage in sports involving overhead motion, there is an overlap between rotator cuff overuse and recurrent anterior subluxation.[9] Young patients with persistent shoulder pain after acromioplasty may be experiencing secondary impingement symptoms as a result of subtle anterior subluxation. They may report a forceful abduction–external rotation injury, a distal traction injury, or "dead arm" symptoms while throwing.

Examination may reveal increased passive external rotation with the arm at 90 degrees of elevation in the scapular plane, underlying multidirectional laxity or generalized ligamentous laxity, or

a positive relocation test. Radiographic evaluation should include specialized views such as the apical oblique or Garth view,[10] the West Point view,[11] and the Stryker notch view.[12] These may demonstrate small Hill-Sachs defects and calcification or fracture of the glenoid rim consistent with recurrent posttraumatic anterior subluxation (Fig. 4).

Treatment includes activity modification and strengthening exercises for the rotator cuff, deltoid, and scapular stabilizers. If

this treatment fails, surgical stabilization may be considered.

Labral or Bicipital Tendon Abnormalities

The tendon of the long head of the biceps traverses the bicipital groove, enters the glenohumeral joint slightly anterior to the supraspinatus insertion, becomes confluent with the superior labrum, and attaches to the supraglenoid tubercle. Because of its course, the biceps tendon may become involved in the subacromial impinge-

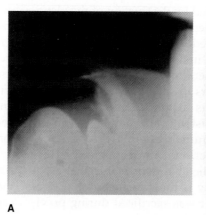
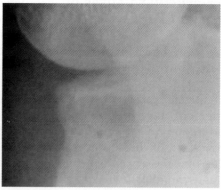

A   B

Fig. 4   **A,** Standing anteroposterior 30-degree tilt radiograph of a patient with continued pain after two arthroscopic acromioplasties and one distal clavicle excision. Physical examination findings were consistent with anterior subluxation. **B,** Stryker notch view revealed calcification at the inferior glenoid margin.

ment process.[1,13] In addition, attritional changes to the tendon within the groove, primary biceps tendinitis, and anterior-to-posterior lesions of the superior labrum ("SLAP" lesions) may result in persistent symptoms after surgery for impingement syndrome.

The physical findings are nonspecific but may include painful resisted forearm supination with the elbow at 90 degrees of flexion. Diagnostic arthroscopy allows visualization of the superior labrum and the biceps tendon. The extra-articular portion of the tendon within the bicipital groove can be visualized by advancing the tendon into the joint with the assistance of a probe or other instrument placed through an anterior portal (Fig. 5). Treatment options include labral repair, labral debridement, and biceps tenodesis.

Extra-articular Causes of Persistent Pain

Persistent Subacromial Impingement

Insufficient supraspinatus outlet decompression may result from residual anterior acromial spurring,[14-17] regrowth of bone or subacromial calcification,[18] inferior projecting acromioclavicular osteophytes,[13] and persistence or regrowth of the coracoacromial ligament.[16,17] Persistent impingement syndrome related to residual supraspinatus outlet narrowing is a common cause of continued shoulder pain after surgery for rotator cuff disease and has been reported in 18% to 79% of patients with failed acromioplasty.[14-17]

Physical examination reveals a positive impingement sign and the impingement reinforcement sign (i.e., Hawkins, or abduction internal rotation ["ABIR"], sign). Substantial reduction in the pain

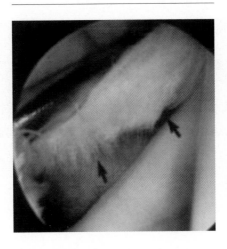

Fig. 5 Arthroscopic image of severe partial tearing of the long head of the biceps in a patient with continued pain after open acromioplasty and cuff repair followed by open distal clavicle excision.

associated with these maneuvers after subacromial injection of lidocaine (i.e., a positive impingement test) helps to confirm the presence of continued subacromial impingement.[1] Radiography should include a supraspinatus outlet view[19] and a 30-degree caudal tilt view[20] to evaluate for continued anterior acromial spurring and a Zanca view[21] (standing anteroposterior view with 15- to 30-degree cephalic tilt) to visualize any inferiorly projecting acromioclavicular osteophytes (Fig. 6).

The results of revision acromioplasty are less reliable than the results of primary acromioplasty.[14-17] Flugstad et al[14] reported the cases of 13 patients who underwent revision acromioplasty with an intact cuff. Six patients described their shoulders as "much better"; the other 7, as "better." Hawkins et al[15] reported the cases of 51 patients in whom acromioplasty had failed. Twelve of these patients underwent repeat acromioplasty, one with a rotator cuff repair. All 12 patients were receiving workmen's compensation.

Only 1 achieved a satisfactory result. Ogilvie-Harris et al[16] evaluated 67 shoulders in 65 patients more than 2 years after an initial acromioplasty for impingement syndrome without a cuff tear. Eighteen of the 65 patients underwent revision rotator cuff surgery (6 rotator cuff repairs and 12 revision acromioplasties). There was a good result in 9 of the 12 patients (75%). Rockwood and Williams[17] reported 67% good or excellent results in 27 patients who underwent revision acromioplasty with an intact or repairable cuff.

Because of the inconsistent results of revision acromioplasty, successful management of patients with persistent subacromial outlet narrowing requires careful patient selection. Nonoperative management should be maximized in all cases. Repeat surgery is reserved for patients with radiographic evidence of continued impingement who obtain pain relief with subacromial lidocaine. In spite of these stringent selection criteria, the results of revision acromioplasty will likely not approach those of primary acromioplasty.

Persistent or Recurrent Rotator Cuff Defect

Evaluation

The presence of a full-thickness rotator cuff defect can be compatible with asymptomatic shoulder function.[22] Furthermore, some authors have reported high percentages of patients with good or excellent results after acromioplasty and cuff repair in spite of arthrographically and ultrasonographically proven persistent or recurrent rotator cuff defects.[23-25] Therefore, when evaluating patients with continued pain and a persistent or recurrent rotator cuff defect after rotator cuff repair, it is important to eliminate other causes of persis-

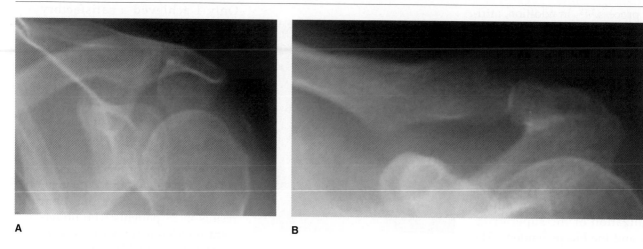

Fig. 6 The 30-degree caudal-tilt radiograph **(A)** and the Zanca view **(B)** are useful adjuncts to the supraspinatus outlet and axillary views when evaluating patients with continued pain after rotator cuff surgery.

tent pain before focusing on the residual rotator cuff defect.

Physical findings are variable and depend on the size of the recurrent rotator cuff defect. Small defects, which primarily affect the supraspinatus tendon, are characterized by an intact anterior (i.e., subscapularis) and posterior (i.e., infraspinatus and teres minor) rotator cuff force couple. The impingement and impingement-reinforcement signs may be positive and accompanied by subacromial crepitus. However, range of overhead elevation, shoulder strength, and function are relatively normal.

Large defects extend anteriorly and/or posteriorly into the subscapularis and infraspinatus–teres minor, respectively. Posterior extension results in weakness of external rotation with the arm at the side and the humerus in neutral rotation. If the posterior rotator cuff insufficiency is severe enough, the patient will be unable to raise the arm overhead, in spite of full passive motion.

The signs of anterior (i.e., subscapularis) rotator cuff insufficiency can be more subtle than the signs of posterior rotator cuff insuf-

ficiency. Increased passive external rotation with the arm at the side is suggestive of subscapularis involvement. Subscapularis insufficiency is verified by a positive "lift off" test.[26] This test is performed by passively resting the back of the patient's hand against the ipsilateral buttock and then asking the patient to actively lift the hand off the back and away from the body without simultaneously extending the shoulder or the elbow (Fig. 7). This requires maximal internal rotation with the subscapularis. Inability to perform this test is indicative of subscapularis insufficiency. However, pain and limitation of passive internal rotation may make interpretation of this test difficult.

Ultrasonography, arthrography, and MR imaging have all been used to evaluate rotator cuff pathology.[27-29] When there has been prior surgery, the presence of subacromial scarring, subacromial bursal thickening, and postsurgical tendon irregularities may complicate the interpretation of the images obtained with these modalities. Therefore, imaging studies must be interpreted with caution

and correlated carefully with the overall clinical impression. In particular, MR imaging of the rotator cuff is not as sensitive or specific as in the shoulder that has not been treated surgically.[30]

Abnormalities of tendon signal intensity in the absence of alterations in signal morphology may

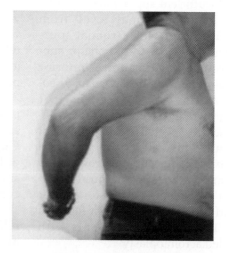

Fig. 7 A patient with an intact subscapularis is able to lift a hand placed on the buttock off the back and away from the body by maximal internal rotation without simultaneously extending the shoulder or elbow.

have no clinical relevance and should be interpreted with caution (Fig. 8, A). However, the presence of a well-defined gap in the tendon with synovial fluid traversing the entire thickness of the tendon into the subacromial space is definitive evidence of a persistent or recurrent defect (Fig. 8, B-D). When a full-thickness defect is present, MR imaging can accurately quantitate the size of the defect in both the anteroposterior and medial-lateral planes and can estimate atrophy in each of the four rotator cuff muscles.

Treatment

In many patients, a persistent cuff defect is accompanied by continued supraspinatus outlet narrowing. DeOrio and Cofield[31] reported the data on 27 patients (27 shoulders) who underwent a second attempt at repair of a rotator cuff tear. Seven patients had physical findings consistent with continued subacromial impingement, and only 12 of the 27 shoulders had undergone an anterior acromioplasty at the time of the initial repair. Neviaser and Neviaser[32] reported on 46 cases of revision cuff repair, in all of which repeat acromioplasty was necessary, presumably because of persistent supraspinatus outlet narrowing. Bigliani et al[33] documented a 90% incidence of inadequate prior acromioplasty in their 31 patients who underwent a repeat repair.

The reported results of revision rotator cuff repair are inconsistent and, in general, inferior to the results of primary cuff repair.[31-33] In the study by DeOrio and Cofield,[31] 7 of the 27 patients (26%) who underwent revision rotator cuff repair required a third operative procedure before study completion and were not, therefore, included in the final results. None of the remaining 20 patients had

excellent results, and only 42% had good results. Bigliani et al[33] reported satisfactory results in 52% of 31 patients who underwent repeat rotator cuff repair. Neviaser and Neviaser[32] reported on 46 revision rotator cuff repairs and critically evaluated return of range of motion in their outcome analysis. Twenty-two patients gained motion (mean, 45 degrees), 22 had no change, and 2 lost motion.

Given the relatively disappointing results of revision acromioplasty and rotator cuff repair, the merits of nonoperative management should not be overlooked. An important component is activity modification, which should involve employment, daily-living, and recreational activities. Physiotherapy, including capsular stretching and strengthening exercises for the remaining portions of the rotator cuff, the deltoid, and the scapular rotators, should be maximized. Revision rotator cuff repair should be considered if nonoperative man-

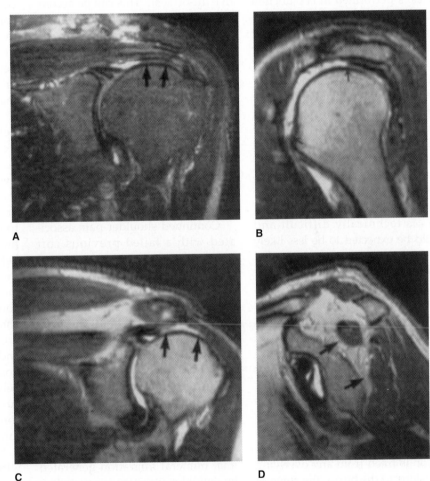

Fig. 8   In the postoperative setting, MR imaging criteria for rotator cuff tears must be more stringent. **A,** Isolated abnormal signal intensity may have no clinical relevance and should be interpreted with caution. The size of a recurrent defect can be quantitated in both the anteroposterior direction **(B)** and the medial-lateral direction **(C)**. The presence of a tendon signal defect traversed by synovial fluid is indicative of a recurrent defect. **D,** Atrophy of individual muscles can be assessed.

agement has failed and the patient is willing to accept the reality of inconsistent results.

The goal of all revision rotator cuff procedures is to achieve a surgical repair that ultimately heals to bone at the operative site and remains intact over the long term. Patients who achieve this goal are most likely to experience the best results with regard to pain, strength, and function.[34] With smaller, more mobile cuff tears, this goal is often attainable. Revision acromioplasty and/or removal of inferior acromioclavicular osteophytes is performed in conjunction with rotator cuff repair when residual supraspinatus outlet narrowing from anterior acromial or inferior acromioclavicular spurring exists.

The rotator cuff tears most likely to rerupture after repair are the large tears with two- or three-tendon involvement, particularly in older patients.[34] In addition, large initial tears are most likely to be difficult to repair, primarily because of poor tissue quality. Therefore, revision of failed repairs of large rotator cuff tears is technically difficult and would be expected to be less likely to result in a permanently healed tendon.

The most important aspects of surgical technique in these difficult cases are tendon identification and mobilization. The subacromial bursa may be abnormally thickened and must not be mistaken for the torn rotator cuff tendon edge. Once the retracted tendon edge has been identified, it is systematically mobilized laterally. First, the superficial surface of the retracted tendon is freed from any overlying adhesions to the bursa, the spine of the scapula, and the deep surface of the posterior deltoid and trapezius. Second, the retracted tendon edge is pulled laterally in order to identify any contracture of the coracohumeral ligament, which is

released if present. Finally, if necessary, any tenodesis effect of the underlying capsule is addressed by stretching the posterior capsule with an intra-articular "metal finger" or by releasing the capsule sharply slightly distal to the labrum. The mobilized tendon is then repaired to bone on the greater tuberosity or at the anatomic neck, slightly medial to the anatomic insertion site.

The subscapularis tendon should routinely be inspected for partial or complete avulsion, especially in patients with a positive preoperative lift-off test. This can be accomplished through a standard superior incision by flexing the humerus to bring the subscapularis into the wound. Alternatively, if preoperative evaluation indicates an isolated subscapularis injury, an anterior deltopectoral approach can be utilized. In either case, the subscapularis tendon is mobilized laterally and repaired to bone. Sufficient mobilization to allow repair may require release of the underlying anterior capsule.

Continued shoulder pain associated with a failed previous cuff repair in an irreparable persistent rotator cuff defect is a potentially difficult problem, which may not have a good solution. The interaction between the deltoid, the rotator cuff, and the coracoacromial arch (anterior acromion, distal clavicle, and coracoacromial ligament) during elevation of the arm is complex and not completely understood. In the presence of an intact and normally functioning rotator cuff mechanism, the potential proximal humeral migration generated by deltoid contraction is resisted by the rotator cuff; the humerus remains relatively centered on the glenoid fossa, and normal overhead elevation is accomplished.[35,36] Under these circumstances, the relative role of the coracoacromial

arch as a humeral-head containment mechanism is minor.

In some cases involving irreparable rotator cuff tears, enough anterior and posterior rotator cuff function remains to effectively resist proximal humeral migration during deltoid contraction. The humeral head again remains relatively centered, and overhead elevation is normal or near normal in range but may be weak. The rotator cuff function lost to the irreparable cuff defect is "compensated" for by the remaining balanced anterior and posterior rotator cuff force couple.[37] The degree to which the coracoacromial arch functions as a humeral-head containment mechanism is variable and is probably dependent on the amount of anterior and posterior rotator cuff remaining.

If the persistent rotator cuff defect is too large, the associated loss of rotator cuff function cannot be compensated for. In this relatively "uncompensated" shoulder, the remaining anterior and posterior rotator cuff mechanism is unable to effectively resist the proximal humeral migration associated with deltoid contraction. Consequently, the coracoacromial arch becomes more important as a humeral-head containment mechanism.[38,39] Incompetence of the coracoacromial arch due to prior acromioplasty and coracoacromial ligament resection combined with a poorly compensated or uncompensated rotator cuff defect may result in severe compromise of overhead shoulder function.[39]

Surgical treatment of a patient with persistent pain and an irreparable rotator cuff defect is potentially difficult and is dependent on the supposed cause of the continued pain as well as the size of the defect. In the presence of continued supraspinatus outlet narrowing, as documented on supraspinatus outlet and 30-degree caudal-tilt radiographs, persistent pain is likely to be the result of continued subacromial impingement. If pain is relieved with subacromial lidocaine and the irreparable rotator cuff defect is compensated for, as evidenced by intact overhead function and relative preservation of the acromiohumeral interval (i.e., an acromiohumeral interval of 7 mm or greater), repeat subacromial decompression without repair should provide acceptable pain relief while preserving overhead function.[40]

Rockwood et al[40] have reported satisfactory results with subacromial decompression and partial cuff debridement in patients with subacromial impingement syndrome associated with chronic irreparable rotator cuff defects. The results were less satisfactory in patients who had undergone prior rotator cuff surgery. However, many of these patients also had iatrogenic deltoid insufficiency. Although more complicated surgical options for management of the irreparable cuff defect have been reported,[41-47] none has been demonstrated to be superior to debridement alone when the defect is well compensated.

Debridement alone for patients with persistent pain associated with an uncompensated irreparable rotator cuff defect is unlikely to either alleviate pain or improve function. If the patient is unable to actively raise the arm overhead preoperatively, even when pain is relieved with subacromial lidocaine, it is unlikely the ability to raise the arm overhead postoperatively will be regained unless some of the lost anterior or, more commonly, posterior rotator cuff function can be reestablished. In fact, repeat subacromial decompression and partial rotator cuff debridement may further compromise shoulder function by removing the

humeral-head containment provided by any remaining portions of the acromion and coracoacromial ligament.[39]

The painful shoulder with an uncompensated irreparable rotator cuff defect and an incompetent coracoacromial arch is currently a problem without a solution. Many techniques have been described to reconstruct massive irreparable rotator cuff defects.[41-47] However, few of them have the potential to restore lost rotator cuff function, as opposed to merely filling the defect. Reconstruction of the superior defect with autograft fascia lata, allograft fascia lata or rotator cuff, or prosthetic material may provide a tenodesis effect, but is not likely to restore function to severely atrophic rotator cuff musculature.[44,45,47] Superior transposition of the teres minor and/or the subscapularis has the potential advantage of improving head depression but has the potential disadvantage of destabilizing the anterior-posterior force couple.[41,46] From a conceptual point of view, transfer of the latissimus dorsi insertion into the posterosuperior humeral head is appealing.[48] It provides a functional musculotendinous unit without sacrificing any remaining anterior or posterior rotator cuff function. In addition, the resultant line of action provides potential head depression. The indications for unipolar latissimus dorsi transfer continue to be defined. The reported results have been variable and seem to be best when the subscapularis is not also deficient.

The role of coracoacromial arch reconstruction in this setting has yet to be established. Wiley[39] described the use of a coracoacromial interpositional iliac-crest autograft in five patients with persistent symptoms associated with irreparable rotator cuff defects and defi-

cient coracoacromial arches after a failed acromioplasty and rotator cuff repair. The results were disappointing, and useful overhead function could not be restored. At least three of these patients had anterior deltoid deficiency, which may have contributed to the poor postoperative elevation. The importance of a functional coracoacromial arch in patients with an uncompensated irreparable rotator cuff defect seems clear. However, additional work is required to define surgical techniques and indications for coracoacromial arch reconstruction or repair.

Acromioclavicular Joint Arthropathy

Acromioclavicular arthropathy is a relatively common cause of persistent pain after acromioplasty with or without cuff repair. Resectional arthroplasty or distal clavicle excision is indicated if the following criteria are met: (1) the acromioclavicular joint is tender to palpation and painful during crossbody adduction, (2) there is radiographic evidence of arthritis, and (3) temporary pain relief follows a local intra-articular injection of lidocaine.

The optimal amount of bone to be resected from the distal clavicle remains somewhat controversial. Displacement of the clavicle along its longitudinal axis, toward the acromion, is primarily controlled by the trapezoid portion of the coracoclavicular ligament.[49] With large displacements, the acromioclavicular ligaments primarily resist anteroposterior displacement of the clavicle, and the coracoclavicular ligament (especially the conoid portion) resists superoinferior displacement.[49] Results of distal clavicle excision may be negatively affected by excessive translation of the distal clavicle in both the anteroposterior and superoinferior planes. Therefore, the amount of bone resected should be sufficient to prevent axial compression or contact between the residual clavicle and the acromion, but not so much as to compromise the capsular and coracoclavicular ligaments.

Resection can be performed arthroscopically or by traditional open techniques. Our current practice in most cases is to arthroscopically remove 1.0 cm of distal clavicle, which results in a final gap distance of 1.2 to 1.5 cm.

Deltoid Insufficiency

Denervation or postoperative detachment of the deltoid after acromioplasty and cuff repair is a devastating complication, which is best managed by prevention (Fig. 9). The axillary nerve exits the quadrilateral space and divides into a posterior branch, which innervates the teres minor and the posterior portion of the deltoid, and an anterior branch, which innervates the middle and anterior deltoid. As the anterior branch courses from posterior to anterior, it lies approximately 4 to 5 cm distal to the lateral edge of the acromion. In this position, the nerve is vulnerable to injury if the surgical incision splits the deltoid beyond the 4- to 5-cm "safe zone."[1] If this occurs, all portions of the deltoid anterior to the deltoid incision can be denervated, which results in substantial functional impairment. Therefore, extreme caution should be used when splitting the deltoid in line with its fibers, so that the length of the split does not exceed 4 to 5 cm.

Postoperative deltoid detachment can be minimized by using a deltoid-preserving approach during acromioplasty and cuff repair.[50] Once the interval between the anterior and middle deltoid fibers has been identified, the deltoid split is

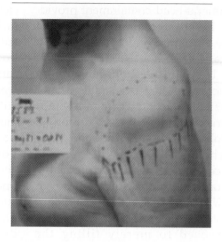

Fig. 9 Deltoid detachment is an operative disaster, as in this patient who underwent radical acromionectomy and sustained postoperative deltoid disruption.

extended proximally into the deltotrapezius aponeurosis, at the anterior edge of the acromion. The incision in the deltotrapezius aponeurosis should be carefully placed so that it leaves a strong tendinous edge on the anterior deltoid to allow secure reattachment. Deltoid reattachment is accomplished by intratendinous repair of the deltotrapezius aponeurosis, which can be supplemented by transosseous sutures through the acromion.

If detachment of the deltoid is recognized early in the postoperative period, repair is much easier and more likely to yield a satisfactory result than if the postoperative detachment is discovered late, when the tendon has retracted and the muscle has atrophied. Therefore, the deltoid repair should be routinely inspected at each postoperative visit. The findings associated with deltoid dehiscence can be subtle. If the patient is requested to gently contract the deltoid while the arm is supported by the examiner, the integrity of the deltoid origin can be verified. Early postoperative failure of the deltoid repair is

often associated with large hematoma formation, which should always raise the index of suspicion for possible deltoid disruption. When deltoid detachment is suspected, operative repair is warranted. If the initial repair was not transosseous, attempting reattachment to bone should be considered. Because the tissue quality is often suboptimal, an abduction brace or pillow may be used for protection.

The surgical management of chronic postoperative deltoid detachment or denervation includes primary repair, local muscle transposition, and distant muscle transfer.[51,52] When the defect is small to moderate in size, primary repair is attempted. Complete closure of larger defects may require anterior transposition of a portion of the middle deltoid. Loss of the entire anterior deltoid due to denervation is a very difficult problem. If the deltoid deficiency is accompanied by a massive, potentially irreparable rotator cuff defect and coracoacromial arch incompetence, arthrodesis may be the most prudent option. If rotator cuff integrity has been maintained, however, bipolar transfer of the latissimus dorsi may be indicated.[52]

Patients who have undergone radical or complete acromionectomy represent a specific subgroup of patients with postoperative deltoid insufficiency that is even more difficult to treat than the group as a whole.[53] Satisfactory results with radical acromionectomy have been reported.[54] However, when deltoid dehiscence occurs after radical or complete acromionectomy, absence of the acromion makes reattachment of the deltoid technically difficult, if not impossible. In addition, radical acromionectomy, by definition, results in coracoacromial arch insufficiency. Postoperative deltoid detachment after radical acromionectomy combined with a persistent uncompensated rotator cuff defect results in severe functional disability, which is probably not salvageable without arthrodesis. For these reasons, radical acromionectomy is unpopular.

Summary

Shoulder pain that persists after rotator cuff surgery may be the result of many causes, both intrinsic and extrinsic to the shoulder. Appropriate evaluation may identify a subset of patients with intrinsic shoulder disorders amenable to surgical correction. When continued pain is the result of persistent subacromial impingement or a persistent rotator cuff defect, the results of revision surgery are inferior to the reported results of primary acromioplasty and cuff repair. The goals of revision rotator cuff repair are a decompressed supraspinatus outlet and a permanently healed tendon. If the rotator cuff defect is irreparable but compensated, satisfactory results can be obtained with repeat subacromial decompression and partial rotator cuff debridement. The combination of an irreparable uncompensated rotator cuff defect and coracoacromial arch incompetence is currently an unsolved problem.

References

1. Neer CS II: Anterior acromioplasty for the chronic impingement syndrome in the shoulder: A preliminary report. *J Bone Joint Surg Am* 1972;54:41-50.

2. Neer CS II: Replacement arthroplasty for glenohumeral osteoarthritis. *J Bone Joint Surg Am* 1974;56:1-13.

3. Neer CS II, Craig EV, Fukuda H: Cuff-tear arthropathy. *J Bone Joint Surg Am* 1983;65:1232-1244.

4. Arntz CT, Jackins S, Matsen FA III: Prosthetic replacement of the shoulder for the treatment of defects in the rotator cuff and the surface of the glenohumeral joint. *J Bone Joint Surg Am* 1993;75:485-491.

5. Pollock RG, Deliz ED, McIlveen SJ, et al: Prosthetic replacement in rotator cuff deficient shoulders. *J Shoulder Elbow Surg* 1992;1:173-186.

6. McLaughlin HL: The "frozen shoulder." *Clin Orthop* 1961;20:126-131.

7. Pollock RG, Duralde XA, Flatow EL, et al: The use of arthroscopy in the treatment of resistant frozen shoulder. *Clin Orthop* 1994;304:30-36.

8. Harryman DT II: Shoulders: Frozen and stiff. *Instr Course Lect* 1993;42:247-257.

9. Jobe FW, Tibone JE, Jobe CM, et al: The shoulder in sports, in Rockwood CA Jr, Matsen FA III (eds): *The Shoulder.* Philadelphia: WB Saunders, 1990, vol 2, pp 961-990.

10. Garth WP Jr, Slappey CE, Ochs CW: Roentgenographic demonstration of instability of the shoulder: The apical oblique projection—A technical note. *J Bone Joint Surg Am* 1984;66:1450-1453.

11. Rokous JR, Feagin JA, Abbott HG: Modified axillary roentgenogram: A useful adjunct in the diagnosis of recurrent instability of the shoulder. *Clin Orthop* 1972;82:84-86.

12. Hall RH, Isaac F, Booth CR: Dislocations of the shoulder with special reference to accompanying small fractures. *J Bone Joint Surg Am* 1959;41:489-494.

13. Neer CS II: Impingement lesions. *Clin Orthop* 1983;173:70-77.

14. Flugstad D, Matsen FA, Larry I, et al: Failed acromioplasty: Etiology and prevention. *Orthop Trans* 1986;10:229.

15. Hawkins RJ, Chris T, Bokor D, et al: Failed anterior acromioplasty: A review of 51 cases. *Clin Orthop* 1989;243:106-111.

16. Ogilvie-Harris DJ, Wiley AM, Sattarian J: Failed acromioplasty for impingement syndrome. *J Bone Joint Surg Br* 1990;72:1070-1072.

17. Rockwood CA Jr, Williams GR: The shoulder impingement syndrome: Management of surgical treatment failures. *Orthop Trans* 1992/93;16:739-740.

18. Lazarus MD, Chansky HA, Misra S, et al: Comparison of open and arthroscopic subacromial decompression. *J Shoulder Elbow Surg* 1994;3:1-11.

19. Neer CS II, Poppen NK: Supraspinatus outlet. *Orthop Trans* 1987;11:234.

20. Cone RO II, Resnick D, Danzig L: Shoulder impingement syndrome: Radiographic evaluation. *Radiology* 1984;150:29-33.

21. Zanca P: Shoulder pain: Involvement of the acromioclavicular joint (analysis of 1,000 cases.) *AJR Am J Roentgenol* 1971;112:493-506.

22. Sher JS, Uribe JW, Posada A, et al: Abnormal findings on magnetic resonance images of asymptomatic shoulders. *J Bone Joint Surg Am* 1995;77:10-15.

23. Blauth W, Gartner J: Ergebnisse postoperativer Arthrographien nach Naht rupturierter Rotatorenmanschetten. *Orthopade* 1991;20:262-265.

24. Calvert PT, Packer NP, Stoker DJ, et al: Arthrography of the shoulder after operative repair of the torn rotator cuff. *J Bone Joint Surg Br* 1986;68:147-150.

25. Wulker N, Melzer C, Wirth CJ: Shoulder surgery for rotator cuff tears: Ultrasonographic 3-year follow-up of 97 cases. *Acta Orthop Scand* 1991;62:142-147.

26. Gerber C, Krushell RJ: Isolated rupture of the tendon of the subscapularis muscle: Clinical features in 16 cases. *J Bone Joint Surg Br* 1991;73:389-394.

27. Ghelman B, Goldman AB: The double contrast shoulder arthrogram: Evaluation of rotary cuff tears. *Radiology* 1977;124:251-254.

28. Mack LA, Gannon MK, Kilcoyne RF, et al: Sonographic evaluation of the rotator cuff: Accuracy in patients without prior surgery. *Clin Orthop* 1988;234:21-28.

29. Iannotti JP, Zlatkin MB, Esterhai JL, et al: Magnetic resonance imaging of the shoulder: Sensitivity, specificity, and predictive value. *J Bone Joint Surg Am* 1991;73:17-29.

30. Owen R, Iannotti JP, Kneeland B, et al: Shoulder after surgery: MR imaging with surgical validation. *Radiology* 1993;186:443-447.

31. DeOrio JK, Cofield RH: Results of a second attempt at surgical repair of a failed initial rotator-cuff repair. *J Bone Joint Surg Am* 1984;66:563-567.

32. Neviaser RJ, Neviaser TJ: Reoperation for failed rotator cuff repair: Analysis of 46 cases. *Orthop Trans* 1989;13:241.

33. Bigliani LU, Cordasco FA, McIlveen SJ, et al: Operative treatment of failed repairs of the rotator cuff. *J Bone Joint Surg Am* 1992;74:1505-1515.

34. Harryman DT, Mack LA, Wang KW, et al: Repairs of the rotator cuff: Correlation of functional results with integrity of the cuff. *J Bone Joint Surg Am* 1991;73:982-989.

35. Poppen NK, Walker PS: Normal and abnormal motion of the shoulder. *J Bone Joint Surg Am* 1976;58:195-201.

36. Kelkar R, Newton PM, Armengol J, et al: Three-dimensional kinematics of the glenohumeral joint during abduction in the scapular plane. *Trans Orthop Res Soc* 1993;18:136.

37. Burkhart SS: Arthroscopic treatment of massive rotator cuff tears: Clinical results and biomechanical rationale. *Clin Orthop* 1991;267:45-56.

38. Flatow EL, Wang VM, Kelkar R, et al: The coracoacromial ligament passively restrains anterosuperior humeral subluxation in the rotator cuff deficient shoulder. *Trans Orthop Res Soc* 1996; 21:229.

39. Wiley AM: Superior humeral dislocation: A complication following decompression and debridement for rotator cuff tears. *Clin Orthop* 1991;263:135-141.

40. Rockwood CA Jr, Williams GR Jr, Burkhead WZ Jr: Debridement of degenerative, irreparable lesions of the rotator cuff. *J Bone Joint Surg Am* 1995; 77:857-866.

41. Cofield RH: Subscapular muscle transposition for repair of chronic rotator cuff tears. *Surg Gynecol Obstet* 1982;154:667-672.

42. Debeyre J, Patte D, Elmelik E: Repair of ruptures of the rotator cuff of the shoulder with a note on advancement of the supraspinatus muscle. *J Bone Joint Surg Br* 1965;47:36-42.

43. Ha'eri GB, Wiley AM: Advancement of the supraspinatus muscle in the repair of ruptures of the rotator cuff. *J Bone Joint Surg Am* 1981;63:232-238.

44. Nasca RJ: The use of freeze-dried allografts in the management of global rotator cuff tears. *Clin Orthop* 1988; 228:218-226.

45. Neviaser JS, Neviaser RJ, Neviaser TJ: The repair of chronic massive ruptures of the rotator cuff of the shoulder by use of a freeze-dried rotator cuff. *J Bone Joint Surg Am* 1978;60:681-684.

46. Neviaser RJ, Neviaser TJ: Transfer of the subscapularis and teres minor for massive defects of the rotator, in Bayley I, Kessel L (eds): *Shoulder Surgery.* Berlin: Springer, 1982, pp 60-63.

47. Parrish FF, Murray JA, Urquhart BA: The use of polyethylene mesh (Marlex) as an adjunct in reconstructive surgery of the extremities. *Clin Orthop* 1978; 137:276-286.

48. Gerber C: Latissimus dorsi transfer for the treatment of irreparable tears of the rotator cuff. *Clin Orthop* 1992;275: 152-160.

49. Fukuda K, Craig EV, An KN, et al: Biomechanical study of the ligamentous system of the acromioclavicular joint. *J Bone Joint Surg Am* 1986;68:434-440.

50. Matsen FA III, Arntz CT: Subacromial impingement, in Rockwood CA Jr, Matsen FA III (eds): *The Shoulder.* Philadelphia: WB Saunders, 1990, pp 623-646.

51. Groh GI, Simoni M, Rolla P, et al: Loss of the deltoid after shoulder operations: An operative disaster. *J Shoulder Elbow Surg* 1994;3:243-253.

52. Itoh Y, Sasaki T, Ishiguro T, et al: Transfer of latissimus dorsi to replace a paralysed anterior deltoid: A new technique using an inverted pedicled graft. *J Bone Joint Surg Br* 1987;69:647-651.

53. Neer CS II, Marberry TA: On the disadvantages of radical acromionectomy. *J Bone Joint Surg Am* 1981;63:416-419.

54. Bosley RC: Total acromionectomy: A twenty-year review. *J Bone Joint Surg Am* 1991;73:961-968.

Management of Chronic Deep Infection Following Rotator Cuff Repair*

BY RAFFY MIRZAYAN, M.D.†, JOHN M. ITAMURA, M.D.†, C. THOMAS VANGSNESS, JR., M.D.†,
PAUL D. HOLTOM, M.D.†, RANDY SHERMAN, M.D.†, AND MICHAEL J. PATZAKIS, M.D.†

*Investigation performed at the Department of Orthopaedic Surgery, University of
Southern California School of Medicine, University Hospital, Los Angeles, California*

Abstract

Background: Deep infection of the shoulder following rotator cuff repair is uncommon. There are few reports in the literature regarding the management of such infections.

Methods: We retrospectively reviewed the charts of thirteen patients and recorded the demographic data, clinical and laboratory findings, risk factors, bacteriological findings, and results of surgical management.

Results: The average age of the patients was 63.7 years. The interval between the rotator cuff repair and the referral because of infection averaged 9.7 months. An average of 2.4 procedures were performed prior to referral because of infection, and an average of 2.1 procedures were performed at our institution. All patients had pain on presentation, and most had a restricted range of motion. Most patients were afebrile and did not have an elevated white blood-cell count but did have an elevated erythrocyte sedimentation rate. The most common organisms were *Staphylococcus epidermidis*, *Staphylococcus aureus*, and Propionibacterium species. At an average of 3.1 years, all patients were free of infection. Using the Simple Shoulder Test, eight patients stated that the shoulder was comfortable with the arm at rest by the side, they could sleep comfortably, and they were able to perform activities below shoulder level. However, most patients had poor overhead function.

Conclusions: Extensive soft-tissue loss or destruction is associated with a worse prognosis. Extensive débridement, often combined with a muscle transfer, and administration of the appropriate antibiotics controlled the infection, although most patients were left with a substantial deficit in overhead function of the shoulder.

Rotator cuff tear is one of the most common afflictions of the shoulder and is commonly treated surgically. The prevalence of infection after open rotator cuff repair has ranged from 0.27 percent[17] to 1.7 percent[11]. Deep infection following rotator cuff repair can be missed because of a low index of suspicion. This may lead to chronic infection of the shoulder, which can result in devastating limitations of function. However, there are few reports in the literature regarding the management of chronic deep infection of the shoulder following surgery[14,17,21].

In this retrospective report, we analyzed the demographic data, clinical and laboratory findings, risk factors, bacteriological findings, and results of surgical management in thirteen patients with deep shoulder infection following rotator cuff surgery.

Materials and Methods

Patient Population

Between 1991 and 1997, thirteen patients were referred to our center for the treatment of chronic deep infection following open rotator cuff surgery. There were seven men and six women. The average age was 63.7 years (range, twenty-six to eighty-one years). The dominant shoulder was involved in eleven patients. Four patients were receiving Workers' Compensation. Five patients were laborers, and eight patients had a sedentary job. The interval between the rotator cuff repair and the referral because of infection averaged 9.7 months (range, three to twenty-five months). An average of 2.4 (range, one to six) procedures were performed prior to referral, and an average of 2.1 (two, three, or four) procedures were performed at our institution. The average duration of follow-up was 3.1 years (range, one to 6.6 years).

Risk Factors

The classification system for osteomyelitis described by Cierny and Mader[3] (Table I) was used since eleven patients had osteomyelitis of the humeral head or the clavicle. One patient was an A-host — that is, there were no risk factors for infection or compromised wound-healing. Eight patients who were B-hosts with systemic compromise were sixty years of age or older, and one of the eight had adult-onset diabetes and coronary artery disease. Three B-hosts with systemic compromise had hypothyroidism, and one of the three also had a primary IgA deficiency. Six B-hosts with systemic compromise were smokers, and two drank alcohol on a daily basis. Four patients were B-hosts with local compromise. Two of these patients had had an ipsilateral mastectomy[4]. One of the two had had a radical mastectomy and axillary lymph-node dissection without radiation or chemotherapy. Chronic lymphedema developed in the involved extremity. The other patient had had a mastectomy followed by three reconstructive breast procedures. The other two B-hosts with local compromise had had two steroid injections each prior to surgery. No documentation of steroid injections could be found for the other patients. Six patients had more than one risk factor.

Surgical Procedures

The surgery included drainage of the infected glenohumeral joint in all thirteen patients and drainage of the acromioclavicular joint in two. Débridement of infected and necrotic bone was carried out in

*No benefits in any form have been received or will be received from a commercial party related directly or indirectly to the subject of this article. No funds were received in support of this study.

†Department of Orthopaedic Surgery, University of Southern California School of Medicine, 1200 North State Street, GNH 3900, Los Angeles, California 90033.

TABLE I

RISK FACTORS ACCORDING TO
THE CIERNY-MADER CLASSIFICATION[3]

	No. of Patients
I. A-host	1
II. B-host	
A. Systemic compromise	
1. Age ≥60 years	
a. No other medical problems	7
b. With type-II diabetes and coronary artery disease	1
2. Hypothyroidism	
a. With primary IgA deficiency	1
b. Without primary IgA deficiency	2
3. Smoking	6
4. Alcoholism	2
B. Local compromise	
1. Mastectomy	
a. With lymphedema	1
b. Without lymphedema	1
2. Steroid injections	2

seven humeral heads, four clavicles, four acromions, and three glenoids. Eleven patients had synovectomy, six had bursectomy, and nine had sinus tract excision. Nonabsorbable sutures were removed in all thirteen patients. The biceps tendon sheath was identified and explored for purulence in four patients. Irrigation with ten liters of fluid, with the last liter containing 100,000 units of bacitracin and 1,000,000 units of polymyxin, was performed in all patients. After the initial débridement, dead spaces were managed with suction drainage in ten of the patients and with insertion of antibiotic-impregnated beads in three. All patients returned to the operating room for serial irrigations and débridements. Intraoperative specimens of fluid, soft tissue, bone shavings, and curetted material from the intramedullary canal were obtained from all thirteen patients and were sent for aerobic, anaerobic, fungal, and acid-fast-bacillus culture. The patients received parenteral antibiotics for six weeks on the basis of the culture results.

Four patients required a latissimus dorsi flap (Figs. 1-A through 1-F), and three required a pectoralis major flap. When available local soft tissue was found to be inadequate for tension-free wound closure with complete obliteration of any residual dead space, the patient was returned to the operating room for muscle flap transfer. The addition of vascularized soft tissue to the wound maximized the chance of successful closure and minimized the possibility of late recurrence. The latissimus dorsi and pectoralis major muscles both offer a generous amount of vascularized tissue for the management of nearly all types of shoulder wounds. Because of its long vascular pedicle and broad dimensions, the latissimus dorsi flap is preferable for larger, more complex wounds[12,19]. Also, there is less deformity and morbidity when the latissimus flap, as opposed to the pectoralis flap, is used. At times, however, it may be better to manage a medially based lesion by rotating a small portion of the pectoralis into it[13,16]. If the thoracodorsal pedicle has been injured during previous dissections, the latissimus muscle may be unusable.

Method of Outcome Evaluation

The Simple Shoulder Test[10] was administered to twelve patients (Table II). Five patients were examined in our clinic, and seven were interviewed over the telephone. The Simple Shoulder Test is a function-based outcome-assessment tool consisting of twelve questions, some of which were derived from the evaluation devised by Neer and the American Shoulder and Elbow Surgeons[10]. It is a quick, practical, and inexpensive method for assessing a patient's satisfaction with treatment. In addition, it indirectly assesses the patient's range of motion by asking such questions as "Can you reach the small of your back to tuck in your shirt with your hand?" and "Can you place a coin on a shelf at the level of your shoulder without bending your elbow?" The questions require a yes-or-no response. Little equipment is needed, and the test can be carried out over the telephone or by mail.

Results

Clinical and Laboratory Findings

All patients had pain on presentation. In addition, eight patients had swelling and erythema. Four patients

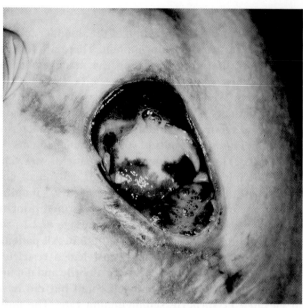

FIG. 1-A

Figs. 1-A through 1-F: A sixty-year-old woman in whom an infection developed following an open rotator cuff repair. She had three risk factors, including an age of sixty years, cortisone injections prior to the rotator cuff surgery, and an ipsilateral mastectomy. Two irrigations and débridements were performed prior to referral for the infection.

Fig. 1-A: Photograph made at the time of presentation, showing a two by three-centimeter open wound with the humeral head exposed.

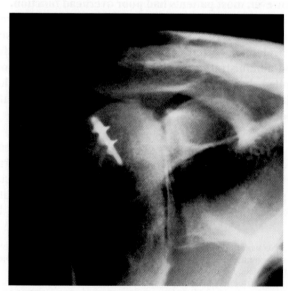

FIG. 1-B

Anteroposterior radiograph of the right shoulder, showing a retained suture anchor.

reported fevers prior to presentation. Nine patients had a draining sinus or a synoviocutaneous fistula (Figs. 2-A through 2-D). The humeral head was exposed in three patients, and the clavicle was exposed in one. All thirteen patients had less than 90 degrees of forward elevation. The average temperature at presentation was 98.0 degrees Fahrenheit (36.7 degrees Celsius) (range, 96.6 to 99.7 degrees Fahrenheit [35.9 to 37.6 degrees Celsius]). The average white blood-cell count was 7700 per cubic millimeter (7.7×10^9 per liter) (range, 4800 to 10,300 per cubic millimeter [4.8 to 10.3×10^9 per liter]) with an average neutrophil count of 58 percent (range, 43 to 77 percent). The erythrocyte sedimentation rate was available for eight patients; it averaged fifty-seven millimeters per hour (range, six to 135 millimeters per

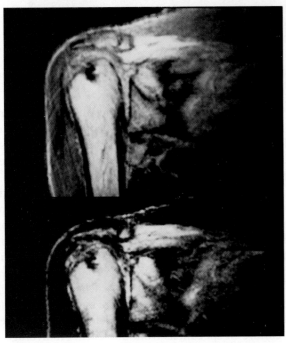

FIG. 1-C

Proton-density magnetic resonance image (top) and T2-weighted magnetic resonance image (bottom) showing involvement of the humeral head and the glenoid.

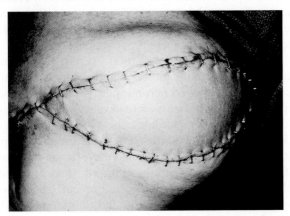

FIG. 1-D

Photograph showing wound coverage with a rotational myocutaneous latissimus dorsi flap following another irrigation and débridement.

TABLE II
RESULTS OF SIMPLE SHOULDER TEST[10]

	No. of Patients Capable of Activity
Shoulder comfortable with arm at rest by side	8
Shoulder allows comfortable sleep	8
Tuck in shirt at small of back	8
Place hand behind head	5
Place coin on shelf at level of shoulder without bending elbow	4
Lift 1 pound (0.5 kilogram) to level of shoulder without bending elbow	3
Lift 8 pounds (3.6 kilograms) to level of shoulder without bending elbow	0
Carry 20 pounds (9.1 kilograms) at side with affected extremity	8
Toss softball underhand 10 yards (9.1 meters)	8
Toss softball overhand 10 yards (9.1 meters)	1
Wash back of contralateral shoulder	6
Work full-time at regular job	5

hour). All but one patient had an abnormal erythrocyte sedimentation rate.

One of the drawbacks of a retrospective study is incomplete information. The only information that was available about the patients was that they had had an open rotator cuff repair. There was no information regarding the size of the original tear, the method of repair, whether the axilla had been shaved, use of perioperative antibiotics, or whether diagnostic arthroscopy had been performed prior to the open procedure.

Intraoperative Findings

All thirteen patients had an infected glenohumeral joint, and two had an infected acromioclavicular joint. Seven patients had osteomyelitis of the humeral head alone, two had osteomyelitis of the humeral head and the glenoid, two had osteomyelitis of the clavicle and the acromion, and two did not have osteomyelitis but had a subdeltoid abscess. Four patients had eburnated cartilage of the humeral head. All thirteen patients were found to have a deficiency of the rotator cuff at the time of the surgery for the infection. Five had immediate repair of the rotator cuff at the time of repeat débridement, which allowed coverage of the glenohumeral joint. One patient had a delayed repair of the rotator cuff six months after the surgery for the infection. Seven patients required a rotational flap to allow for coverage of the joint.

Culture Results

Staphylococcus aureus (five patients) and *Staphylococcus epidermidis* (four patients) were the most common organisms isolated, followed by Propionibacterium

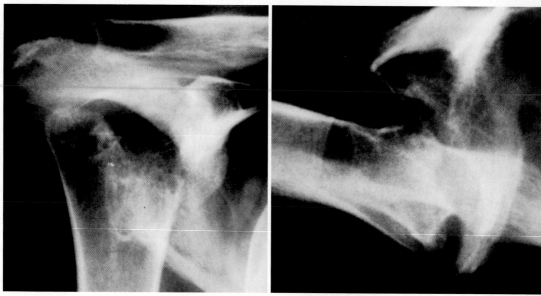

FIG. 1-E   FIG. 1-F

Anteroposterior and axillary radiographs made at one year. There were no signs of infection, and the patient had no pain with the arm at rest by the side, could sleep comfortably, and could perform activities that did not require overhead function.

species (three), diphtheroids (one), coagulase-negative *Staphylococcus aureus* (one), and streptococcal species (one). Three patients had a polymicrobial infection. Three patients had no growth on intraoperative culture, but purulent material was noted intraoperatively.

Functional Results

At an average of 3.1 years, all patients were free of infection.

The results of the Simple Shoulder Test are presented in Table II. Eight patients stated that the shoulder was comfortable with the arm at rest by the side, they could sleep comfortably, and they were able to perform activities below shoulder level. Three patients could lift a one-pound (0.5-kilogram) weight and none could lift an eight-pound (3.6-kilogram) weight to the level of the shoulder without bending the elbow. Eight patients could throw underhand, but only one could throw overhand.

Of the five patients who were examined in our office at the time of follow-up, two had reflex sympathetic dystrophy and two had a deficient deltoid. All four of these patients stated that the shoulder was uncomfortable with the arm at rest by their side and that it did not allow them to sleep comfortably at night. At the time of follow-up, none of the four patients who had been receiving Workers' Compensation preoperatively had returned to work, while all eight who had not been receiving Workers' Compensation had returned to work.

Discussion

Chronic deep shoulder infection following rotator cuff repair is a rare and debilitating complication[15]. In a review of forty reports published between 1982 and 1995, Mansat et al.[11] found that, of 2948 rotator cuff repairs, thirty-one (1.1 percent) were complicated by deep infection. In their own series of 116 cuff repairs, Mansat et al.[11] reported a deep infection in two patients (1.7 percent). Settecerri et al.[17] reported an infection rate of 0.27 percent (eight of 2927) after open rotator cuff repairs performed at the Mayo Clinic. Eight additional patients who had had the index procedure at other institutions were referred for treatment. Propionibacterium species grew on culture of specimens from five patients; *Staphylococcus epidermidis* and *Staphylococcus aureus* grew on culture of specimens from four each; and *Peptostreptococcus magnus*, Corynebacterium, and both *Staphylococcus epidermidis* and Propionibacterium species grew on culture of specimens from one each. An average of 3.5 operative procedures were required to eradicate the infection. At the time of follow-up, six of the sixteen patients were pain-free, five had mild pain, and five had moderate pain. Nearly half were able to actively elevate the arm beyond 90 degrees. The results of that study were similar to those of the present study with respect to the findings on culture and the functional outcomes.

Recently, Torres and Wright[21] reported on three cases of postoperative infection and a synovial cutaneous fistula after failed acromioplasty and rotator cuff repair. All three patients were seventy years of age or older. Similar to our findings, the average duration of infection was 10.2 months; however, unlike our patients, the patients had a normal erythrocyte sedimentation rate on presentation. In all three patients, dehiscence at the site of the rotator cuff repair was found at the time of irrigation and débridement. The wounds were closed primarily by elevation of skin flaps and other portions of the rotator cuff. The shoulders were immobilized for six weeks. At an average of

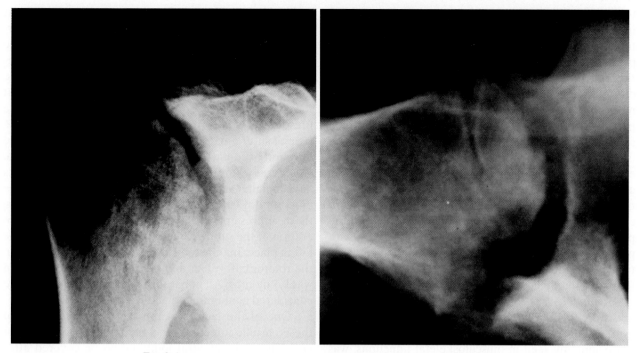

FIG. 2-A   FIG. 2-B

Figs. 2-A through 2-D: A sixty-year-old man in whom an infection developed following an open rotator cuff repair.
Figs. 2-A and 2-B: Anteroposterior and axillary radiographs of the right shoulder, made at the time of presentation, demonstrating loss of joint space and erosive changes of the humeral head and the glenoid.

nineteen months, the patients were free of infection and pain, shoulder elevation averaged 130 degrees, and external rotation averaged 50 degrees. The success in controlling the infection in these patients, as well as in ours, was apparently due to complete excision of the fistulous tract, wide resection of infected tissues, and restoration of the soft-tissue envelope. Torres and Wright reported that, in all three patients, the rotator cuff was easily mobilized and rerepaired, the deltoid was directly closed, and skin edges were sutured without tension; therefore, a flap was not required.

Several factors increase the risk of postoperative infection. One of these factors is an age of greater than sixty years[1,22]. Eight patients in our series were sixty years of age or older. Six patients had a known underlying medical condition that could have predisposed them

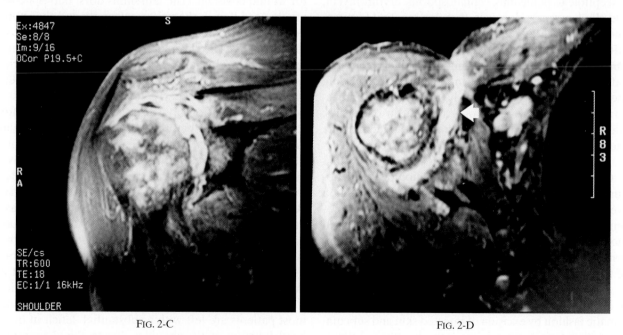

FIG. 2-C   FIG. 2-D

Coronal and axial T1-weighted magnetic resonance images with contrast medium, demonstrating osteomyelitis of the humeral head and the glenoid as well as a synoviocutaneous fistula (arrow).

to infection. Chaudhuri et al.[4] reported on five patients in whom septic arthritis of the shoulder developed after surgery and radiation therapy for breast cancer. All patients had chronic lymphedema. The authors believed that radiation therapy may damage local tissues. In addition, local host-defense mechanisms may be compromised by the lymphatic stasis and lymphedema. Four patients had a delay in diagnosis and treatment, which resulted in a poor outcome. Two patients in our series had a mastectomy, and one of them had chronic lymphedema. Six patients were habitual smokers, and two consumed alcohol daily. Although the number of patients in our series is too small for us to draw significant conclusions, the recording of a detailed history and the performance of an examination prior to surgery with particular attention paid to the above factors may help to identify patients who are at risk for deep infection following shoulder surgery.

Staphylococcus epidermidis and *Staphylococcus aureus* were the most common infecting organisms. However, an unusual organism, Propionibacterium, which is not commonly seen in musculoskeletal infections, was the third most commonly isolated organism. Propionibacterium species are anaerobic, gram-positive, non-spore-forming bacilli[7]. They are the dominant anaerobic organism isolated from normal skin flora[18]. They are often found in lipid-rich areas, such as hair follicles and sebaceous glands, and in moist areas, such as the axilla[2]. Propionibacterium species are rarely associated with infections; descriptions of musculoskeletal infections with this organism have been limited to isolated case reports[6]. The vast majority of blood isolates appear to be skin contaminants and are detected only after prolonged incubation of blood cultures[2]. The organisms are susceptible to penicillins, cephalosporins, erythromycin, and clindamycin[20]. However, they are resistant to nitro-imidazoles such as metronidazole[23]. Since most of the infecting organisms are present in the normal skin flora, careful preparation and draping can prevent contamination. There is no consensus in the literature regarding the routine shaving of axillary hair. Since Propionibacterium species were commonly isolated in our series, additional studies need to be carried out to identify the usefulness of shaving the axilla prior to surgery.

The presentation of our patients was similar to that in other studies of patients with infection of the glenohumeral joint[9,22]. The patients were afebrile and had a normal white blood-cell and neutrophil count on presentation. The erythrocyte sedimentation rate was almost always elevated and is the most useful laboratory test for diagnostic purposes and for following the course of treatment.

The key to infection control is radical débridement of infected necrotic tissue. This was carried out in a systematic fashion by excision of infected skin and subcutaneous tissue, sinus tract, bursa, capsule, synovial tissue, tendon, and bone. Postoperative function depends on residual muscle power[19]. Therefore, every attempt must be made to maintain the deltoid attachment, the tuberosities, and the rotator cuff. However, eradication of the infection should be the primary goal. If the deltoid is detached, it should be repaired primarily with absorbable monofilament sutures. Elek and Conen[5] showed that fewer bacteria are required for infection to occur in the presence of suture material. They concluded that the type of suture material, the infecting organism, and the duration of contact influence the adherence of bacteria. Compared with monofilament sutures, braided sutures have a higher surface area for bacterial adhesion. Since most rotator cuff repairs are done with braided sutures, these sutures must be evaluated carefully during the operation. If the sutures are not contaminated, they can be left in place. In our study, the average duration between the rotator cuff repair and the referral for the infection was 9.7 months. All nonabsorbable braided sutures were considered contaminated and were removed.

One of the factors in the success of treatment of these chronic infections was the presence of a rotator cuff. The glenohumeral joint should be covered after all nonviable tissues have been removed during serial débridements. If the rotator cuff cannot be repaired primarily, the glenohumeral joint is left exposed or is covered only by thin subcutaneous tissue that is not adequate in the presence of an infected joint. Inadequate soft-tissue coverage leads to breakdown of the skin and subcutaneous tissue, leading to the formation of sinus tracts. Muscle coverage can seal off the joint and improve the biological environment by bringing in a fresh blood supply and promoting host defense mechanisms for control of the infection. This was the case in our seven patients who were managed with a rotational flap for wound coverage. The latissimus dorsi flap is a commonly used flap in the upper extremity and the shoulder because of its large arc of rotation and the size of the muscle[12,19]. The clavicular head of the pectoralis major muscle can be safely rotated to cover the superior aspect of the clavicle and shoulder without detachment of the sternocostal head[13,16].

The presentation of a deep shoulder infection following surgery may be subtle and often leads to a delay in diagnosis. Delay in treatment results in the worst outcome[1,8,14]. Patients with deep shoulder infection usually report pain and restricted motion of the shoulder, which often are regarded as expected postoperative symptoms. The lack of systemic symptoms may make the physician less suspicious of an infection. One must have a high index of suspicion for infection, especially if symptoms do not resolve in an expected time frame. The risk factors for an infection should also be kept in mind when making a diagnosis. Chronic deep infection following rotator cuff repair can be controlled, although most patients are left with a substantial deficit in overhead function of the shoulder due to this devastating complication.

References

1. **Bettin, D.; Schul, B.;** and **Schwering, L.:** Diagnosis and treatment of joint infections in elderly patients. *Acta Orthop. Belgica,* 64: 131-135, 1998.

2. **Brook, I.:** Anaerobic gram-positive non-sporulating bacilli. In *Mandell, Douglas and Bennett's Principles and Practice of Infectious Diseases,* edited by G. L. Mandell, J. E. Bennett, and R. Dolin. Ed. 4, pp. 2206-2209. New York, Churchill Livingstone, 1995.

3. **Calhoun, J. H.; Cierny, G., III; Holtom, P.; Mader, J.;** and **Nelson, C. L.:** Symposium: current concepts in the management of osteomyelitis. *Contemp. Orthop.,* 28: 157-185, 1994.

4. **Chaudhuri, K.; Lonergan, D.; Portek, I.;** and **McGuigan, L.:** Septic arthritis of the shoulder after mastectomy and radiotherapy for breast carcinoma. *J. Bone and Joint Surg.,* 75-B(2): 318-321, 1993.

5. **Elek, S. D.,** and **Conen, P. E.:** The virulence of Staphylococcus pyogenes for man. A study of the problems of wound infection. *British J. Exper. Pathol.,* 38: 573-586, 1957.

6. **Estoppey, O.; Rivier, G.; Blanc, C. H.; Widmer, F.; Gallusser, A.;** and **So, A. K.:** Propionibacterium avidum sacroiliitis and osteomyelitis. *Rev. Rheumat., English Ed.,* 64: 54-56, 1997.

7. **Finegold, S. M.:** Anaerobic bacteria: general concepts. In *Mandell, Douglas and Bennett's Principles and Practice of Infectious Diseases,* edited by G. L. Mandell, J. E. Bennett, and R. Dolin. Ed. 4, pp. 2156-2173. New York, Churchill Livingstone, 1995.

8. **Gelberman, R. H.; Menon, J.; Austerlitz, M. S.;** and **Weisman, M. H.:** Pyogenic arthritis of the shoulder in adults. *J. Bone and Joint Surg.,* 62-A: 550-553, June 1980.

9. **Leslie, B. M.; Harris, J. M.;** and **Driscoll, D.:** Septic arthritis of the shoulder in adults. *J. Bone and Joint Surg.,* 71-A: 1516-1522, Dec. 1989.

10. **Lippitt, S. B.; Harryman, D. T., II;** and **Matsen, F. A., III:** A practical tool for evaluating function: the Simple Shoulder Test. In *The Shoulder: A Balance of Mobility and Stability,* pp. 501-518. Edited by F. A. Matsen, III, F. H. Fu, and R. J. Hawkins. Rosemont, Illinois, American Academy of Orthopaedic Surgeons, 1993.

11. **Mansat, P.; Cofield, R. H.; Kersten, T. E.;** and **Rowland, C. M.:** Complications of rotator cuff repair. *Orthop. Clin. North America,* 28: 205-213, 1997.

12. **Minami, A.; Ogino, T.; Ohnishi, N.;** and **Itoga, H.:** The latissimus dorsi musculocutaneous flap for extremity reconstruction in orthopaedic surgery. *Clin. Orthop.,* 260: 201-206, 1990.

13. **Palmer, R. S.,** and **Miller, T. A.:** Anterior shoulder reconstruction with pectoralis minor muscle flap. *Plast. and Reconstr. Surg.,* 81: 437-439, 1988.

14. **Pfeiffenberger, J.,** and **Meiss, L.:** Septic conditions of the shoulder — an up-dating of treatment strategies. *Arch. Orthop. and Trauma Surg.,* 115: 325-331, 1996.

15. **Post, M.:** Complications of rotator cuff surgery. *Clin. Orthop.,* 254: 97-104, 1990.

16. **Rosenberg, L.,** and **Mahler, D.:** Extended rotation-transposition of the pectoralis major myocutaneous flap in the repair of lesions over the shoulder. *British J. Plast. Surg.,* 34: 322-325, 1981.

17. **Settecerri, J. J.; Pitner, M. A.; Rock, M. G.; Hanssen, A. D.;** and **Cofield, R. H.:** Infection following open repair of the rotator cuff. *Orthop. Trans.,* 20: 949, 1996-1997.

18. **Socransky, S. S.,** and **Manganiello, S. D.:** The oral microbiota of man from birth to senility. *J. Periodontol.,* 42: 485-496, 1971.

19. **Stern, P. J.,** and **Carey, J. P.:** The latissimus dorsi flap for reconstruction of the brachium and shoulder. *J. Bone and Joint Surg.,* 70-A: 526-535, April 1988.

20. **Sutter, V. L.,** and **Finegold, S. M.:** Susceptibility of anaerobic bacteria to antimicrobial agents. *Antimicrob. Agents and Chemother.,* 10: 736-752, 1976.

21. **Torres, J. A.,** and **Wright, T. W.:** Synovial cutaneous fistula of the shoulder after failed rotator cuff repair. *Orthopedics,* 22: 1095-1097, 1999.

22. **Vincent, G. M.,** and **Amirault, J. D.:** Septic arthritis in the elderly. *Clin. Orthop.,* 251: 241-245, 1990.

23. **Wexler, H. M.; Molitoris, E.;** and **Finegold, S. M.:** In vitro activities of three of the newer quinolones against anaerobic bacteria. *Antimicrob. Agents and Chemother.,* 36: 239-243, 1992.